BOOKS BY THE SAME AUTHOR

1. Advanced Public Administration
2. Public Administration: Theory and Practice
3. Public Financial Administration
4. Public Health Policy and Administration
5. Public Personnel Administration: Theory and Practice
6. Administration and Management of NGOs: Text and Case Studies
7. Panchayati Raj in India: Theory and Practice
8. Urban Development and Management
9. Management Techniques: Principles and Practices
10. Encyclopaedia of Disaster Management (Set in 3 Vols.)
11. Management of Hospitals: Hospital Administration in the 21st Century (Set in 4 Vols.)
12. Hospital Core Services
13. Hospital Managerial Services
14. Hospital Preventive and Promotive Services
15. Hospital Supportive Services
16. Health Care System and Management (Set in 4 Vols.)
17. Health Care Management and Administration
18. Primary Health Care Management
19. Health Care Organisation and Structure
20. Health Care, Policies and Programmes
21. Nursing Services: Management and Administration
22. Distance Education in 21st Century
23. Encyclopaedia of Higher Education in 21st Century
24. Human Values and Education
25. Stress Management
26. Population Policy and Family Welfare Administration
27. International Administration
28. International Civil Service : Principles, Practice and Prospects
29. Social Welfare Administration (2 Volumes)
30. Family Planning Programme and Beyond
31. Education Policy and Administration
32. Human Resource Development in 21st Century
33. Disaster Management
34. Slum Improvement through Participatory Urban Based Community Structures
35. Development Planning and Administration
36. Public Health Administration
37. Hospital Administration: Theory and Practice
38. Principles, Problems and Prospects of Co-operative Administration
39. Personnel Administration in Co-operatives
40. Public Personnel Administration and Management
41. Right to Information and Good Governance
42. Health Education: Theory and Practice
43. School Health Education
44. Good Governance: An Integral Approach
45. Disaster Administration and Management

IN PRESS

46. Education of Lifestyle and Lifetime Diseases
47. Health Education of Communicable and Non-Communicable Disease
48. Health Education Administration : From International Level to Village Level
49. Education for Healthy Urban Cities
50. Environment and Value Education
51. Women Health Education
52. Rural Health Education

WOMEN HEALTH EDUCATION

DR. S.L. GOEL

Editor, The Indian Journal of Public Administration, New Delhi
Former Vice-President, Executive Council,
Indian Institute of Public Administration, New Delhi
Professor of Public Administration (Retd.)
Panjab University, Chandigarh
Emeritus Fellow, University Grants Commission
Director, State Bank of India (Local Board), Chandigarh
Director, National Horticulture Board, Ministry of Horticulture,
Government of India, New Delhi
Formerly Member UGC, Member Distance Education Council
and Member All India Board of Management, AICTE

and

DR. ARUNA GOEL

Professor of Sanskrit, Panjab University, Chandigarh,
Member, University Grants Commission,
Member, Indian Institute of Advanced Study, Shimla,
Member, Sahitya Academy, Government of India, New Delhi (Sanskrit Board)

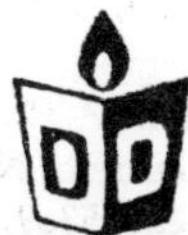

DEEP & DEEP PUBLICATIONS PVT. LTD.
F-159, Rajouri Garden, New Delhi-110027

WOMEN HEALTH EDUCATION

ISBN 978-81-8450-116-2

Typeset by S.S. COMPOSERS,
3190, Mohindra Park, Shakur Basti, Delhi-110034.

Printed in India at MAYUR ENTERPRISES,
WZ Plot No. 3, Gujjar Market, Tihar Village, New Delhi-110018.

Published by DEEP & DEEP PUBLICATIONS PVT. LTD.,
F-159, Rajouri Garden, New Delhi-110027.
Phones: 25435369, 25440916
E-mail: ddpbooks@yahoo.co.in • ddpubs@gmail.com
Showroom:
2/13, Ansari Road, Daryaganj, New Delhi-110002 • Telefax: 23245122

Contents

Preface

Women in developing countries face many health challenges because of ignorance, superstition and other social norms.

Ministry of Health and Family Welfare in Annual Report, 2003-04, GOI, New Delhi indicates that in the decades, the life expectancy of the population in India has shown remarkable improvement from 41 at birth in 1961 to the present day of 65 years. Yet, over a 100,000 women in India continue to die of pregnancy related causes every year. The maternal Mortality Ratio in India is 407 per 100,000 live births (SRS, RGI, 1998). The major causes of these deaths have been identified as hemorrhage (both *ante* and *post-partum*), toxemia (Hypertension during pregnancy), anemia, obstructed labour, puerperal sepsis (infections after delivery) and unsafe abortion.

Maternal Mortality is a cause of great concern. However, reliable estimates of maternal mortality are not available. Any intervention to check it will only be effective if we know reasonably accurate data on maternal mortality. An expert group has been constituted in the Department of Family Welfare, which is looking into the modalities of carrying out a survey for collection of data on Maternal Mortality. A pilot survey for this has already been completed.

Department of Women and Child Development, HRD, GOI clearly states that as the new millennium begins, it is apparent that many definite gains have been made. Women in India have learnt to articulate and voice their concerns. They have come to realize that they have to lead, be in decision-making bodies and develop mechanisms that will ensure change and progress in the social, political and economic spheres.

At the Beijing Conference countries from all over the world made commitments to take action at the national and international levels with regard to 12 critical areas of concern for women. The aim has been to create awareness that women are entitled to equality in all fields of life and to mobile all sectors of society to actively.

The foundation for establishing gender equality in India has been laid through the struggles of women across rural and urban areas, individually and collectively; through programme and policy interventions by government and social organization, and by the legislative framework set-up in the last century.

Policies and programmes, as well as partnerships with the voluntary sector have all made a single, united effort—that of empowering women. Women are being given encouragement and support to become self-reliant.

A review of the status of the Beijing Platform for Action has yielded several insights into the past and the future direction this process must take. It is important to take stock at this point and plan cautiously and carefully for the coming years as we enter this new millennium.

Recently India has taken major steps to improve healthcare services for women by adopting a target-free and community-based approach for reproductive and child healthcare. The goal is to provide easily accessible healthcare facilities to women for their health requirements at every stage of their life cycle.

INTERVENTIONS

Reduction of maternal mortality is an important goal. The Department of Family Welfare has took several new initiatives, during the Ninth Plan period, to make the programme broad-based and client friendly. The focus was, accordingly, shifted from individualized vertical interventions to a more holistic and integrated life cycle approach giving more focused attention to the reproductive healthcare. The maternal health programme which is a component of the Reproductive and child health programme aims at reducing maternal mortality to less than 100 by the 2010. The major interventions includes:

Essential Obstetric Care

Essential obstetric care intends to provide the basic maternity services to all pregnant women. The RCH programme aims at providing at least 3 antenatal check ups during which weight and blood pressure check, abdominal examination, immunization against tetanus, iron and folic acid prophylaxes as well as anaemia management are provided to the pregnant women. Data from the Rapid Household Survey (RHS) 1998-99 indicate that at the national level 67.2 per cent pregnant women received at least one check up but only 10.6 per cent had three antenatal check ups. In Uttar Pradesh and Bihar, the content and quality of antenatal care was poor as compared to Haryana and Tamil Nadu.

We may keep in mind that the most important factor for the health of women is health education. The creation of awareness is integral to social development. The possibility for the power of communication to liberate the minds and potential of people to critical awareness is real in every field linked to human development, and the generation of public will hinges on effective communication of information and ideas that relate to people's needs, aspirations and capacities for progress in thought and action. In this sense, getting the development process started is largely the task of information, education and communications.

The authors in their book, "Family Planning Programme and Beyond" mentions that written communication are usually the mainstay of the formal communications system of the organization, perhaps because the fluidity and impermanence of oral communication, whether conducted face to face or by telephone, does not lend itself to planning or control. However, in the field of Family Welfare Administration, formal communication is not sufficient. It has to be supplemented to a great extent by informal communication. Informal communication is based on a sharing of interests or affinities among individuals. The importance of informal communication to the social welfare administrator is to help him to communicate information that cannot be transmitted through formal channels, i.e. it provides opportunities to communicate with organisation members who cannot be reached directly through the formal channels of hierarchy. It helps in making of internal and external communication. Therefore, there is a great need to train the family welfare administrators in the art of informal communication, as according to Ordway Tead, "Communication is the touching of mind by mind, of person with person, whether it be one man, to a thousand . . . it can include conversation, interview, dialogue, visual technique carefully used." Terry has viewed eight factors as essential to make communication effective. These are: (i) Inform yourself fully; (ii) Establish a mutual trust in others; (iii) Find a common ground of experience; (iv) Use mutually known words; (v) Have regard for context; (vi) Secure and hold the receiver's attention; (vii) Employ examples and visual aids; and (viii) Practice delaying relations.

According to Millet, seven factors make communication effective, i.e. it should be clear, consistent with the expectation of the recipient adequate, timely, uniform, flexible and acceptable. Mr. Eric R. Ram in his article "Information is Power" in *World Health,* January-February, 1989 has rightly said that we have to employ all credible channels of communication, including the traditional methods of story-telling and drama, in order to reach all people, Films, Radio and Television whenever available can be useful but we have to recognise their limitations; they are useful in creating awareness among people in their communities, but to bring about a real change in health practices people have to decide for themselves and take responsibility for their own health.

Since information about how to use a method may be new and hard to understand, there is a need to make it easy to remember how to use Family Planning. Six Key Points in helping clients remember are:

(a) Brevity

The less a client has to remember, the easier it will be to remember. Therefore, providers need to select the most important matters to tell the clients so that these are registered in their mind.

(b) Organisation

Information organised into categories is easier to remember. The way the information is organised should be described to the client.

(c) First Thing First

The instructions presented first are best remembered.

(d) Simplicity

Use short sentences and simple words that clients understand. Avoid technical words and scientific explanations that have no practical use to clients.

(e) Repetition

Repeat the most important information and they will be remembered better.

(f) Specificity

Instructions can be remembered and followed more easily, if they are concrete and specific rather than abstract and vogue.

ESSENTIALS AND ASPECTS OF MASS MOTIVATION CAMPAIGN

Essentials

D.R. John Hubley quoted by Gloria Gorden in his Article, "Let's Communicate" in *World Health* (January-Feb. 1989) has rightly described the essentials of Communication—

- Promote actions which are realistic and feasible within the constraints faced by the community.
- Build on ideas, concepts and practices that people already have.
- Repeat and reinforce information overtime, using different methods.
- Use existing channels of communication such as songs, drama and story-telling, and be adaptable.
- Entertain and attract the attention of the Community.
- Use clear, simple language with local expressions and emphasize short-term benefits of action.
- Provide opportunities for dialogue and discussion to allow learner participation and feedback on understanding and implementation.
- Use demonstrations to show the benefits of adopting practices.

World conference to review the achievements of UN decade for women, July 1985, Nairobi felts that education is the basis for the full promotion and improvement of the status of women. It is the basic tool that should be given to women in order to fulfil their role as full members of society. Governments should strengthen the participation of women at all levels of national educational policy and in formulating and implementing plans, programmes and projects. Special measures should be adopted to revise and adapt women's education to the realities of the developing world. Existing and new services should be directed to women as intellectuals, policy-makers, decisions-makers, planners, contributors and beneficiaries, with particular attention to the UNESCO Convention against Discrimination in Education (1960). Special measures should also be adopted to increase equal access to scientific, technical and vocational education, particularly for young women, and evaluate progress made by the poorest women in urban and rural areas.

Special measures should be taken by Governments and the international organizations, especially UNESCO to eliminate the high rate of illiteracy by the year 2000, with the support of the international community. Governments should establish targets and adopt appropriate measures for this purpose. While the elimination of illiteracy is important to all, priority programmes are still required to overcome the special obstacles that have generally led to higher illiteracy rates among women than among men. Efforts should be made to promote functional literacy, with special emphasis on health, nutrition and viable economic skills and opportunities in order to eradicate illiteracy among women and to produce additional material for the eradication of illiteracy. Programmes for legal literacy in low-income urban and rural areas should be initiated and intensified. Raising the level of education among women is important for the general welfare of society among women is important for the general welfare of society and because of its close link to child survival and child spacing.

The causes of high absenteeism and dropout rates of girls in the educational system must be addressed. Measures must be developed, strengthened and implemented to ensure that women have equal opportunity to acquire education, support from the Government, employment and equitable participation in upbringing of children and maintenance of home.

In this book, we have stressed the need of educating the women so that they become responsible for their own health. This requires a definite policy approach and action. It is hoped that this book having nine chapters would be useful to all those interested in women health as on their health depends the health of the family, society and the universe.

Chandigarh

S.L. GOEL
ARUNA GOEL

CHAPTER I

UNDERSTANDING DEMOGRAPHY AND VITAL STATISTICS ABOUT WOMEN

"... the principle which regulates the existing social relations between the two sexes—the legal subordination of one sex to the other—is wrong in itself, and now one of the chief hindrances to human improvement; ... it ought to be replaced by a principle of perfect equality, admitting no power or privilege on the one side, nor disability on the other."

—J.S. Mill and Hariet Taylor Mill

Understanding Demography and Vital Statistics about Women

CONSTITUTIONAL GUARANTEES TO INDIA'S WOMEN

The concern in safeguarding the rights and privileges of women found its best expression in the Constitution of India. The Constitution of India was ahead of its time, not only by the standards of the developing nations but also of many developed countries, in removing every discrimination against women in the legal and public domain of the Republic. Let us examine a few provisions:

Fundamental Rights

Article 14: "The State shall not deny to any person equality before the law or the equal protection of the laws within the territory of India."

Article 15(1): "The State shall not discriminate against any citizen on grounds only of religion, race, caste, sex, place of birth or any of them."

Article 15(3): "Nothing in this article shall prevent the State from making any special provision for women and children."

This article empowers the state to make affirmative discrimination in favour of women.

Article 16(2): "No citizen shall, on grounds only of religion, race, caste, sex, descent, place of birth, residence or any of them, be ineligible for, or discriminated against in respect of, any employment or office under the State."

Directive Principles of State Policy

Article 39: "The State shall, in particular, direct its policy towards securing—

(a) that the citizens, men and women equally, have the right to an adequate means of livelihood;

(b) that there is equal pay for equal work for both men and women; and

(c) that the health and strength of workers, men and women, and the tender age of children are not abused and that citizens are not forced by economic necessity to enter vocations unsuited to their age or strength."

Article 42: "The State shall make provision for securing just and humane conditions of work and for maternity relief."

Article 51A(e) imposed a fundamental duty on every citizen to renounce the practices derogatory to the dignity of women.

In our opinion, the national objective of integrating women into the process of development at all levels and the constitutional guarantees given to them require social acceptance of the multiple roles of women as home-makers, mothers, and socially and economically productive individuals. It is therefore imperative that society in general and the state in particular provide the necessary conditions and support to enable women to perform their various roles successfully. Marriage and motherhood which contribute to the continuation of the nation should not become disabilities in the gainful participation of women in the economic process. Without the type of supportive services and institutionalized aids suggested here, these dual roles will continue to impose tremendous strain on the physical and mental resources of women and affect the welfare and development of children.[1] We therefore recommend the adoption of a well-defined policy, through a Government Resolution, to fulfil the Constitutional directives and government's long-term objective of total themselves. In the absence of a Well-defined social structure and the identity of traditional culture it is unfortunate to watch young girls from well-to-do families going out in unorthodox and provocative outfits. They can be seen showing thumbs to single motorists for a lift even where buses or 'specials' are available to them; they can also be seen bunking classes and adventuring into a cinema hall in the afternoons or a fast food joint in the company of rich car or motorcycle borne jazzy clothed boys in jeans and costly sun glasses with a cigarette in hand. "It is my life" would be the reaction of an average girl who would retort by telling how conservative and out of times you are. Terrace or garden parties are not very uncommon where a small drink or beer is just about right. The nucleus of a permissive society where 'not-mare-than-this' relationship determines the initial indulgence, lies here. Most of the crimes in this segment of society are the aftermath of natural jealousy, frustration or at times to cover up the exposure of deceit.

Parents who cry foul when something happens are equally to blame since they choose to close their eyes when the girls go out of the houses in outfits almost inviting trouble or when they pass off the misadventure of their boys as childish errands. It is one thing to say that the men should exercise restraint but an entirely different thing to presume all men to be the disciplined lot. The disciplined are no threat any was justify the wrong, the fact to be considered is that if someone dares to bare as a matter of personal liberty, she should be able to accept the consequences too. Instinctively, the human male, unless checked by the society will accost a human female. The ways to woo, however, will differ involvement of women in national development. The policy will have to be implemented carefully so that women are not excluded from any occupation except those from which they are debarred by law, without specifying clearly the basis of unsuitability. It is also necessary to create a cell in the Ministry of Labour and Employment, at both the Central and State levels, to deal with problem of women.[2]

DEMOGRAPHY AND VITAL STATISTICS

Women Population

There has been a slight increase in the total female population of the country, from 407.1 million (48.1 percent of total population) in 1991 to 495.7 million (48.3 per cent) in 2001. While the percentage increase of 0.2 is very marginal, increase in term of absolute numbers was 88.6 million as against 77.1 million between 1981 and 1991. The grown rate of female population for the 1991-2001 decade was 21.79 percent, which was 0.86 percentage points higher than that of the total population. Yet, the demographic imbalances between women and men continue to exist till date. (Refer Table 1.1)

TABLE 1.1

Sex Ratio (1981-2001)

Census	*Sex Ratio*
1981	934
1991	927
2001	933

Note: Sex Ratio: Females per thousand males.
Source: Census of India, 2001, Provisional Population Totals, Registrar General and Census Commissioner, GOI, New Delhi.

If demographic balances were affected by economic factors, then poor states of Orissa, Bihar or Madhya Pradesh would have recorded the worst sex ratios. On the contrary, it is the prosperous states of Haryana, Punjab and Delhi that are among the worst. Better sex ratios are noted among the southern states, some hill regions and states with large tribal populations. Kerala (1071) Pondicherry (1007) are the only States/UTs where sex ratio is tilted in favour of the females.

Comparison over the decade 1991 to 2001 based on rank analysis shows that ranks of Maharashtra, Madhya Pradesh, Punjab, Goa, Gujarat and Himachal Pradesh have droppted by 2 or more places, while it has improved in the States of West Bengal, Manipur, Arunachal Pradesh, Mizoram, Meghalaya and Nagaland.

TABLE 1.2

Rank 2001	*States/UTs*	*Adult 2001*	*Sex Ratio 1991*	*Rank 1991*	*Differences 2001-1991*
1.	Sikkim	858	860	2	2
2.	Haryana	869	862	3	7
3.	Punjab	886	883	6	3
4.	Arunachal Pradesh	888	829	1	59
5.	Uttar Pradesh	895	867	5	28
6.	Nagaland	899	865	4	34
7.	Bihar	916	899	7	17
8.	Madhya Pradesh	917	926	12	-9
9.	Maharashtra	923	931	12	-8
10.	Rajasthan	925	908	9	17
11.	Assam	926	910	10	16
12.	Gujarat	927	936	14	-9
13.	West Bengal	929	907	8	22
14.	Mizoram	932	911	11	21
15.	Tripura	947	940	15	7
16.	Goa	964	967	19	-3
17.	Karnataka	966	960	18	6
18.	Meghalaya	974	947	16	27
19.	Orissa	976	972	20	4
20.	Andhra Pradesh	980	972	21	8
21.	Himachal Pradesh	981	980	23	1
22.	Manipur	981	955	17	26
23.	Tamilnadu	992	978	22	12
24.	Kerala	1071	1049	24	22
	India	934	923		11

Source: Annual Report of Women and Child Development Department, Ministry of HRD (Government of India).

TABLE 1.3

Life Expectancy at Birth (1981-2001) (In Years)

Year	*Female*	*Males*
1981-85	55.7	55.4
1989-93*	59.7	59.0
1996-2001	65.3	62.3

* Based on the Sample Registration System.

Source: *Ibid*. Estimates.

Sex Ratio in 6+ Age group : Ranks in 1991 and 2001 and Decadal Differences (1991-2001) among States

This clearly points to the fact that economic growth may not necessarily bring about an improvement in the status of women. This, in turn, can be attributed to the discrimination the girl child faces and the consequential problems of poor health and nutritional status. Added to these are the problems of female fortified and female infanticide, the incidence of which is on an increase.

Expectation of Life

The life expectancy at birth among females has been steadily improving over the years from 23.3 in 1901 to 65.3 in 2001 and has surpassed that of men since the eighties. Male life expectancy in 2001 is 62.3 years. The urban female life expectancy is higher at 68. The rural urban difference is the highest in Madhya Pradesh (8.6) and the lowest in Kerala (1.0).

The life expectancy indicator highlights that number of older women will be on the rise. Many of them will be widows and living alone given the increasing tendency of nuclearisation of families. The absence of social security measures for them on the one hand and the declining support structures from family and society on the other, indicate the plight of these already low status aged women.

Female Infant Mortality Rate

In many States, the number of infant deaths among girls exceed that of boys due to discriminatory child care practices. The worst case is that of Haryana, where the gender difference in IMR is 19. This is followed by Punjab, Rajasthan and Tamil Nadu. Contrarily in Orissa, where infant mortality rates are the highest (96), girls have marginally higher chance of survival than boys.

Maternal Mortality Rate

In India the Maternal Mortality Rate (MMR), which is calculated as the number of maternal deaths per 100,000 live births, is among the highest

TABLE 1.4

Maternal Mortality Rate (1990-1998)

(Per lakh live births)

Year	*Maternal Mortality Rate*
1980	468
1993	437
1998	407

Source: Ibid.

in the world and therefore a matter of great concern. It has come down from 468 in 1980 to 407 in 1988.

There is wide range of variation in MMR across regions and States —from 28 in Gujarat to 707 in Uttar Pradesh.

Mean Age at Marriage

Similarly, the effective mean age at marriage for females has also increased from 18.3 years in 1981 to 19.5 years in 1997. The Child Marriage Restraint Act, 1976 which raised the age of marriage for girls from 15 to 18 years has no doubt, helped reduce child/early marriages and the consequent early pregnancies and birth of premature babies at the same time, education and employment of women/girls has also played a very important role in raising the age of marriage.

TABLE 1.5

Mean Age at Marriage (1981-1997)

(in years)

Year	*Females*	*Males*
1981	18.3	23.3
1991	19.5	23.9
1997	19.5	N.A.

Source: Sample Registration System Bulletins for respective years, Registrar-General and Census Commissioner, GOI, New Delhi.

Women's Health and Family Welfare

Lack of adequate resources prevents women belonging to poorer households from availing health services for themselves. Undernourished, ill-fed and overworked, most women from such households are extremely vulnerable to ailments and diseases, which do not get properly diagnosed and treated. Poor sanitation, unhygienic surroundings, difficulty in procuring safe drinking water are some of the factors that affect the general health of women.

Every second woman in India suffers from some degree of anaemia. 2 percent of them are severely anaemic, while 35 and 15 percent have mild and moderate anaemia levels respectively. Here again, the inter-State differences are very pronounced.

While the Birth Rate has declined by 7.8 points from 33.9 in 1981 to 26.1 in 1999, the Death Rate has also declined by 3.8 points from 12.5 in 1981 to 8.7 in 1999. (Refer Tables 1.6 and 1.7)

However while the female Death Rate has come down by 4.4 points from 12.7 in 1981 to 8.3 in 1999, the male death rate has come down by 3.4 points, i.e. from 12.4 in 1981 to 9.0 in 1991.

TABLE 1.6

Birth Rate (1981-1999)

(per thousand)

Year	*Birth Rate*
1981	33.9
1991	29.5
1999	26.1

Source: *Ibid.*

TABLE 1.7

Death Rate (1981-1999)

(per thousand)

Year	*Females*	*Males*	*Total*
1981	12.7	12.4	12.5
1991	9.7	10.0	9.8
1999	8.3	9.0	8.7

Source: *Ibid.*

Female Literacy

Literacy or the ability to read and write is the first step towards formal education. Female literacy has been steadily improving over the years. The proportion of women who are literate has increased by 15 percent over the last decade from 39.29 percent in 1991 to 54.16 percent in 2001. Yet, even today, 193 million women are illiterate in India.

TABLE 1.8

(In Percent)

Census	*Females*	*Males*	*Persons*	*Male-female gap in literacy rate*
1981	29.76	6.38	43.57	26.62
1991	39.29	64.13	52.21	24.84
2001	54.16	75.85	65.38	21.69

Note: The literacy rates relate to the population aged seven years and above. The 1991 census rates exclude Jammu and Kashmir.

Source: Census of India, 2001: Provisional Population Totals, Registrar General and Census Commissioner, GOI, New Delhi

TABLE 1.9

Enrolment of Girls in Graduate/Post-Graduate/Professional Courses (1990-91 to 1999-2000)

(Figures in Million)

Levels	*1990-91*		*1996-97*		*1999-2000*	
	Women	*Total*	*Women*	*Total*	*Women*	*Total*
Graduate	1.14	3.29	1.82	4.87	2.66	6.51
(B.A./B.Sc./B.Com.)	(34.7)		(37.4)		(40.9)	
Post-Graduate	0.12	0.35	0.17	0.54	0.22	0.55
(M.A./M.Sc./M.Com.)	(32.8)		(30.5)		(39.6)	
Ph.D./D.Sc./D.Phil.	0.01	0.03	0.01	0.04	0.02	0.05
	(26.2)		(29.2)		(35.4)	
B.E./B.Sc (Eng)/B. Architecture	0.03	0.24	0.05	0.33	0.08	0.36
	(10.9)		(14.9)		(22.0)	
M.B.B.S.	0.03	0.08	0.04	0.12	0.05	0.14
	(34.3)		(35.4)		(37.8)	
Total	1.32	3.99	2.09	5.90	3.03	7.61
	(33.0)		(35.3)		(39.8)	

Source: Selected Educational Statistics for respective years, Department of Education, Ministry of Human Resource Development, GOI, New Delhi.

Gender gap in literacy continues to be very high at 22 percentage points. The gaps are even more glaring among disadvantaged groups such as scheduled castes and tribes. Among scheduled castes (SCs), 50 percent males are literate while only 24 percent females can read and write. Similarly, among scheduled tribes (STs), 41 percent and 18 percent, males and females respectively are literate.

Urban-rural differences are significant, with urban females almost matching up to rural male literates, especially among SC/STs. The female literacy rate for rural areas is only 47, while it is 73 in urban locations. Bihar and Jharkhand, the two poor literacy states in rural areas (30) perform relatively better in urban areas. They are at third and eighth ranks respectively.

The gross enrolment ratio for girls both at primary and middle levels have also increased from 64.1 in 1980-81 to 85.2 in 1999-2000 in respect of primary level and from 28.6 to 49.7 in respect of middle level during the same period. Between 1990-91 and 1999-2000, the GER of girls at the middle level has also increased from 47.8 to 49.7.

The number of women in higher education which includes colleges, universities, professional colleges of engineering, medicine, technology, etc. has also increased form 1.32 million (33.0 percent) in 1990-91 to 3 million (39.8 percent) in 1999-2000 (Table 1.9). The number of women enrolled has shown an increase in both absolute and relative terms.

Work and Employment

While the female work participation rate increased from 19.7 per cent in 1981 to 25.7 per cent in 2001, still it is much lower than the male work participation rate in both urban and rural areas (Table 1.10). There are wide regional variations amongst the major states, ranging from as high as 34 per cent in Mizoram to as low as 4 per cent in Punjab, as per the 1991 Census. (State-wise data for the 2001 Census is not yet available). (Table 1.10)

Women's share in the organised work-force has also shown an increasing trend, from 2.8 million (12.2 per cent) in 1981 to 4.8 million (17.2 per cent) in 1999. Between 1991 and 1999, rise in the percentage points of women was 3.1 in contrast, the share of men has been declining. However, women's participation in the organised sector is still very low, as compared to men. (Table 1.11)

Similarly, women's employment in the public sector has also recorded an increase from 1.5 million (9.7 per cent) in 1981 to 2.8 million (14.5 per cent) in 1999 (Table 1.12). However, it is still much lower than that of men. (Table 1.12)

Just as in the case of women in Public Sector, they also hold a low-key with only 14.6 per cent of the total 10.7 million employees in Government in 1997. No doubt, there has been an increasing trend in the representation of women in Government, as it rose from 11.0 to 14.6 per cent between 1981 and 1997, but at the same time, their representation can be rated as very low, when compared to the number of educated women. (Table 1.13)

Decision-making

(i) Administrative

The representation of women in the decision-making levels through the Premier Services viz., the Indian Administrative Service (IAS) and Indian Police Services (IPS), which stood at only 5.4 per cent in 1987 increased marginally to 7.6 per cent in 2000. However, the figure is still very low, requiring not only affirmative action but also special interventions to help raise the number of women at various decision-making levels. (Refer Table 1.14)

(ii) Political

The 73rd and 74th Constitutional Amendments in 1993 have brought forth a definite impact on the participation of woman, in terms of absolute numbers, in grassroot democratic institutions viz. Panchayati Raj Institutions (PRIs) and Local Bodies (Table 1.15). In fact, these amendments have helped women not only in their effective participation but also in decision-making in the grassroots democracy of the 475 Zilla Parishads in the country, 158 are being chaired by women. At the Block Level, out of 51,000 members of Block Samitis, 17,000 are women. In addition, nearly

TABLE 1.10

Works Participation Rates by Sex (1981-2001)

(In per cent)

Census	*T/R./U*	*Females*	*Males*	*Persons*
1981	Total	19.7	52.6	36.7
	Rural	23.1	53.8	38.8
	Urban	8.3	49.1	30.0
1991	Total	22.3	51.6	37.5
	Rural	26.8	52.6	40.1
	Urban	9.2	48.9	30.2
2001	Total	25.7	51.9	39.3
	Rural	31.0	52.4	42.0
	Urban	11.6	50.9	32.2

Source: Census of India, 1991, Series 1 and Census of India, 2001: Provisional Population Totals, Registrar General and Census Commissioner, GOI, New Delhi.

TABLE 1.11

Women in the Organised Sector (1998-99)

(Figures in Million)

Year	*Women*	*Men*	*Total*
1981	2.8 (12.2)	20.1	22.9
1991	3.8 (14.1)	23.0	26.7
2001	4.8 (17.2)	23.3	28.1

Source: Director-General of Employment and Training, Ministry of Labour, GOI, New Delhi.

TABLE 1.12

Women in the Public Sector (1981-99)

(Figures in Million)

Year	*Women*	*Men*	*Total*
1981	1.5 (9.7)	14.0	15.5
1991	2.4 (12.3)	16.7	19.1
2001	2.8 (14.5)	16.6	19.4

Source: Director-General of Employment and Training, Ministry of Labour, GOI, New Delhi.

TABLE 1.13

Women in the Government (1981-97)

(Figures in Million)

Year	*Women*	*Men*	*Total*
1981	1.2 (11.0)	9.7	10.9
1997	1.6 (14.6)	9.1	10.7

Source: Director-General of Employment and Training, Ministry of Labour, GOI, New Delhi.

TABLE 1.14

Representation of Women in Premier Services (1987-2000)

Service	*1987*		*1997*		*2000*	
IAS	339 (7.5)	4.204	512 (10.2)	4,991	535 (10.4)	5159
IPS	21 (0.9)	2418	67 (2.2)	3045	110 (3.3)	3301
Total	360 (5.4)	6622	579 (7.2)	8036	645 (7.6)	8460

Note: Figures within parentheses indicate percentage to total.
Source: Department of Personnel and Training, GOI, New Delhi.

TABLE 1.15

Women in Panchayati Raj Institutions (1995-2001)

(Figures in thousand)

Year	*Women*	*Men*	*Total*
1995	318 (33.5)	630	948
2001	725 (26.6)	1997	2722

Source: Ministry of Rural Development, GOI, New Delhi.

one-third of the mayors of the municipalities are women. In the elections to PRIs held between 1993 and 1997, women have achieved participation even beyond the mandatory requirement of $33^{1/3}$ per cent of the total seats in states like Karnataka (43.45 per cent). Kerala (36.4 per cent) and West Bengal (35.4 per cent), However, the all India figure for women show that their representation in 2001 is still low.

TABLE 1.16

Representation of Women in Parliament (1998-2001)

Year	*Females*	*Males*	*Total*
1998	59 (7.2)	761	820
1999	67 (8.5)	723	790
2001	70 (8.5)	750	820

Note: Figures within parentheses indicate percentage to total.
Sources: 1. Election Commission of India.
2. National Informatics Centre, Parliament House, New Delhi.

Although the number of women in Parliament has increased from 59 in 1998 to 70 in 2001, their share continues to be very low representing only 8.5 per cent (Table 1.16) of the total members in Parliament in 2001.

The number of women in the Central Council of Ministers continues to remain extremely low, but with a marginal increase of 0.8 percent between 1995 and 2001 (Table 1.17). Of these, 2 are of Cabinet rank and 6 are of the rank of Minister of State, and of these, 2 are holding Independent Charge. These trends point out very clearly to the need for affirmative action besides addressing these issues in a systematic and expeditious way so that women's concerns gain political prominence and a fairly representative number of women are in position not only at grassroot level, but also at the state and national levels.

TABLE 1.17

Representation of Women in the Central Council of Ministers (1985-2001)

Year	*Females*	*Males*	*Total*
1985	4 (10.0)	36	40
2001	8 (10.8)	66	74

Source: National Information Centres, Parliament House, New Delhi.

To sum up, Table 1.18 presents the status of women including that of the girl child along with the progress made by them over a period of two development decades (1981-2001) as reflected in the 21 Selected Gender Development Indicators. (Table 1.18)

A quick review of the progress made by women has not only focused light on the gains but also brought forth to surface certain critical areas of concern relating to women by Draft Tenth Plan requiring attention of the

TABLE 1.18

The 21 Selected Gender Development Indicators: 1981-2001

Sl. No.	Indicators	Women	Men	Total	Women	Men	Total
1	2	3	4	5	6	7	8
	Demography and Vital Statistics						
1.	Polulation (in million in 1981 and 2001)	330.0	353.4	683.4	495.7	531.3	1027.0
2.	Decennial Growth (1981 and 2001)*	24.93	24.41	24.66	21.79	20.93	21.34
3.	Sex Ratio (1981 and2001)**	934	—	—	933	—	—
4.	Life Expectancy at Birth (in years in 1981-85 and 1996-01)	55.7	55.4	—	65.3	62.3	—
5.	Mean Age at Marriage (in years in 1981 and 1991)	18.3	23.3	—	19.5	23.9	—
	Health and Family Welfare						
6.	Birth Rate (per thousand in 1981 and 1999)	—	—	33.9	—	—	26.1
7.	Death Rate (per thousand in 1981 and 1999)	12.7	12.4	12.5	8.3	9.0	8.7
8.	Infant Mortality Rate (per thousand live births in 1988 and 1999)	93.0	96.0	94.5	70.8	69.8	70.0
9.	Child Mortality Rate (per thousand live births under 5 years of age in 1985 and 1997)	40.4	36.6	—	24.5	21.8	—
10.	Maternal Mortality Rate (per one lakh live births in 1980 and 1998)	468	—	—	407	—	—
	Literacy and Education						
11.	Literacy Rates (1981 and 2001)*	29.76	56.38	43.57	54.16	75.85	65.38
12.	Gross Enrolment Ratio (1980-81 and 1999-2000)						
	Classes I-V	64.1	95.8	80.5	85.2	104.1	94.9
	Class VI-VIII	28.6	54.3	41.9	49.7	67.2	58.8
13.	Dropout Rate (1980-81 and 1999-2000)*						
	Class I-V	62.5	56.2	58.7	42.3	38.7	40.3
	Class VI-VIII	79.4	68.0	72.7	58.0	52.0	54.6

(Contd.)

TABLE 1.18 *(Contd.)*

1 2	3	4	5	6	7	8
Work and Employment						
14. Work Participation Rate (1981 and 2001)*	19.7	52.6	36.7	25.7	51.9	39.3
15. Organised Sector (No. in million in 1981 and 1999)	2.80 (12.2%)	20.05	22.85	4.83 (17.2%)	23.28	28.11
16. Public Sector (No. in million in 1981 and 1999)	1.5 (9.7%)	14.0	15.5	2.8 (14.5%)	16.6	19.4
17. Government (No. in million in 1981 and 1997)	1.2 (11%)	9.7	10.9	1.6 (14.6%)	9.1	10.7
Decision-Making						
18. Administration (No. in IAS and IPS in 1987 and 2000)	360 (5.4%)	6262	6622	645	7815	8460
19. PRIs (No. in thousand in 1995 and 2001)	318 (33.5%)	630	948	725 (26.6%)	1997	2722
20. Parliament (No. in 1998 and 2001)	59 (7.2%)	761	820	70 (8.5%)	750	820
21. Central Council of Ministers (No. in 1985 and 2001)	4 (10%)	36	40	8 (10.8%)	66	74

Sources: Census of India 1991; Census of India, 2001.
Draft: Tenth Plan (2000-01), p. 237.

Government during the Tenth Plan. They include: increasing burden of poverty; unequal access to primary healthcare, under malnutrition, high rates of illiteracy and lack of training; lack of access and control on assets and resources; inequalities in sharing of power and decision-making; lack of access to information and media; increasing violence against women, adolescent and the girl child persisting discrimination against the girl child, etc. Keeping these Issues/Concerns in view, the Tenth Plan suggests the following approach not only to strengthen, but also to speed up, the on going process/efforts of empowering of women.

Strategies in the Five Year Plans

Over the years the planning strategies on women and children in the country has evolved from 'welfare' to 'development' to 'empowerment'.

The approach in the First Five Year Plan (1951-56) was to provide adequate services to 'promote the welfare of women' so that they can play their 'legitimate role in the family and the community'. It was noted, 'the position and functions of women differ to a great extent in different communities, and therefore, community welfare agencies will have to work out their programmes and activities according to the specific requirements in which they work'. The Plan document further noted that special organizations on the part of the Central or State Governments for promotion of the welfare of women had not yet been developed and therefore stressed that 'the major burden of organizing activities for the benefit of vast female population has to be borne by the private agencies'. The Central Social Welfare Board (CSWB) was set-up in 1953 to promote voluntary organizations at various levels, especially at the grassroots, to take up welfare-related activities for women.

The Second, Third, Fourth and Fifth Plans, including the four years of Plan holiday that preceded the Fourth Plan continued the same approach for the welfare of women. The concept of women's development was mainly 'welfare' oriented and was clubbed with other categories of welfare such as the old and the disabled. The schemes of Condensed Course of Education and Women and Socio-Economic Programme were introduced during the Second Plan (1956-61) and that of Working Girl's Hostel and Short Stay Home in the Fourth Plan (1969-71). These were the only women specific schemes of the Department during the first twenty-eight years of the planning history.

The end of the Fourth Plan has seen the release of the monumental repot of Committee on Status of Women in India entitled 'Towards Equality which revealed that the dynamics of development has adversely affected a large section of women and created new imbalances and disparities. The Report led to a debate in Parliament and the emergence of new consciousness of women as critical inputs for national development rather than as targets for welfare policies'. A Women's Welfare and Development Bureau was set-up in 1976 under the Ministry of Social Welfare to initiate necessary policies, programmes and measures for women. Four separate

Working Groups on Employment of Women, Adult Education Programmes for Women, Women in Agriculture and Rural Development were set-up to chalk out strategies for action in all these areas.

These led to a definite shift in the approach from 'welfare' to 'development' in the Sixth Plan (1980-85), which recognized women as participants of development and not merely as objects of welfare. The Plan adopted a multi-disciplinary approach with a special thrust on the three core sectors of health, education and employment. Accordingly priority was given to implementation of programmes for women under different sectors of agriculture and its allied activities of dairying, poultry, animal husbandry, handlooms, handicrafts, small scale industries, etc. Women's Employment Programme was introduced in 1982 with assistance from Norwegian Development Agency (NORAD).

SEVENTH PLAN: OBJECTIVES AND STRATEGIES

The long-term objectives of the developmental programmes for women would be to raise their economic and social status in order to bring them into the mainstream of national development. Due recognition has to be accorded to the role and contribution of women in the various socio-economic, political and cultural activities.

In the Seventh Plan, the basic approach would be to inculcate confidence among women and bring about an awareness of their own potential for development, as also special measures would be initiated for strict enforcement of the Dowry Prohibition Act and also to prevent harassment and atrocities on women. Voluntary agencies and educational institutions would be fully involved in launching organized campaigns to combat these evils. An integrated multi-disciplinary approach would be adopted covering employment, education, health, nutrition, application of science and technology and other related aspects that is extend facilities for income-generating activities and to enable women to participate actively in socio-economic development. The educational programmes will be restructured and the school curricula will be modified to higher secondary and higher education courses, formal as well as non-formal. It will be given high priority.

The Seventh Plan (1985-90) continued the stress on generation of both skilled and unskilled employment of women through proper education and vocational training. Two new schemes of Support to Training and Employment (STEP) and Awareness Generation Programme for Rural and Poor Women (AGP) were introduced. Three landmark reports, namely Shram Shakti, the Report of the National Commission on Self-Employed Women and Women in Informal Sector, National Perspective Plan on Women (1988-2000) and SAARC Guidebook on Women in Development were prepared during this period. The Department of Women and Child Development was set-up in 1985 to serve as the nodal point for women and children within the National Machinery.

Alongwith women, major initiatives were taken to focus on girl child for breaking the vicious continuum, of girl child and woman, so that girls can get the much required space for physical and mental development before being asked to take up the responsibilities of wife and mother. Spatial expansion and enrichment of child development services took place through programmes in different sectors. Much emphasis was also given on human development through advocacy, mobilization and community empowerment.

Recognizing the role and contribution of women in development, the Eighth Plan (1990-95), adopted the strategy to ensure that 'benefits' of development from different sectors do not bypass women and special programmes are implemented to complement the general development programmes. Two new schemes, which were introduced during this period, were Mahila Samridhi Yojana and Indira Mahila Yojana. The other major developments during this plan period were setting up of National Commission for Women and National Credit Fund for Women known as Rashtriya Mahila Kosh, and the 73rd and 74th Constitutional Amendments wherein one-third of seats of rural and urban self-governing institutions were reserved for women. The Government declared its commitment to the development of 'every child', which was manifested in the two National Plan of Action adopted in 1992, one for the Children and the other exclusively for the Girl Child.

Special initiatives for the well-being of women during the Eighth Plan (1992-97)—

- Setting up of National Commission for Women in 1992 to safeguard the interests of women.
- Setting up of Rashtriya Mahila Kosh in 1993 to meet the credit needs of poor and assetless women.
- Adoption of the National Nutritional Policy in 1993 to fulfil the constitutional commitment of improving the nutritional status of people in general and in particular that of the children, adolescent girls, expectant and nursing mothers.
- Launching of the schemes of Mahila Samriddhi Yojana in 1993 which sought to empower women by institutionalizing their savings so that they could have greater control over household resources (now being revamped).
- Launching of Indira Mahila Yojana in 1995, advocating an integrated approach for women's empowerment through Self-Help Groups.
- Proposal for setting up of National Resource Centre for Women (in progress).
- Formulation of a draft National Policy for the Empowerment of Women.[3]

THE STRATEGY FOR THE NINTH PLAN[4]

Empowerment of Women being one of the primary objectives of the Ninth Plan, every effort will be made to create an enabling environment where women can freely exercise their rights both within and outside home, as equal partners along with men. This will be realised through early finalisation and adoption of the 'National Policy for Empowerment of Women' which laid down definite goals, targets and policy prescriptions along with a well defined Gender Development Index to monitor the impact of its implementation in raising the status of women from time to time.

An integrated approach will be adopted towards empowering women through convergence of existing services, resources, infrastructure and manpower available in both women-specific and women-related sectors with the ultimate objective of achieving the set goal. To this effect, the Ninth Plan directs both the 'Centre and the States' to adopt a special strategy of 'Women's Component Plan' through which, not less than 30 per cent of funds/benefits are earmarked in all the women-related sectors. It also suggests a special vigil to be kept on the flow of the earmarked funds/ benefits through an effective mechanism to ensure that the proposed strategy brings forth a holistic approach towards empowering women.

While organising women into Self-Help Groups marks the beginning of a major process of empowering women, the institutions thus developed would provide a permanent forum for articulating their needs and contributing their perspectives to development. Recognising the fact that women have been socialised only to take a back seat in public life, affirmative action through deliberate strategies will be initiated to provide equal access to and control over factors contributing to such empowerment, particularly in the areas of health, education, information, life-long learning for self-development, vocational skills, employment and income generating opportunities, land and other forms of property including through inheritance, common property, resources, credit, technology and markets, etc. To this effect, the newly elected women members and the women Chairpersons of Panchayats and the Local Bodies will be sensitised through the recently launched special training package to take the lead in ensuring that adequate funds/benefits flow towards the empowerment of women and the girl child.

APPROACH TO THE TENTH PLAN—PATH AHEAD

In the context of having laid down National Policy, approach to the Tenth Plan for empowering women will be very distinct from that of the earlier Plans, as it now stands on a strong Platform for Action with definite goals, targets and a time frame. Further, as the process of empowering women initiated during the Ninth Plan is expected to continue through and beyond the Tenth Plan, there can be no better approach than translating the recently adopted National Policy for Empowerment of Women (2001) into action through—

- Creating an environment, through positive economic and social policies, for the development of women to enable them to realize their full potential;
- Allowing the *de-jure* and *de-facto* enjoyment of all human rights and fundamental freedoms by women on par with men in all spheres—political, economic, social, cultural and civil;
- Providing equal access to participation and decision-making for women in social, political and economic life of the nation;
- Ensuring equal access to women to healthcare, quality education at all levels, career and vocational guidance, employment, equal remuneration, occupational health and safety, social security and public office, etc.;
- Strengthening legal systems aimed at the elimination of all forms of discrimination against women;
- Changing societal attitudes and community practices by active participation and involvement of both men and women;
- Mainstreaming a gender perspective into the development process;
- Eliminating discrimination and all forms of violence against women and the girl child; and
- Building and strengthening partnerships with civil society, particularly women's organization, corporate and private sector agencies.

The Operational strategy, as prescribed in the Policy, direct all the Central Ministries and State Departments to draw up Bound Action Plans for translating the Policy into a set of concrete actions through a participatory process of consultations with all the concerned, both in the governmental and non-governmental sectors. Accordingly, the first step in this direction will be to prepare a National Plan of Action for implementation of the Policy by the nodal Department of Women and Child Development through identifying its partners; specifying Action Points in all the women-related development sectors; developing an in-built mechanism for effective coordination and monitoring of the implementation of the Policy; besides evaluating/assessing the impact of the implementation of Policy in improving the status of women, based on a Gender Development Index.

The Plans of Action thus prepared will clearly specify—(i) the measurable goals to be achieved along with the time targets, preferably in consonance with the time frames set by the other women-related national policies; (ii) commitment of resources; (iii) earmarking of the benefits under WCP; (iv) fixing of responsibilities for implementation of the Action Points; and (v) identification of structures and mechanisms to ensure effective review, monitoring, and impact assessment of all the related policies, Plans of Action and programmes in raising the status of women, adolescent girls and girl children on par with their counterparts. As the time target set for achieving the goals in the Policy goes beyond the Tenth Plan, the following measurable/monitorable goals set in the Tenth Plan (Approach Paper) having a direct bearing on the empowerment of women and the girl child, will be adopted in the proposed Action Plans:

- Reduction of poverty ratio by 5 percentage points by 2007 and by 15 percentage points by 2012;
- Proving gainful (high-quality) employment of the addition to the labour force over the Tenth Plan period;
- All children in school by 2003; all children to complete 5 years of schooling by 2007;
- Reduction of gender gaps in literacy and wage rates by at least 50 percent by 2007;
- Reduction in the decadal rate of population growth between 2001 and 2011 to 16.2 percent;
- Increase in Literacy rate to 75 percent within the Plan period;
- Reduction of IMR to 45 per 1000 live births by 2007 and to 28 by 2012;
- Reduction of MMR to 2 per 1000 live births by 2007 and to 1 by 2012; and
- All villages to have sustained access to potable drinking water by 2007.

To translate the above Goals into action, the Tenth Plan reaffirms the major strategy of mainstreaming the gender perspectives in all sectoral policies and programmes and plans of action. This will help achieve the ultimate goal of eliminating gender discrimination and creating an enabling environment of gender justice, which would encourage women and girls to act as catalysts, participants and recipients in the country's development process. Further, women specific interventions will be undertaken to bridge the existing gaps.

Acknowledging the fact that women's equality in power sharing and active participation in decision-making, both in administrative and political spheres, is a very strong instrument to achieve the goals of empowerment, the Tenth Plan will initiate all necessary steps to guarantee equal access and full participation to women in decision-making bodies, including the legislative, executive, judicial, corporate, statutory bodies and their advisory Commissions/Committees, Boards, etc. Affirmative action such as reservations/quotas, including in the higher political, administrative and legislative bodies, will also be considered, if necessary, on a time bound basis. Introduction of women friendly personnel policies will be an additional feature during the Tenth Plan to encourage women to participate effectively in all the administrative decision-making processes.

The process of organizing women into Self-Help Groups (SHGs), started during the Ninth Plan to provide them a permanent forum for articulating their needs and contributing their perspectives to development, has made tremendous progress as it brought into action more than a million SHGs all over the country. Experience has already shown that these Groups have been very effective institutions at grassroot level in facilitating access to women, be it for financial or material resources or services or for information. Therefore, the Tenth Plan will continue to encourage SHG mode to act as the agents of social change, development and empowerment of women.

To adopt a Sector-specific Three-Fold Strategy for empowering women, based on the prescriptions of the National Policy for Empowerment of Women. They include:

Social Empowerment

To create an enabling environment through various affirmative development policies and programmes for development of women besides providing them easy and equal access to all the basic minimum services so as to enable them to realise their full potentials.

Economic Empowerment

To ensure provision of training, empowerment and income generation activities with both 'forward' and 'backward' linkages with the ultimate objective of making all potential women economically independent and self-reliant.

Gender Justice

To eliminate all forms of gender discrimination and thus, allow women to enjoy not only the *de-jure* but also the *de-facto* rights and fundamental freedom on par with men in all spheres, viz. political, economic, social, civil, cultural, etc.

SOCIAL EMPOWERMENT

Create an enabling environment through adopting various affirmative developmental policies and programmes for development of women, besides providing them easy and equal access to all the basic minimum services so as to enable them to realize their full potentials through—

- Providing easy and equal access to ensure basic minimum services of primary healthcare and family welfare with a special focus on the under-served and under-privileged segements of population through universalising Reproductive and Child Health (RCH) services.
- Achieving the goals set by the National Population Policy (2000) with regard to reducing Infant Mortality Rate (IMR) to 30 per thousand and Maternal Mortality Rate (MMR) to 100 per lakh live births by 2010.

- Supplementing healthcare and nutrition services through the Pardhan Mantri Gramodaya Yojana (PMGY) to fill the critical gaps in the existing primary healthcare infrastructure and nutrition services.
- Tackling both macro and micro nutrient deficiencies through nutrition supplementary feeding programmes with necessary support services like health check ups, immunization, health and nutirition education and nutrition awareness, etc.
- Consolidating the progress made under female education and carrying it forward for achieving the set goal of 'Education for Women's Equality' as advocated by the National Policy on Education, 1986 (revised in 1992).
- Providing easy and equal access to and free education for women and girls at all levels and in the field of technical and vocational education and training in up coming and job-oriented trades.
- Increasing enrolment/retention rates and reducing dropout rates by expanding the support services through mid day meals, hostels and incentives like free supply of uniforms, text books, transport charge, etc.
- Extending the existing network of regional vocational training centres to all the states and Women's Industrial Training Institutes and Women's Wings with General Industrial Training Institutes with residential facilities in all districts and sub-districts and provision of training in marketable trades.
- Encouraging the media to project positive images of women and the Girl Child; change the mind set of the people and thus promotes the balanced portrayals of women and men.
- Gender sensitizing both the administrative and enforcement machinery and ensuring that the rights and interests of women are taken care of, besides involving them in planning, implementation and monitoring of processes.

ECONOMIC EMPOWERMENT

Ensure provision of training, employment and income generation activities with both 'forward' and 'backward' linkages with the ultimate objective of making all women economically independent and self-reliant through—

- Organising women into Self-Help Groups under various poverty alleviation programmes, viz. Swarnajayanti Gram Swarozgar Yojana (SGSY), Swarnajayanti Shahari Rozgar Yojana (SJSRY), Rashtriya Mahila Kosh (RMK), Support for Training and Employment Programme (STEP), Training-*cum*-Production Centres for Women (NORAD), etc. and offering them a range of economic options along with necessary support measures to enhance their capabilities and earning capacities with an ultimate objective of making them economically independent and self-reliant.

- Ensuring that women in the Informal Sector who account for more than 90 per cent are given special attention with regard to improving their working conditions as the same continued to be very precarious, without even minimum or equal wages, leave aside other legislative safeguards.
- Making concerted efforts to ensure that the benefits of training and extension in agriculture and its activities of horticulture, small animal husbandry, poultry, fisheries, etc. reach women in proportion to their numbers; and also issue of Joint Forest for husband and wife under the Social Forestry and Joint Forest Management programmes
- Ensuring that the employers fulfil their legal obligation towards their women workers in extending child facilities, maternity benefits, special leave, protection from occupational hazards, allowing formation women workers' associations/unions, legal protection/aid, etc.
- Re-training/upgrading the skills of women displaced from traditional sectors due to advancement of technology so that they can take up jobs in the new and expanding areas of employment and formulating appropriate policies and programmes to promote alternative opportunities for wage/self-employment in traditional sectors like khadi and village industries, handicraft handlooms, sericulture, small scale and cottage industries
- Initiating affirmative action to ensure at least 30 per cent of reservation for women in services in the Public Sector as their representation in 1999 was only 14 per cent, along with required provisions for upward mobility.
- Increasing access to credit for women either through the establishment of new micro-credit mechanisms or micro-financial institutions catering to women strengthening existing arrangements in these areas along with an expansion of the limited coverage of RMK.

GENDER JUSTICE

Eliminate all forms of gender discrimination and, thus, enable women to enjoy not only *de-jure* but also *de-facto* rights and fundamental freedom on par with men in all spheres, viz. political, economic, social, civil, cultural, etc. through:

- Complete eradication of female foeticide and female infanticide through effective enforcement of both the Indian Penal Code, 1860 and the Pre-Natal Diagnostic Technique (Regulation and Prevention of Misuse) Act, 1994 with most stringent measures of punishment so that a very harsh path is set for the illegal practitioners.
- Adopting measures that take into account the reproductive rights of women to enable them to exercise their reproductive choices.
- Working out strategies, in close collaboration with the Ministry of Labour, to ensure extension of employment opportunities and thus, remove inequalities in employment—both in work and accessibility.
- Initiating interventions at the macro-economic level to amend existing legislations to improve women's access to productive assets and resources.
- Ensuring that the value added by women in the Informal Sector as workers and producers is recognised through redefinition/re-interpretation of conventional concepts of work and preparation of Satellite and National Accounts
- Defining the Women's Component Plan (WCP) clearly and identifying the schemes/programmes/projects under each Ministry/Department which should be covered under WCP and ensuring the adoption of women-related mechanisms through which funds/benefits flow to women from these sectors.
- Initiating action for enacting new women-specific legislations; amending the existing women-related legislation, if necessary, based on the review made and recommendations already available to ensure gender justice, besides, reviewing all the subordinate legislations to eliminate all gender discriminatory references.
- Expediting action to legislate reservation of not less than 1/3rd seats for women in the Parliament and in the State Legislative Assemblies and thus ensure women in proportion to their numbers reach decision-making bodies so that their voices are heard.
- Arresting the ever-increasing violence against women and the Girl Child including the Adolescent girls on top priority with the strength and support of a well-planned Programme of Action prepared in consultation with all the concerned, especially the enforcement authorities; implementing effectively with the strength of the Law and Order Authorities both at the centre and state levels and assessing the situation.
- Expediting standardisation of a Gender Development Index based on which the gender segregated data will be collected at national, state and district levels; compiled/collated and

analysed to assess the progress made in improving the status of women at regular intervals with an ultimate objective of achieving equality on par with men.

- Initiating/accelerating the process of societal reorientation towards creating a Gender-Just Society.

Effective Monitoring

Lack of gender disaggregated data on various Development Indicators, both at the state and district levels has been a major problem in monitoring the progress made in improving the status of women towards achieving 'Equality' on par with men. Realising this problem, the Tenth Plan will take immediate steps to expedite standardisation of the Gender Development Index based on which the; gender segregated data will be collected at national, state and district levels; compiled/collated and analysed so as to make Assessment Reports on the progress of the status of women at regular intervals which should be comparable not only at the national level, but also at international levels. In fact, the nodal Department of Women and Child Development, in collaboration with CSO which is already engaged in collecting and publishing gender-based data and other primary and secondary data collecting Agencies like Registrar General of India, National Sample Survey Organisation (NSSO) and concerned Ministries/Departments should develop Women's Information Network, System to ensure that the gender disaggregated data flows into on a regular basis. This would help make an assessment of the efforts in achieving the ultimate goal of Gender Justice. Also the efforts initiated by the Planning Commission in collaboration with States/UTs and with the assistance of UNDP, Delhi to bring out both national and state level human development reports should allocate a separate Chapter on Gender, besides continuing these reports on biennial basis. Over and above this technical monitoring, the National Council for Women, being set-up under the Chairpersonship of the Prime Minister and the Parliamentary Committee on Empowerment of Women set-up in 2000 will oversee and review from time to time the progress made by women in achieving gender equality/gender justice on par with men.

To sum up, if Gender Justice is to be ensured, women need to be empowered socially, economically and politically. If women are to be empowered socially, it is necessary to make everyone of them literate, reach them information and generate awareness, equip them with legal literacy and help them in every way to realise their own potential. If women are to be empowered economically, it is necessary to equip them with vocational skills; provide employment and income generation, extend free channels of micro-credit, provide management/entrepreneurial skills, social security and thus allow them greater visibility. If women are to be empowered politically, the immediate need is to adopt to different forms of affirmative discriminations so that women in a proportionate numbers reach critical places to ensure that their voices are heard. In fact, it is the empowerment strategy that has emerged as the most challenging task not only for those who are working for women, but also for women themselves.[5]

Legislative Measures

To make the *de-jure* equality into a *de-facto* one, the State has enacted both women-specific and women-related legislations to safeguard the rights and interests of women, besides protecting against social discrimination, violence and atrocities and also to prevent social evils like child marriages, dowry, rape, practice of *Sati,* etc. Efforts of the Government have been to review and amend these legislations from time to time to take care of the interests of women in the changing situations and societal demands/obligations. The National Commission for Women was attending to this responsibility since its inception in 1992 as it was mandated to. Of the total 41 legislations having direct/indirect bearing on women, the Commission has reviewed and suggested certain amendments in 32 Acts and forwarded the same to the Government for necessary action. The recommendations of the Commission in respect of 14 Acts were further examined in detail in 2000 by a Task Force on Women and Children headed by Shri K.C. Pant, Deputy Chairman, Planning Commission. To start with, the nodal Department of Women and Child Development has initiated action to move amendments in respect of 4 women-specific legislations, viz. The Immoral Traffic (Prevention) Act, 1956; The Dowry Prohibition Act, 1961; The Indecent Representation of Women (Prohibition) Act, 1986 and The Commission of Sati (Prevention) Act, 1987, besides drafting a Bill on Domestic Violence against Women (Prevention). This draft Bill is now awaiting the approval of the Parliament.

While the impact of various developmental policies, plans and programmes implemented over the last few decades have brought forth a perceptible improvement in the socio-economic status of nation and violence continue to persist even today.[6]

LEGISLATIVE SUPPORT FOR WOMEN

Women-specific Legislations

- The Immoral Traffic (Prevention) Act, 1956@
- The Dowry Prohibition Act, 1961 (28 of 1961)@
- The Indecent Representation of Women (Prohibition) Act, 1986@
- The Commission of Sati (Prevention) Act, 1987 (3 of 1988)@

Women-related Legislations

- The Guardians and Wards Act, 1860 (8 of 1890)*
- Indian Penal Code, 1860**
- The Christian Marriage Act, 1872 (15 of 1872)*
- The Indian Evidence Act, 1872 (yet to be reviewed)

- The Married Women's Property Act, 1874 (3 of 1874)*
- The Workmen's Compensation Act, 1923**
- The Legal Practitioners' (Women) Act, 1923@
- The Indian Succession Act, 1925 (39 of 1925)*
- The Child Marriage Restraint Act, 1929 (19 of 1929)*
- The Payments of Wages Act, 1936**
- The Muslim Personal Law (Shariat) Application Act, 1937*
- The Factories Act, 1948@
- The Minimum Wages Act, 1948@
- The Employees' State Insurance Act, 1948@
- The Plantation Labour Act, 1951**
- The Cinematograph Act, 1952**
- The Special Marriage Act, 1954*
- The Hindu Marriage Act, 1955 (28 of 1989)*
- The Hindu Adoptions and Maintenance Act, 1956*
- The Hindu Minority and Guardianship Act, 1956*
- The Hindu Succession Act, 1956*
- The Maternity Benefit Act, 1961 (53 of 1961)@
- The Beedi and Cigar Workers (Conditions of Employment) Act, 1966**
- The Foreign Marriage Act, 1969 (33 of 1969)*
- The Indian Divorce Act, 1969 (4 of 1969)*
- The Medical Termination of Pregnancy Act, 1971 (34 of 1971)*
- Code of Criminal Procedure, 1973**
- The Bonded Labour System (Abolition) Act, 1976@
- The Equal Remuneration Act, 1976@
- The Contract Labour (Regulation and Abolition) Act, 1979.
- The Inter-State Migrant Workmen (Regulation of Employment and Conditions of Service) Act, 1979@
- The Family Courts Act, 1984@
- Juvenile Justice Act, 1986*
- The Child Labour (Prohibition and Regulation) Act, 1986**
- National Commission for Women Act, 1990 (20 of 1990)*
- The Infant Milk Substitutes, Feeding Bottles and Infant Foods (Regulation of Production, Supply and Distribution) Act, 1992*
- The Pre-Natal Diagnostic Technique (Regulation and The Prevention of Misuse) Act, 1994*

* Reviewed by National Commission for Women (NCW).
** Reviewed by the Task Force on Women and Children.
@ Reviewed by both NCW and the Task Force on Women and Children.

CRITICAL APPRAISAL

Planning Women's Participation in their Own Welfare

Women should themselves exert pressure to get the due benefits for their welfare. They should unite to form voluntary organizations to help themselves and ultimately the nation. It was rightly stated in the National Plan of Action for Women that:

Women voluntary organizations are best suited for motivation in the field of health, family planning and nutrition. There is therefore, every need for creating a conductive climate, so that they can render the needed service effectively.[7]

In this implementation process, women themselves will have to be the most forceful agents for change and active participants in the dynamic role. The contemporary social situation of women in India should not be frustrating and disheartening but should be rather challenging and it is the men and women of India, particularly the women who have to face the challenge. It has been demonstrated by the women in the field that they are as capable and efficient as men in carrying out various kinds of work and have even much more endurance for hardships than is commonly believed. All of us who are associated with the development of the country in any capacity, must renew our dedication to the cause of women which would lead to national development and modernization. There is also a need of making realistic policies for women impowerment.

Policies should be made in Consonance with the Objectives

By goal or objective is meant the end towards which action is directed. Since a policy is a guidance for action, it is reasonable to expect that a policy indicates the direction towards which action is guided, either explicitly or implicitly. For this reason, students of policy sciences often define public policies as a programme of goals and objectives.

Absence of Contradictions and Inconsistencies

It is necessary for public administrators to help in making policies purposeful and goal-oriented, and to assist in defining goals and objectives clearly, in making them concrete and also quantifiable if possible and in removing, to the extent possible, any contradictions and inconsistencies.

Temporal Dimensions

The modern world is rapidly changing. So, our policies must not remain constant but should change with the change in times. A UN report suggests the following three points:

(a) It is a well-known fact that a public policy, in order to be effective, must not be too little or too late;
(b) Time sequence is an essential part of a successful policy. An effective policy should comprise not only what a government should do but also when to do one thing after another. Timing is often an essential factor for the success or failure of a policy; and
(c) Synchronization is another timing element.

Feasibility, Probability and Possibility

Policies which are not based on the technical, economic, administrative and perhaps also proposed political feasibility should be avoided unless it is the specific wish of the policy-makers to adopt such policies. It is important to note that feasibility, probability and possibility are all relative terms. If the policy-makers have reason to believe that what they plan will change the circumstances in favour of the planned objectives, then they are justified in the planning for what may appear to be 'Improbable' or even 'Impossible' to the experts who assume that the circumstances will remain constant. For the developing countries, estimates by experts on feasibility, probability and possibility are often poorly informed guess-work, in part owing to lack of sufficient or decisive evidence and in part owing to a high degree of uncertainty. In a UN document which warns against 'paper planning' and blind commitments to the blatantly impossible, it is stated:

"From the previous extremes of seeking the impossible, the planners may go so far in emphasizing the possible that they will think mainly of short-run feasibility. In this effort, they will often be encouraged by economists who have become accustomed to fighting utopia with myopia, that is with 'hard nosed' calculations of small benefits that might be obtained quickly. The result can easily be that instead of planning for the impossible, they will focus upon most possible and feasible of all, namely, the inevitable. This is the fallacy of epiphenomenal planning. Here the main advantage is that the planners can take credit for any minor progress that might have taken place."

Relevant Forecasts and Projections

According to a U.N. report, "Forecasting and projection are important for public policy-making mainly for two reasons. First, as just indicated, policy is a guidance for action that lies necessarily in the future. Therefore, no rational approach to policy-making is possible without some basis for making assumptions about the future. Forecasting and projection can assist policy-makers in this respect. Secondly, public policies should be used. If at all possible, to avoid crisis rather than to meet crisis situations. Unless a government is capable of making useful forecasts and projections, it is not in a position to avoid crisis and may have to devote most of its resources to crisis management. At the same time, a government which is under constant pressure from immediate crisis may not be able to devote its attention and resources to the future in order to prevent the recurrence of crisis. This is a vicious circle which a government should break, and it can succeed in doing so only by assigning suitable priority to forecasting the future."

Appropriate Administrative Machinery

Within the central policy cluster there should also be special arrangement for ensuring that appropriate administrative machinery is established for:

(a) policy and plan implementation,
(b) reporting and feed-back,
(c) evaluation and control, and
(d) the adjustment and revision of policies, plans and programmes.

This would ensure effective relationships between policy formulation and policy implementation.

Understanding the Implications of Policy

Policies must be interpreted and explained, to all members of the organisation. What people do not understand they cannot use correctly and are likely to distrust. Therefore, there is a need to explain it to all persons to whom it applies.

Environmental Considerations

Policy is based on actual information or factual data which can be collected from a number of sources by applying different methods. But, before the data can be changed into a policy, many factors have to be taken into consideration, e.g. policies must be made in accordance with the provisions of the constitution and the laws enacted by the legislature; these must also be made in accordance with the social, political, cultural, economic and ethical environment prevailing in the country; these must also be linked with the agencies interested in the same policy to have maximum utility and effectiveness; these must also be made in accordance with the opinion of the public otherwise they would not cooperate with the government in their execution.

Positive Role of Parliamentary Committee on Empowerment of Women

A Joint Committee of the Parliament on Empowerment of Women has been constituted to keep women's issues under constant review and monitoring and to watch progress in pursuance of plans of action evolved at international and national levels. The functions of the Committee on Empowerment of Women are:

- To consider the reports submitted by the National Commission for Women and to report on the measures that should be taken by the Union Government for improving the status/conditions of women in respect of matters within the purview of the Union Government including the Administrations of the Union Territories;
- To examine the measures taken by the Union Government to secure for women equality, status and dignity in all matters;
- To examine the measures taken by the Union Government for comprehensive education and adequate representation of women in Legislative bodies/services and other fields;

- To report on the working of the welfare programmes for women;
- To report on the action taken by the Union Government and Administrations of the Union Territories on the measures proposed by the Committee; and
- To examine such other matters as may seem fit to the Committee or are specifically referred to it by the House or the Speaker and the Rajya Sabha or the Chairman of Rajya Sabha.

The Committee on the status of women, 1974 believed that:

(a) Equality of women is necessary, not merely on the grounds of social justice, but as a basic condition for social, economic and political development of the nation;

(b) In order to release women from their dependent and unequal status, improvement of their employment opportunities and earning power has to be given the highest priority;

(c) Society owes a special responsibility to women because of their child-bearing function. Safe bearing and rearing of children is an obligation that has to be shared by the mother, the father and society;

(d) The contribution made by an active housewife to the running and management of a family should be admitted as economically and socially productive and contributing to national savings and development;

(e) Marriage and motherhood should not become a disability in women fulfiling their full and proper role in the task of national development. Therefore, it is important that society, including women themselves, must accept their responsibility in this field;

(f) Disabilities and inequalities imposed on women have to be seen in the total context of a society, where large sections of the population—male and female, adults and children—suffer under the oppression of an exploitative system. It is not possible to remove these inequalities for women only. Any policy or movement for the emancipation and development of women has to form a part of a total movement for removal of inequalities and oppressive social institutions, if the benefits and privileges won by such action are to be shared by the entire women population and not be monopolised by a small minority; and

(g) If our society is to move in the direction of the goals set by the Constitution, then special temporary measures will be necessary to transform *de-jure* into *de-facto* equality.

"We realise that changes in social attitudes and institutions cannot be brought about very rapidly. It is, however, necessary to accelerate this process of change by deliberate and planned efforts. Responsibility for this acceleration has to be shared by the State and the community, particularly that section of the community which believes in the equality of women. We, therefore, urge that community organisations, particularly women's organisations should mobilise public opinion and strengthen social efforts against oppressive institutions like polygamy, dowry, ostentatious expenditure on wedding and child marriage, and mount a campaign for the dissemination of information about the legal rights of women to increase their awareness. This is a joint responsibility which has to be shared by community organisations, legislators who have helped to frame these laws and the Government which is responsible for implementing them."

CONCLUSION

Report on the Status of Women rightly mentions that development in its wider perspective covers all aspects of community life. The accepted goals of national development such as maximum production, full employment, and attainment of economic equality and social justice apply equally to men and women. Their realization in an egalitarian society is not, however, possible, unless special efforts are made to assist the underprivileged groups. Our constitution therefore stresses the urgent need for promoting the educational and economic interests of the weaker sections of the people; and as women are handicapped by social customs and traditions, they need special attention to help them to play their full and proper role in a national life.[8]

"The great occupation of women should be to beautify life; to cultivate, for her own sake and that of those who surround her, all her faculties of mind, soul, and body; all her powers of enjoyment, and powers of giving enjoyment; and to diffuse beauty, elegance, and grace, everywhere. If in addition to this the activity of her nature demands more energetic and definite employment, there is never any lack of it in the world. If she loves, here natural impulse will be to associate her existence with him she loves, and to share his occupations; in which, if he loves her (with that affection of equality which along deserves to be called love) she will naturally take as strong an interest, and he as thoroughly conversant, as the most perfect confidence on his side can make her."[9]

Dr. (Miss) Mira Seth, the then Member, Planning Commission, Government of India, delivered the convocation address at the annual convocation of the Banasthali Vidyapith (Deemed University). She said that the Parliament legislation has been an instruments of giving equality and status to women in our country and this has taken the place of the ancient Vedic, Paurnaic, Shastra and Smriti injunctions. Our Parliament has enacted sixteen laws from the Hindu Marriage Act, 1955 to the Commission of Sati (Prevention) Act, 1987 for giving legal sanction to this principle of equality.

In the development processes and the Five Year Plans of our country, they give emphasis to the instrument of education as one of the major tools for empowering women. The focus on educational planning for women has shifted from their traditional role as housewives and mothers to non-traditional roles as producers, partners and partakers in the national development.[10]

Ms. Terjani Vakil, Former Chairman and Managing Director, Export-Import Bank of India, delivered the Convocation address at the Banasthali Vidyapith, Banasthali (Rajasthan). She said, "Keep a space for yourself as a person. Think about what you are, what you want to be, what is your personal *raison de etre* for living. What interests you, what pleases you, do that. Keep a time and space for yourself in your life. For you are an individual, a human being and not just someone's wife, mother, daughter. I would want you to think about this."[11]

Notes and References

1. ICSSR—Status of Women in India—A Synopsis of the Report of the National Commission, New Delhi, 1975, pp. 84-85.
2. *Ibid.*
3. GOI, Planning Commission, Ninth Five Year Plan, p. 336.
4. *Ibid.*, pp. 321-22.
5. GOI, Planning Commission, Draft Tenth Five Year Plan, 2002-07, New Delhi, Chapter 2.11.
6. National Plan of Action for Women, p. 71.
7. *Ibid.*
8. ICSSR, Status of Women in India, *op. cit.*, p. 116.
9. John Stuart Mill and H.T. Mill, Early Essays on Marriage and Divorce, Alice and Rossi (ed.) Essays on Sexual Equality, p. 225.
10. AIU, *University News*, July 22, 1996, pp. 18-19.
11. AIU, *University News*, April 13, 1990, p. 12.

CHAPTER 2

WOMEN DEVELOPMENT AND EMPOWERMENT: ESSENTIAL FOR WOMEN HEALTH

"Women's expectations and hopes for a greener, cleaner, responsive and representative politics have gone up. They will send out more clearly and energetically the message of women's empowerment and social development. For that reservation needs to be accompanied by considerable amount of affirmative action programme."

—India Panchayati Raj Report, 2001,
Vol. II, NIRD, Hyderabad, India, pp. 302-03

Women Development and Empowerment: Essential for Women Health

"Real Change in India will come when women begin to affect the political deliberations of the nation."

—*Gandhiji*

Women especially rural women, urban women living in slums and tribal women are faced even today with large number of problems which do not allow them to develop. Problems of poverty, ill-health, social customs keep her busy. She can never imagine to move foreward.

Snehlata Panda in her Article, "Reservation for Women in Union and State Legislatures: A Perspective" in IIPA, Oct.-Dec., 2001 rightly states that the Constitution of India empowers the State to "adopt measures of positive discrimination in favour of women to assist them to overcome cumulative socio-economic educational and political oppression faced for centuries." But in reality women are invisible in the national mainstream, they are harassed in the family, society, the work place, vindicating the absolute incompetence of the laws which have been enacted to protect women's rights and recognise their rights as human rights. An Inter-parliamentary Union Report in February 1997 revealed that women hold 7.2 per cent seats in the Lok Sabha, 7.8 per cent in the Rajya Sabha. Even as ministers they hold mostly unimportant posts like health education, welfare, child development, etc., the gender specific allocation of jobs in offices and in manual labour is but an extension of the domestic role of women arising from a mindset which sans transformation in tandem with the amendments in law relating to women. Women's representation in the Parliament or state legislative assemblies has never been more than 10 per cent despite the fact that they constitute 50 per cent of the total population. The fact that women in India are no way better in their social position than the social

CHART 2.1

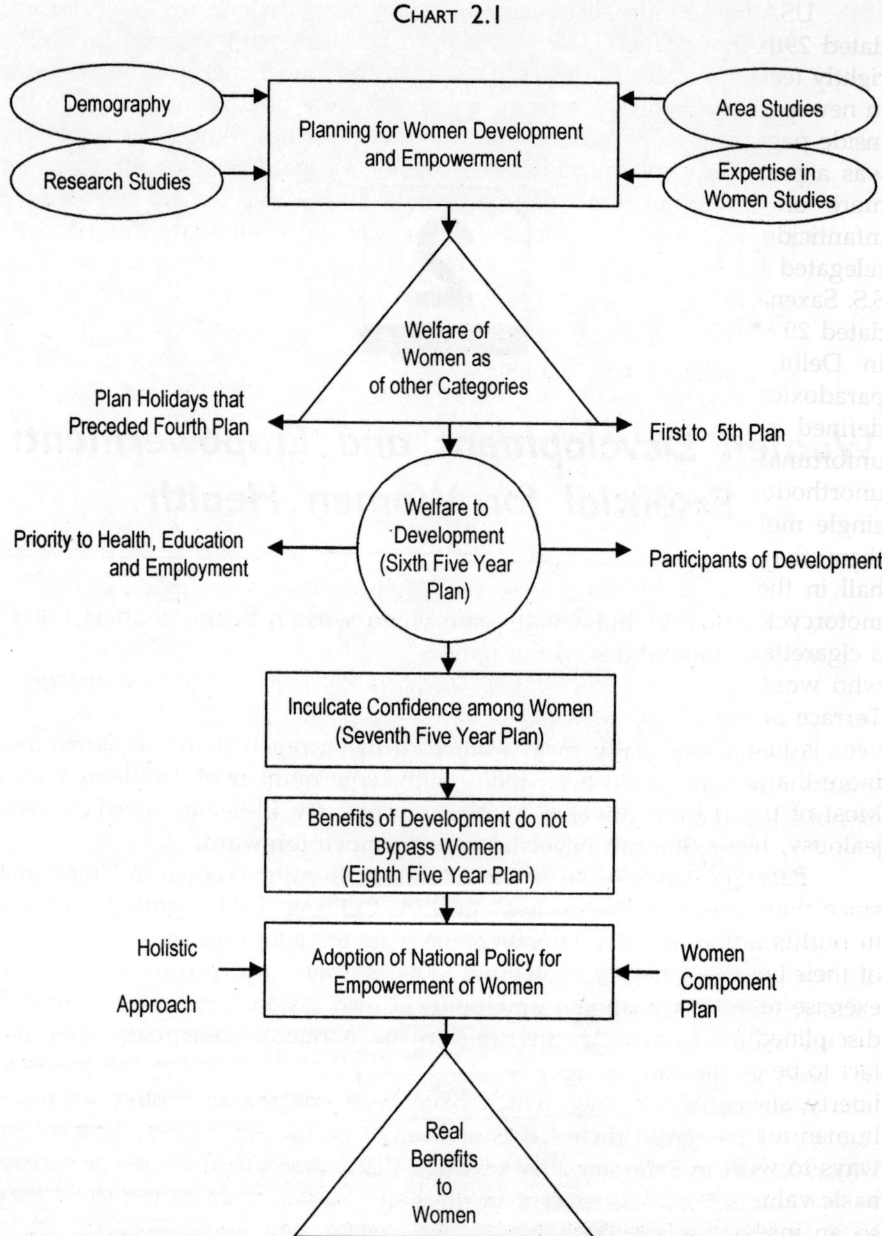

categories for whom reservation has been provided in the Union and state legislatures has never been seriously viewed. Therefore, in the Constituent Assembly reservation for women was defeated with an ideological presumption that the working of democracy in the normal course would ensure the representation of all sections of Indian society including women and reservation would underestimate the strength of women to compete as equals.

USA-based journalist Seema Sirohi in her Article in the *Daily Tribune* dated 29th June 2003, "Dowry Needs to be Dealt with and not Ignored", rightly feels that cases of dowry harassment no longer merit prime positions in newspapers. Even stories of dowry deaths were now being pushed to the inside pages, reflecting a clear shift in social priorities. Where earlier dowry was a principal concern, now even women's organisations were focusing more on the other emerging problems like child abuse and female infanticide. I was not comfortable with the idea of allowing dowry to be relegated to the background. In cities, women themselves invite violence. S.S. Saxena in his Article, "Why is Delhi Unsafe for Women" in *The Tribune* dated 29.6.2003 puts the blame on women themselves for many problems. In Delhi, a major contribution to perpetuate crimes against women paradoxically comes from the women themselves. In the absence of a well-defined social structure and the identity of traditional culture it is unfortunate to watch young girls from well to do families going out in unorthodox and provocative outfits. They can be seen showing thumbs to single motorists for a lift even where buses or 'specials' are available to them; they can also be seen bunking classes and adventuring into a cinema hall in the afternoons or a fast food joint in the company of rich car or motorcycle borne jazzy clothed boys in jeans and costly sun glasses with a cigarette in hand. "It is my life" would be the reaction of an average girl who would retort by telling how conservative and out of times you are. Terrace or garden parties are not very uncommon where a small drink or beer is just about right. The nucleus of a permissive society where 'not-more-than-this' relationship determines the initial indulgence, lies here. Most of the crimes in this segment of society are the aftermath of natural jealousy, frustration or at times to cover up the exposure of deceit.

Parents who cry foul when something happens are equally to blame since they choose to close their eyes when the girls go out of the houses in outfits almost inviting trouble or when they pass off the misadventure of their boys as childish errands. It is one thing to say that the men should exercise restraint but an entirely different thing to presume all men to be the disciplined lot. (the disciplined are no threat any was justify the wrong, the fact to be considered is that if someone dares to bare as a matter of personal liberty, she should be able to accept the consequences too. Instinctively, the human male, unless checked by the society will accost a human female. The ways to woo, however, will differ depending upon the male's sense for the basic value. No one can, not even stringent laws, can guarantee this, more so an insensitive society.

Traces of such a 'way of life' do not remain confined to only to rich, educated and the well-to-do sections of the urban population in Delhi. It encourages others to ape the same in varying degrees. As a result, even the less enterprising and not so bold, fall into the trap either due to innocence or the inability to suppress the temptation of an occasional filing. The consequences and the gravity of these encounters also depend on the extent of the distortions in the general perception and the attitude of the young, lack of education and erosion of respect for the parental authority.

Tragically, in a society, surviving with loose knots of cultural heritage and discipline, uncontrolled urge to fall for cheap temptations and base thrills would naturally overshadow and erode the virtues of self-control, caution, restraint and discretion.

S.R. Bakshi and Kiran Bala feel that patriarchal values and formative structure established some two thousand years ago still persist though in different garb. Motherhood and the ideal of a faithful self-sacrificing wife are projected through the media and the education system. The reality of subordinate position of women is indicated through adverse sex ratio of girls, the growing domestic violence, increasing number of dowry deaths and rape cases.

The relative case with which Indian women secured juridical equality, entered professions and occupied positions of power has led to a myth that Indian women enjoy a very high status in society; they are able to balance their two roles very efficiently and that they wield power naturally. This myth has been eroded during the last ten to fifteen years. There is a growing awareness that men and women suffer from discrimination and deprivation. The problems of educated urban women become more serious since the discrimination and disabilities operate in a more subtle and covert ways. Thus, the dual existence of women holding high positions and yet undergoing various types of suffering continue.

One very hopeful development which has occurred during the last ten years is the emergence of women's movement wherein women have started raising their voice against inequality, patriarchal values and in egalitarian social structure. The new leadership, we hope, will not only expose the myth of the high position of Indian women but will adopt more positive steps to raise the status of women.

J.S. Mul in his book, "The Subjection of Woman" states that one of the greatest disabilities the Indian women suffers from, under the present order is the difference in the standard of morality for men and women. Society ostracizes women for any moral lapse while the man is allowed to escape for the same offence. We believe in a high standard of morality but we also believe that the standard should be the same for both. We, therefore, recommend that an identical standard of morality be insisted on for both man and woman—one that harmonizes social welfare with industrial freedom.

Mrs. Rajshree N. Varhadi rightly feel that violence against women both violates and impairs or nullifies the enjoyment by women of human rights and fundamental freedoms. Taking into account the Declaration on the Elimination of Violence against Women and the work of Special Rapporteurs, gender-based violence, such as battering and other domestic violence, sexual abuse, sexual slavery and exploitation and international trafficking in women and children, forced prostitution and sexual harassment, as well as violence against women, resulting from cultural prejudice, racism and racial discrimination, xenophobia, pornography, ethnic cleansing, armed conflict, foreign occupation, religious and anti-

CHART 2.2

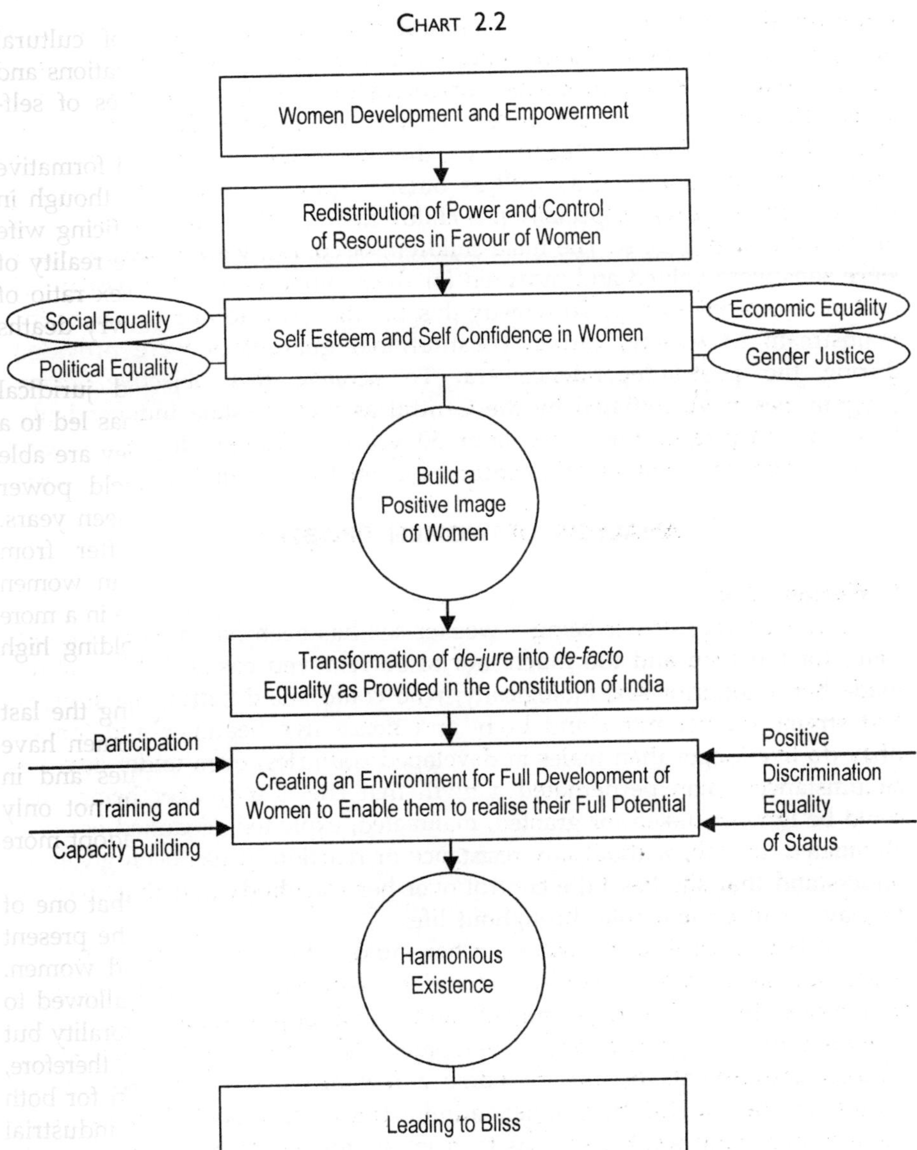

religious extremism and terrorism are incompatible with the dignity and the worth of the human person and must be combated and eliminated. Any harmful aspect of certain traditional, customary or modern practices that violated the rights of women should be prohibited and eliminated. Governments should take urgent action to combat and to eliminate all forms of violence against women in private and public life, whether perpetrated or tolerated by the State or private persons.

Anitha Kaul in her Article, "Women and Children" feels that women were discriminated against in all walks of life, and denied equal opportunities with men. This was reflected in unequal access of women and girls to education, health, nutrition and employment. They, not only had no control over the productive resources such as land, house and other assets, but also had no role to play in decision-making. The system was such that they were relegated to the marginal position with men dominating the domestic as well as outside spheres. While this was the situation the children, especially girl children, were either totally neglected or discriminated against. The male children, of course, were taken seriously since sons were valued and nurtured for their importance in the patriarchal and male-centred society. To remedy this situation and to bring them to the mainstream of society, certain constitutional guarantees were provided during the post-independence era. To achieve this objective, many programmes were initiated by the Central as well as state independents. However, inspite of this, even after 50 years of independence, the gap between men and women still continues in relation to equal opportunities.

ANALYSIS OF WOMEN PROBLEMS

I. Weaker Sex

The concept of her being a weaker sex has been hammered into her 'self', for too long and too much, not to be removed easily. While nature made her a superior sex, biologically, who could stand better, the stresses and strains on her mind and body and hence live healthier and longer (they do live longer than males in developed countries) even under adverse circumstances, man perpetuated a myth that she is a weaker being and could be ignored, taken for granted, maltreated, exploited, assaulted or even eliminated, at will, without any resistance or reaction. It has been given to understand that she has little control over her own body and that she has to play a subservient role throughout life.

It is this sense of weakness in her mind, which makes her suffer at every step, at the alter of family and society. Wherever it has been possible to remove this 'inferiority-complex' and equal opportunities have been provided for her growth and development, she has simply excelled in various departments of life. To name a few areas, she has excelled as doctor, teacher, architect, planner, administrator, and politician, etc. The myth of her being weaker-sex has to crumble, for her proper development and her rightful contribution to the society.

2. Role Differentiation

Even "Atharvaveda contains rituals to ensure the birth of a son preference to that of a daughter." The process of rejecting a female child starts, in many cases before birth, with female foeticide. While talking of female infanticide one researcher says, "If by some strange miracle the female baby survival, she is tolerated but never allowed to develop at expense of her brothers." This attitude of rejection has an immense impact on the female psyche and growth of their personality. Vidu Mohan rightly feels that they live in perpetual feeling of guilt of being a burden on parents. The parents also use double standards and different codes of rearing a boy and a girl. The girl is taught and reared differently from a boy. She is given food having less nutritional in value; in behaviour responses she is taught to give in social behaviour, she is taught withdrawal, she is made to talk in a hush fashion, she is given toys like dolls and kitchen article, not pistols. In earlier stages she is asked to shoulder household responsibilities like serving food, cleaning, etc. in these environmental role differentiation, people start believing that girls by nature are dependent, indecisive, timid,. shy, nervous and affiliative.

3. Psycho-social Perspective

In understanding the female psyche, we have to understand the growth of the 'self'. In the growth of self also some sex-role linked attitudes are developed. The attitude of passivity in women takes a form of fatalism-learned dependency of helplessness established early in life. In a situation of inequality and powerlessness, these characteristics can lead to subservience and to complex psychological problems.

4. Unsatisfactory Environment for Working Women

Though more and more women are taking up work, yet they have also faced a lot of role conflict. Earlier they were supposed to belong only to home and its responsibilities. Today the working woman is tom by the conflict that if she goes to work, she is neglecting her home and children. She feels, it is her responsibility to do both the jobs efficiently. Though more and more women are taking up work, yet they have also faced a lot of role conflict. Earlier they were supposed to belong only to home and its responsibilities. Today the working woman is torn by the conflict that if she goes to work, she is neglecting her home and children. She feels, it is her responsibility to do both the jobs efficiently. In this process she develops feeling of guilt of not devoting full time to her children and home. As a result, she doubles her effort. This furthering of effort tells upon her mental and physical well being. In the cases where the wife dehtands the husband to share household chores, tension starts mounting and family disputes take place. Usually in such situations the in-laws blame the woman for this. Thus, instead of reducing her workload she increases her conflict and guilt. The in-laws like to get the salary of the working daughter in-law, but they do not like to share her household burden. Mr. N. Mukherjee in working mother Femina, 1985 observed, "with inflexible standards to meet at both home and work, the working woman is thus always chasing an impossible ideal. Our society is in a phase of transition, where old traditions and norms are being modified due to current needs. In a society in transition. In which tradition is undergoing change but the modern value has not been accepted fully, a great deal of confusion in social, moral norms and cultural standards is to be expected."

5. Crimes

Women in India face some of the most heinous crimes committed against them, such as rape, flesh trade, foeticide, female infanticide, child abuse, wife battering, dowry deaths, sati, financial exploitation, sexual exploitation of working women and female students. Law is there to prevent all this, yet we find women opposed, exploited, cheated, uneducated, financially dependent, mentally cloister, morally run down and physically violated. A country's socio-economic growth cannot take place if half of its population is down trodden.

We may conclude with some important suggestions which are essential for lessening gender discrimination.

(i) Increasing General and Functional Literacy,
(ii) Provision of Adequate Health Service,
(iii) Provision of Nutritional Service,
(iv) Ensuring Human rights due to them,
(v) Making law enforcing machinery strongest, and
(vi) Ensuring prompt action.

PLANNING WOMEN'S PARTICIPATION IN THEIR OWN WELFARE

Women should themselves excert pressure to get the due benefits for their welfare. They should unite to form voluntary organisations to help themselves and ultimately the nation. It was rightly stated in the National Plan of Action for Women that: "Women voluntary organisations are best suited for motivation in the field of health, family planning and nutrition. There is therefore, every need for creating a conducive climate, so that they can render the needed service effectively."

The women's voluntary organisations in the form of Mother's Club in the Republic of Korea have been quite useful in raising the status of women. By mid-1977. nearly 70,000 such clubs had been organised. The clubs provide opportunities for village women to get together to talk about health education of children and improvement of environment. The club helps in family planning, vaccination and treatment of emergency cast. The mother's club are a genuinely grass-root community net work which owes little to outside administrators or planners. J.C. Abeede in his article on "Women Power in Korea" observes that mother's clubs are helping to change age-old social attitudes towards women. He says, "The growth of women's clubs in Korea has coincided with considerable changes in social attitudes towards women. The trend is towards greater recognition of women contribution to the community, better communication between husband and wife, and more open discussion of family planning matter . . . it seems clear that the enhanced status of women and the growth of mother's clubs have gone hand-in-hand and are contributing significantly to the development of rural communities in Korea.

Such clubs should be set-up in other countries as well. These, state go would help mobilise voluntary resources lying idle and if not used can be a source of destruction. In the developing countries like India, voluntary organisations are urban-based and serve the urban area. These organisations must create a strong base by setting up such clubs and diffuse information to them to be passed among the members of the community. This would bring about a socio-economic revolution and contribute substantially to modernization and development.

The women have shown a significant progress in ensuring their rights and privileges in social, economic, educational and administrative fields. In fact, in certain areas like expectation of life at birth, women have already proved to be better than the men at the same time. However, there is long way for Indian women to traverse before their achieve the equality at par with men.

There is a proposal to reserve 33 percent of the seats in legislative bodies from amongst the women. 73rd and 74th Constitution Amendments have already provided for the reservation of females in rural and urban elected bodies. In the ultimate analysis, women themselves will have to be the most forceful agents for change and active participation in the development efforts. Consistent and persistent efforts are needed to liquidate the limitations still suffered by women to work shoulder to shoulder to improve the standard of living of the Indian masses so that opportunities for living a richer and fruitful life would be .available to both women and men.

Preeti Singh in an Article, "Being Single, and Loving it" in *The Tribune* dated 6.7.2003 feels that over the years a single woman no longer remains alone. She gradually gathers a family of admirers and friends around her. Due to her independent nature, financial freedom and creative living, she gradually becomes a beacon of hope to other women who happen to find themselves single after a painful marriage and divorce.

Komal V. Singh in an Article, "Frowning fathers give way to doting dads" feels that one does not need research to prove that children of loving and involved fathers have a better shot at life. New-age dads realise their children need them to survive and thrive. They carve out time to enter their world and walk their turf. Parental warmth in early childhood has a direct bearing on the social development of the young ones. Fathers have as much role as mothers to play in the kids development. Besides, they are just as capable as their wives of caring for their children. Fathers who are affectionate and liberal with hugs and cuddles arm children with a lifetime insurance of being socially well-equipped. Such children invariably grow up to be good workers, good friends and good spouses. Experiencing a strong sense of bonding with daddy, besides mommy, leads to the development of a sense of security that helps. Society today has given a clarion call for emotionally attuned fathers who are there, building a lifetime bond of special moments and memories with their children. The day has dawned when masculinity is connected to fatherhood. Becoming a father enhances a man. It takes a man to be a dad, after all. There is a certain macho appeal to being a doting dad. And the world just loves to smile at such men.

At this stage a few lines from the poem titled Shabola, written by the great Bengali poet Rabindranath Tagore which embodied women's voice of protest maybe quoted:

"Why must you curtail her rights
And keep women from conquering her own fate
Oh Divine Ruler?
Why should we stand forlorn by the way side!
With bowed heads.
Waiting for our weary patient dreams.
To be fulfiled on some
Auspicious Day?
Must we always stay into vacant space?
Can we not choose for ourselves
The paths to our fulfilments?

Yes, this is a right time for women to choose the path to fulfil their dreams and aspirations in the 21st century. At this juncture it can be said that women have just begun this journey . . . a journey for better survival or more freedom. The path is difficult to pave the way. . . . But journey has certainly begun and is sure to achieve success.

Empowerment of women is one of the most important key factors for the welfare and development of any society. Of late, the government has also subscribed to the idea that without empowering women, the development of society is not possible in the right direction and at a desired pace. So, the government has started many Women Empowerment Programmes (WEP) at national as well as at state level.

Empowerment of women is a slow but continuous process. Women must come up to play their role in planning, decision-making and implementation. The scenario has been changing slowly in cities but the same has not been happening in rural areas and urban slums. For making WEPs successful at grass-root level, in rural areas and urban slums, where it is required the most positive discrimination is required.

One more very important fact, requiring the attention of NGOs and other implementing agencies for WEP's is that there are two big segments amongst the women. One segment is that which is aware of its rights but closes its eyes towards its duties. And another bigger segment of women is that which knows its duties without asking for its rights and thus suffering silently. This gap has to be bridged. Unless and until a balance between rights and duties is struck, WEPs cannot be successful.

Empowerment as a concept was first brought at the International Women's Conference in 1985 at Nairobi. The conference concluded that empowerment is a redistribution of power and control of resources in favour of women through positive intervention.

The Programme of Action 1992 has comprehensively given the below mentioned parameters of empowerment of women:

- Enhance self-esteem and self-confidence in women.
- Build a positive image of women by recognizing their contribution to the society, polity and economy.
- Develop in them an ability to think critically.
- Foster decision-making and action through collective process.
- Enable women to make informed choices in areas like education, employment and health especially reproductive health.
- Ensure equal participation in the developmental process.
- Provide information, knowledge and skill for economic independence.
- Enhance access to legal literacy and information related to their rights and entitlements in the society with a view to enhance their participation on an equal footing in all areas.

The special attention given to the needs and problems of women to enable them to enjoy and exercise their Constitutional equality of status, along with other specific provisions relating to the hitherto suppressed sections of our society have led many scholars to describe the Indian Constitution as a 'social' document embodying the objectives of a social revolution. There is no doubt that the Constitution contemplates attainment of an entirely new social order by making deliberate departures in norms and institutions of democratic governance from the inherited social, political and economic systems. In doing so the Constitution assigns primacy to law as an instrument of directed social change. It thus demands of the legislature, the executive and the judiciary, continuous vigilance and responsiveness to the relationship between law and social transformation in contemporary India.

We believe:

1. that equality of women is necessary, not merely on the grounds of social justice, but as a basic condition for social, economic and political development of the nation;
2. that in order to release women from their dependent and unequal status, improvement of their employment opportunities and earning power has to be given the highest priority;
3. that society owes a special responsibility to women because of their child-bearing function. Safe bearing and rearing of children is an obligation that has to be shared by the mother, the father and society;
4. that the contribution made by an active housewife to the running and management of a family should be admitted as economically and socially productive and contributing to national savings and development;

5. that marriage and motherhood should not become a disability. In women's fulfiling their full and proper role in the task of national development. Therefore, it is important that society, including women themselves, must accept their responsibility in this field;
6. that disabilities and inequalities imposed on women have to be seen in the total context of a society, where large sections of the population—male and female, adults and children—suffer under the oppression of an exploitative system. It is not possible to remove these inequalities for women only. Any policy or movement for the emancipation and development of women has to form a part of a total movement for removal of inequalities and oppressive social institutions, if the benefits and privileges won by such action are to be shared by the entire women population and not be monopolized by a small minority, and
7. that if our society is to move in the direction of the goals set by the Constitution, then special temporary measures will be necessary, to transform *de-jure* into *de-facto* equality.[1]

The World Summit held during Nov. 25-28, 1996 at Trinidad and Tobago was the First Conference of Ministers Responsible for Women Affairs. 45 Commonwealth Countries participated and very useful decisions were taken regarding the implementation of Commonwealth Plan of Action on gender and development, gender management systems, gender integration into politics and conflict resolution, integration of gender concerns into macro economic policies and women's human rights. The next meeting was held at Edinburgh in 1997. However, rigorous efforts are being made throughout the world and various schemes/programmes have been launched to minimize the gender bias, and offer ample opportunities to bring women at par with men in respect to education, employment, human rights and decision-making roles, etc. Still Status of women varies from country to country and even within a country. It varies with the arbitration in the locality (rural/urban), religion, caste and community. It manifests in terms of level of education, occupation, income, restrictions imposed in their activities and financial independence understand the Indian scenario, history that there were distinct stages of rise and fall of in the status of women.[2]

Empowerment of women's being one of the nine primary objectives of the Ninth Plan, every effort will be made to create an enabling environment where women can freely exercise their rights both within and outside home, as equal partners along with men. This will be realized through early finalization and adoption of the 'National Policy for Empowerment of Women' which laid down definite goals, targets and policy prescriptions along with a well defined Gender Development Index to monitor the impact of its implementation in raising the status of women from time to time.

An integrated approach will be adopted towards empowering women through convergence of existing services, resources, infrastructure and manpower available in both women-specific and women-related sectors with the ultimate objective of achieving the set goal. To this effect, the Ninth Plan directs both the Centre and the States to adopt a special strategy of 'Women's Component Plan' through which, not less than 30 per cent of funds/benefits are earmarked in all the women-related sectors. It also suggests a special vigil to be kept on the flow of the earmarked funds/ benefits through an effective mechanism to ensure that the proposed strategy brings forth a holistic approach towards empowering women.

While organising women into Self-Help Groups marks the beginning of a major process of empowering women, the institutions thus developed would provide a permanent forum for articulating their needs and contributing their perspectives to development. Recognising the fact that women have been socialised only to take a back seat in public life, affirmative action through deliberate strategies will be initiated to provide equal access to and control over factors contributing to such empowerment, particularly in the areas of health, education, information, life-long learning for self-development, vocational skills, employment and income generating opportunities, land and other forms of property including through inheritance, common property, resources, credit, technology and markets, etc. To this effect, the newly elected women members and the women Chairpersons of Panchayats and the Local Bodies will be sensitised through the recently launched special training package to take the lead in ensuring that adequate funds/benefits flow towards the empowerment of women and the girl child.

COMMITMENTS OF THE NINTH PLAN (1997-2002)

Objective

- Empowering women as the agents of social change and development

Strategies

- To create an enabling environment for women to exercise their rights, both within and outside home, as equal partners along with men through early finalisation and adoption of "National Policy for Empowerment of women."
- To expedite action to legislate reservation of not less than 1/3rd seats for women in the Parliament and in the State Legislative Assemblies and thus ensure adequate representation of women in decision-making.
- To adopt an integrated approach towards empowering women through effective convergence of existing services, resources,

infrastructure and manpower in both women-specific and women-related sectors.

- To adopt a special strategy of "Women's Component Plan" to ensure that not less than 30 percent of funds/benefits flow to women from other developmental sectors.
- To organise women into Self-help group and thus mark the beginning of a major process of empowering women.
- To accord high priority to reproductive child healthcare.
- To universalise the on-going supplementary feeding programmes—Special Nutrition Programme (SNP) and Mid-Day Meals (MDM).
- To ensure easy and equal access to education for women and girls through the commitments of the Special Action Plan of 1998.
- To initiate steps to eliminate gender bias in all educational programmes.
- To institute plans for free education for girls upto college level, including professional courses.
- To equip women with necessary skills in the modern upcoming trades which could keep them gainfully engaged besides making them economically independent and self-reliant.
- To increase access to credit through setting up of a 'Development Bank for Women Entrepreneurs in small and tiny sectors.[3]

Women who number 498.7 million according to 2001 census prepresent 48.2 per cent of country's population of 1,027.01 million. The development of women has always been the central focus in developmental planning, since Independence. Though there have been various shifts in policy approaches in the last 50 years from the concept of welfare in the 70s, to development in the 80s, and now the empowerment in the 90s, the Department of Women and Child Development, since its inception has been implementing special programmes for holistic development and empowerment of women with welfare programme, particularly in the sectors of health, education, rural and urban development, etc. Initiatives undertaken in the area of women's empowerment include:[4]

- Welfare and Support Services,
- Employment and Training,
- Socio-economic Programme,
- Swayamsidha,
- Swa-shakti Project,
- Balika Samriddhi Yojna,
- Plan of Action to combat Sexual Exploitation of Women and Children,
- Declaring 2001 as Women's Empowerment year,

- Instituting National Commission for Women,
- Rashtriya Mahila Kosh,
- National Institute of Public Cooperation and Child Development,
- Central Social Welfare Board,
- Food and Nutrition Board, and
- Information and Mass Education.

The Constitution of India has guaranteed equality before law and equal protection of law (Art. 14) and prohibits discriminatory provisions for women and children (Art. 15). It has made provisions to prohibit traffic in human beings and provides for just and human conditions of work along with maternity relief (Art. 23 and Art. 42). It is a constitutional duty of every citizen to renounce practices derogatory to the dignity of women (Art. 51A).

To quote J.P. Singh Indisputably, India is committed to the cause of empowerment of women. However, the journey towards progress is long and arduous. In a world of challenge and competition, both the state and the society have to constantly attune themselves to the changing needs. It is recognized that the development of the country is not possible if women, comprising half of the human resource, as labour force and citizens, stay away from the national development process. Women's participation in the political process of development is of crucial importance from the consideration of both equity and development. India has heralded the new millennium by pronouncing the year 2001 as Women's Empowerment Year. In terms of political empowerment, nearly seven lakh women occupy positions as members and chairpersons of grass-roots democratic institutions in India, following the reservation clause in 73rd and 74th.

Amendment providing one-third seats at district, taluk, village and municipal level for women. This is for the first time in our history that an opportunity has been provided for such substantial entry of women in public life and large numbers have come forward to tackle the challenge of leadership at all levels of Panchayats. In fact, right from the days of freedom struggle the Indian women have been consistently encouraged to take part in the active politics. But due to the vitiated political milieu, resulting from increasing politicization and criminalisation of politics, the level of political participation of women has been adversely affected despite the fact that there has been a marked increase in the level of literacy and political awareness of women.[5]

It is recognized that the goals of poverty alleviation are difficult to achieve without the full and active participation of women, who constitute a large section of the workforce in the country. Women's empowerment is critical to the process of development of the community and, therefore, bringing them into the mainstream of development has been a major concern of the Government.

Towards this end and in order to empower women, an enabling environment, with requisite policies and programmes, institutional mechanisms at various levels and adequate financial resources has been created. The Ministry of Rural Development has special components for women in its programmes and funds are earmarked as 'Women's Component' to ensure flow of adequate resources for their development.[6]

The 73rd and 74th Amendments to the Constitution passed by the Parliament in 1992 and ratified in 1993 provide for 33 per cent reservation among elected representatives to the local governments. This has been hailed as a watershed achievement in empowerment of women, as over one million rural women have joined village panchayat posts as sarpanch or adhyaksha or members of community administration.

POLICY FOR THE EMPOWERMENT OF WOMEN

In order to address the concerns of women in society, the Government of India has established the Department of Women and Child Development within the Ministry of Human Resource Development. A National Policy for the Empowerment of Women, 2001, provides the framework for addressing women's issues. The objectives of the policy are as follows:

- Creating an environment through positive economic and social policies for full development of women to enable them to realize their full potential.
- The *de-jure* and *de-facto* enjoyment of all human rights and fundamental freedom by women on equal basis with men in all spheres—political, economic, social, cultural and civil.
- Equal access to participation and decision-making of women in social, political and economic life of the nation.
- Equal access to women to healthcare, quality education at all levels, career and vocational guidance, employment, equal remuneration, occupational health and safety, social security and public office, etc.
- Strengthening legal systems aimed at elimination of all forms of discrimination against women.
- Changing societal attitudes and community practices by active participation and involvement of both men and women.
- Mainstreaming a gender perspective in the development process.
- Elimination of discrimination and all forms of violence against women and the girl child.
- Building and strengthening partnerships with civil society, particularly women's organizations.

COMMITMENTS OF THE TENTH PLAN TO EMPOWER WOMEN

The Approach

To continue with the major strategy of 'Empowering Women' as Agent of Social Change and Development.

Strategies

To adopt a Sector-specific 3-Fold Strategy for Empowering Women, based on the prescriptions of the National Policy for Empowerment of Women. They include:

Social Empowerment

To create an enabling environment through various affirmative developmental policies and programmes for development of women besides providing them east and equal access to all the basic minimum services so as to enable them to realize their full potentials.

Economic Empowerment

To ensure provision of training, employment and income-generation activities with both 'forward' and 'backward' linkages with the ultimate objective of making all potential women economically independent and self-reliant.

Gender Justice

To eliminate all forms of gender discrimination and thus, allow women to enjoy not only the *de-jure* but also the *de-facto* rights and fundamental freedom on part with men in all spheres, viz. political, economic, social, civil, cultural, etc.[7]

Programmes

In keeping with its past and present policy objectives, the Government has launched a number of programmes focussed on women. In 1993, the Women in Agriculture programme were initiated which aimed at 'training' women farmers with small holdings, in allied activities such as animal husbandry, dairying, horticulture, fisheries, etc. In 1998, a scheme was started that aimed at empowering women in rural areas. It was called *Swashakti-Rural* Women Development and Empowerment Project. In 2001 the government launched *Swayamsidha*-Integrated Women Empowerment that aims at holistic empowerment of_empowerment and convergence of various schemes. In 2002, *Swadhar* aimed at women in distress such as destitute widows, women Prisoners released from jail but without a family, women survivors of natural disasters was launched. Assistance under this programme includes food, clothing, healthcare, measures of social and economic rehabilitation through education, awareness, etc. In the international arena, India has ratified the International Convention on Elimination of All Forms of Discrimination Against Women (CEDAW) 1993 and endorsed the Mexico Plan of Action, 1975; the Nairobi Forward Looking Strategies, 1985; the Beijing Declaration as well the Platform for Action.[8]

Status of Women

"That society would be highly developed and prosperous where women have their rightful place", expounds Manu. The Status of women varies enormously from one part of the world to another. However, nowhere do women enjoy equal status with men. In the developing countries like Africa, the Middle-East, Asia and Latin America, the status of women is so low as cannot be imagined by women in the developed countries.

The woman is the pivot around which the family, the society and humanity itself revolves. It is well said that the hand that rocks the cradle, rules the world. Women play a significant role in the development of their offspring. Truly, if a man is educated one person is educated but if the woman is educated, the whole family is educated.

Sumitra Mahajan, Minister of State, Department of Women and Child Development in her message in "Year of Achievements and New Initiatives" mentioned that the women have a high place in our society and this cannot be just an ornamental position. As much as we worship shakti, we have to recognize the innate power of women to nurture their families and to build a new community, based on participation and equality. In recognition of this, we have instituted the STREE SHAKTI PURUSKAR named after five eminent women of the Indian history, namely, Devi Ahilya Bhai Holkar, Rani Laxmi Bai, Mata Jijabai, Rani Gaidinliu Zeliang and Kannagi and will be given to honour the women who have triumphed over difficult circumstances and fought for and established the rights of women in various fields.[9]

Status is a relative term. In sociological expression, it denotes neither rank nor hierarchy but only position *vis-a-vis* others in terms of rights and obligations.[10] In the ultimate analysis, status is "the conjunction of positions a woman occupies, as a worker, student, wife, mother. The power and prestige attached to these positions and the rights and duties she is expected to exercise.[11]

Women's status can then be analysed in terms of their participation in decision-making, access to opportunities in education, training, employment and income.[12] In recent years, there has been an increasing recognition of the interface between women's ability to control their fertility and their exercise and enjoyment of other options in life.

In ancient India, women enjoyed a high place of respect in the society as mentioned in Rigveda and other scriptures.[13] Volumes can be written about the status of our women and their heroic deeds from the Vedic period to the modern times. But later on, because of social, political and economic changes, women lost their status and were relegated to the background. Many evil customs and traditions stepped in, which enslaved the women and tied them to boundaries of the house. The untold miseries and sufferings of women of the 19th century awakened the conscience of mankind. Many reformers like Raja Rammohan Roy, Swami Dayanand, Justice Ranade, Mahatma Gandhi, and other championed the cause of the emancipation of women. The Constitution of India also prohibits any discrimination on grounds of sex. Many laws have also been enacted by the Government of India to protect the rights of women.

Anna Kajumulo Tibaijuka, Executive Director (UNCHS), says: 'Where women are not involved in public decision-making, the quality of services deteriorates. It is time for change from the practice of leaving women to do only the dirty work. We are aware that women have been instrumental in the urban social movements that aim at improving urban poor neighbourhoods. They do this because they want to protect their families' health and create livable communities. These numerous women's initiatives must be recognized. By involving them in governance structures and by addressing the things they care about, in urban policy, planning and management. Women and men have specific and different needs, in areas such as transport, public spaces, the implementation of by-laws, and security. These must all be addressed.[14]

B.K. Chaturvedi has stated in his foreword, "The need to improve the access of women to national resources and to ensure their rightful place in the mainstream of economic development has been emphasized time and again at various fora at national and international levels. Keeping this in view, the year 2001 will be celebrated as the year of women's empowerment.[15]

Jagmohan, Minister of Urban Development and Poverty Alleviation, GOI, suggests the need of involving women in urban affairs affecting their lives. To quote him: "As we know the problems and challenges facing humanity are global but they occur and have to be dealt with at the local level. Women have the equal right to freedom from poverty, discrimination, environmental degradation and insecurity. To fight these problems and to meet the challenges of sustainable human development, it is crucial that women be empowered and involved in local government as decision-makers, planners and managers."[16]

Women's Empowerment is critical to the socio-economic progress of the community. Bringing women into the mainstream of national development has therefore been a major concern of the Government.[17]

The Members of International Union of Local Authorities (IULA), Representating Local Governments World-wide, firmly believe that:

1. Democratic local self-government has a critical role to play in securing social, economic and political justice for all citizens of every community in the world and that all members of society, women and men, must be included in the governance process;
2. Women and men as citizens have equal human rights, duties and opportunities, as well as the equal right to exercise them. The right to vote, to be eligible for election and to hold public office at all levels are human rights that apply equally to women and men;
3. The problems and challenges facing humanity are global but occur and have to be dealt with at the local level. Women have the equal right to freedom from poverty, discrimination, environmental degradation and insecurity. To fight these

problems and to meet the challenges of sustainable human development, it is crucial that women be empowered and involved in local government as decision-makers, planners and managers.

4. Local government is in a unique position to contribute to the global struggle for gender equality and can have a great impact on the status of women and the status of gender equality around the world, in its capacities as the level of governance closest to the citizens, as a service provider and as an employer.
5. The systematic integration of women augments the democratic basis, the efficiency and the quality of the activities of local government. If local government is to meet the needs of both women and men, it must build on the experiences of both women and men, through an equal representation at all levels and in all fields of decision-making, covering the wide range of responsibilities of local governments.
6. In order to create sustainable, equal and democratic local governments, where women and men have equal access to decision-making, equal access to services and equal treatment in these services, the gender perspective must be mainstreamed into all areas of policy-making and management in local government.
7. Women have the right to equal access to the services of local governments, as well as the right to be treated equally in these services and to be able to influence the initiation, development, management and monitoring of services. The provision of services such as education, welfare, etc., governments should aim to see women and men as equally responsible for matters related both to the family and to public life and avoid perpetuating stereotypes of women and men.
8. Women have the equal right to sound environment, living conditions, housing, water distribution and sanitation facilities, as well as to affordable public transportation. Women's needs and living conditions must be made visible and taken into account at all times in planning.
9. Women have the right to equal access to the territory and geographical space of local governments, ranging from the right to own land, to the right to move freely and without fear in public spaces and on public transport.
10. Local government has a role to play in ensuring the reproductive rights or women and the rights of women to freedom from domestic violence and other forms of physical, psychological and sexual violence and abuse.

G. Palanithurai rightly says: Women have come to positions in the local bodies as provision has been made in the Constitution. The outlook of the society towards the women has started changing. But there are hurdles in the process of empowering women. Steps are being taken by the women on their own to overcome the hurdles. It is a long-drawn process. A structure which had been created over centuries to work against the interest of women cannot be altered overnight. To fight against the existing structure, an organised movement involving masses is imperative. In order to make the women achieve result in their positions, a number of interventions are necessary.

The ongoing experiments and experiences suggest that periodical training, orientation and sensitisation can help the women leaders to perform the assigned role in a better way. When the women leaders are responding to the socio-political challenges in this society, they are to be supported by the organisations and institutions which are working for empowerment of women. Wherever such interventions are available, potential and achievements of the women leaders are substantial and impressive. Government will respond to the needs of these women leaders only when they are supported by social organizations and groups.[18]

The 9th Plan working group challenges before elected panchayat women was clear that the component plan had to be hitched to decentralised planning if the promises made to the women were to be actualized. It was no longer enough for plans; programme, allocation and schemes to be made in the government offices at central or even state level. They had to be made by women, where they were situated and where schemes that the women needed and demanded, how much funds were required to be allocated, how they were to be spent, how monitoring was to be done.

Elected women have therefore to fight on several fronts at the same time. They have to fight for their own place in the sun, in the panchayats *vis-a-vis* the patriarchal forces arranged against them and at the same time, they have to fight the political and bureaucratic state agencies for according a greater role in governance to the panchayats.[19]

Mr. R. Pakhriswamy, Chairperson, Thiruvarur, District Panchayat, Tamil Nadu made the following recommendation in a round table conference (2001) mentioned earlier:[20]

1. Responsibility for ensuring security of Women and Dalits—who face threats from anti-social elements—must be taken by PRIs through the help of political parties. At present there is absolutely no support to PRIs from these parties.
2. Existing revenue share for scheduled caste and scheduled tribe groups and women must be increased and implemented through Panchayats.
3. 20% of funds allocated to MLAs (Members of Legislative Assembly) and MPs (Members of Parliament) must be transferred to Panchayats for women's social and economic upliftment.

4. Elementary education, up to Std. V, must be entrusted to Panchayats and they should be empowered to appoint teachers at the ratio of 1:10.
5. Local cess must be levied based on land revenue demand.
6. Revenue collection from mines, minerals and royalties from non-conventional energies should be entrusted to Panchayats.
7. Protection of water resources must be entrusted to PRIs. This must include assessment of pollution levels and its impact on water sources, fisheries and the coast—the results of which should be announced in the gazette at the district level. And the 'polluter' must pay compensation.
8. The whole idea of Self Help Groups (SHGs) and the current way of implementing development programmes through them has to be re-looked at. This is because SHGs no longer attempt self-employment for their members. Instead they have become moneylenders—for high interests! Also involving SHGs in development programmes through NGOs has created clashes among village panchayats and gram sabhas, as village panchayats do not have adequate finances for local development.
9. The 3-tiers of panchayats must have inter-linkages, DPC's (District Planning Committee) functions must be strengthened and planning from below must be entrusted to them.

"Indisputably, India is committed to the cause of empowerment of women. However, the journey towards progress is long and arduous. In a world of challenge and competition, both the State and the society have to constantly attune themselves to the changing needs. It is recognised that the development of the country is not possible if women, comprising half of the human resource, as labour force and citizens, stay away from the national development process Women's participation in the political process of development is of crucial importance from the consideration of both equity and development.

Essential Steps for Women Empowerment

The main efforts required in the context of the Constitution 73rd Amendment is to break the hegemony of male Chauvinism in the rural areas.

The rural women cannot achieve empowerment on their own and need support from outside. We must make efforts to ensure the following among women:

(i) Creating a positive and dignified self-image and self-confidence in dealing with all matters and in all relationships.
(ii) Ensuring equal participation based on equity and social justice.
(iii) Developing ability and maturity to think critically.

(iv) Take part in decision-making and participation.
(v) Assert when women issues are ignored.
(vi) Equality and equity for women are non-negotiable
(vii) Political power is essential.

Women's entry into the functioning of Panchayati Raj at all levels particularly at decision-making levels will usher an era of equality and prosperity to the villages and empowerment of the women leading to rural development on moral values.

Ultimately it provides women with the opportunity to transform the legal, political, economic and social system as per the vision of the 21st Century to realize their demand for an equitable, environmentally clean and peaceful world where there would be no difference based on sex, creed, faith, etc. This would make 21st century really fruitful.

Government, as they stand today would not be able to usher in gender equality in governance as male dominance does not want to yield to promote equality of sex. Women themselves, through their entry into the Politico-legal structures of the nation, must fulfil this task with devotion, determination and without fear. In other words, unless women become government this equality cannot take place. Hence, mechanism by which women can enter effectively, participate and lead the administration, organize and mobilize opinion on national and International issues, and influence policy, are the urgent need of the day. This would then lay the foundation of equality for the future.

What is needed urgently is interventions at the policy level by women themselves. Why is women's participation in policy and decision-making important and how does one go about improving it? This has to be seen in the present context of women's marginalisation through development policies and the ineffectiveness of constitutional and legal provisions for gender equality.

The formulation of development policies and special programmes for women have the effect of relegating them to a minority category of beneficiaries and not actors and decision-makers for their welfare and improvement. Women, who constitute half of the country's population certainly deserve a better deal than spasmodic doles of mercy. They have to have a say not only in things that concern them directly but in all matters that affect the society in so far as they also have the status of citizens.[21]

The planners, policy-makers and administrators responsible for the improvement of the status of women should not be satisfied only with effective planning and policy-making, but should think of the vehicle or administrative structure through which plans and policies are to be implemented. Myron Weinner has rightly pointed out: "India's forte is one of the crisis management. Instincts of leadership are to cope, rather than innovate, and to work within an existing frame-work not only of institutions but of ideas as well."

Thus, with the help of well designed administrative machinery using modern management methods we should try to put the policy into action. In this implementation process, women themselves will have to be the most forceful agents for change and active participants in the development effort, wherever they have the opportunity to play a dynamic role. The contemporary social situation of women in India should not be frustrating and disheartening but should be rather challenging and it is the men and women of India, particularly the women have to face the challenge. It has been demonstrated by the women in the field that they are as capable and efficient as men in carrying out various kinds of work and have even much more endurance for hardships than is commonly believed. All of us who are associated with the development of the country in any capacity, must renew our dedication to the cause of women which would lead to national development and modernization.

The National Commission on self-employed women and women in formal sector has rightly mentioned that although at the Planning level, there is consciousness about women's low status and the need to focus on women's needs in development, but at the implementation level, this awareness percolates very slowly. The delivery system is based on a stereotyped concept of women's development where women are object of piety or welfare and are given some benefits in a sporadic and haphazard manner. . . . If the political leadership decides that women's problems have to be tackled on a priority basis, the entire planning processes, implementing mechanism and monitoring system will be geared in no time.

POLICIES AND PROGRAMMES: A REVIEW

Development of women has been receiving attention of the government right from the very First Plan (1951-56). But, the same has been treated as a subject of 'welfare' and clubbed together with the welfare of the disadvantaged groups like destitute, disabled, aged, etc. the Central Social Welfare Board (CSWB), set-up in 1953, acts an Apex Body at national level promote voluntary action at various levels, especially at the grass-roots, to take up welfare-treated activities for women and children. The Second to Fifth Plans (1956-79) continued to reflect the very same welfare approach, besides giving priority to women's education, and launching measures to improve maternal and child health services, supplementary feeding for children and expectant and nursing mothers.

The shift in the approach from 'welfare' to 'development' of women could take place only in the Sixth Plan (1980-85). Accordingly, the Sixth Plan adopted a multi-disciplinary approach with a special thrust on the three core sectors of health, education and employment. In the Seventh Plan (1985-90), the developmental programmes continued with the major objective of raising their economic and social status and bringing them into the mainstream of national development. A significant step in this direction was to identity/promote the 'Beneficiary-Oriented Schemes' (BOS) in various developmental sectors which extended direct benefits to women.

The thrust on generation of both skilled and unskilled employment through proper education and vocational training continued. The Eight Plan (1992-97), with human development as its major focus, played a very important role in the development of women. It promised to ensure that benefits of development from different sectors do not by-pass women, implement special programmes and to monitor the flow of benefits to women from other development sectors and enable women to function as equal partners and participants in the development process.

The Ninth Plan (1997-2002) made two significant changes in the conceptual strategy of planning for women. Firstly, 'Empowerment of Women' became one of the nine primary objectives of the Ninth Plan. To this effect, the Approach of the Plan was to create an enabling environment where women could freely exercise their rights both within and outside home, as equal parterns along with men. Secondly, the Plan attempted 'convergence of existing service' available in both women-specific and women-related sectors. To this effect, it directed both the center and the states to adopt a special strategy of 'Women's Component Plan' (WCP) through which not less than 30 per cent of funds/benefits flow to women from all the general development sectors. It also suggested that a special vigil be kept on the flow of the earmarked funds/benefits through an effective mechanism to ensure that the proposed strategy brings forth a holistic approach towards empowering women.

To ensure that other general developmental sectors do not by-pass women and benefits from these sectors continue to flow to them, a special mechanism of monitoring the 27 BOS for women was put into action in 1986, at the instance of the Prime Minister's Office (PMO). The same continues to be an effective instrument till today.

SUGGESTIONS TO STRENGTHEN WOMEN EMPOWERMENT

Women empowerment is not something which can be handed over to women. This is a process which involves sincerity, earnestness and capacity and capability on the part of both men and women. It is a challenging task in village India as even today, if a woman is to travel to her parents' house or go somewhere, she must be accompanied by some male members of the family. She cannot take an independent decision. She feels even subordinate to her son. Let us discuss ways and means to improve the process of women empowerment.

1. Low Status: Need of Research and Affirmative Action

Most of the women in a family feel inferior to male members of the family. From olden times, women act as workers and do not take part in decision-making. This attitude needs change to make women as part and parcel of the family by carving out an important place for her. Swami Vivekananda repeatedly stressed the need for cultivating the faith in one self: "The ideal of faith in ourselves is of the greatest help to us. If faith in ourselves had been more extensively taught and practised, I am sure a very large portion of the evils and miseries that we have would have vanished. Throughout the history of mankind, if any motive power has been more potent than another in the lives of all great men and women, it is that of faith in themselves. Born with the consciousness, that they were to be great they come great. Prof. V.C. Kulandaiswamy, Former Vice-Chancellor, Indira Gandhi National Open University, New Delhi, delivered the convocation address at the Eleventh Convocation of the Avinashilingam Institute for Home Science and Higher Education for Women (Deemed University), Coimbatore. He said, "Women's studies should (therefore) concentrate on the nature of opportunities that now emerge for women to prepare themselves for playing an equal role—not necessarily identical role—with men in the affairs of the society. The research studies should consider the areas of disability, the handicaps, the impediments and the prejudices that women face and devise ways of educating and enabling men and women to remove them."[22]

2. Low Morale: Need of Creating Positive attitude

At present women posses low morale which is a depressing situation where she does not get a sense of belongingness. We must develop positive attitude in her by enlightening her about her creative potential for contributing to the overall development of self, family and society. Dr. (Miss) A.S. Desai, Chairperson, University Grants Commission, delivered the Convocation Address at the annual convocation on the S.N.D.T. Women's University, Mumbai. She said, "While education for women is a necessary condition for social development, it has to be accompanied by increasing levels of awareness with respect to the place of women in a patriarchal society, the means to change their position and role, as also to assure that women's rights are seen as an important and major component of human rights.

All this leads us to consider the importance of empowerment of women achieved through both education and greater social awareness. No one, ever in history, has achieved rights without a struggle. Women have to unite across caste, class, ethnicity and religion, if change has to be brought. Political empowerment is now made possible for women at the local levels through the 73rd and 74th Amendments to the Constitution. It has brought a million women opportunity to participate in decision-making and policies at the village, block and district levels as also in the urban municipal corporations. Educated women have a major social obligation to participate in this great experiment, uniquely launched in our country by reserving one-third of the seats at this level. Expanding women's education will serve no purpose if women do not participate in policy and decision-making.[23]

3. Dependence upon Men since Childhood: Need of Indepenence from Early Stages

In Indian villages, girls remain dependent upon father, brother or cousin and this very feeling continue in their married life. We must give capacity building training to girls in schools to be independent. It does not mean breaking the linkages of family rather it leads to strengthening the bond on an equal platform.

4. Change of Attitude of Men towards Capability of Women

Men have built an impression through observation that women are inferior and they cannot face emerging situations. This attitude has to be changed through positive examples from our country and abroad. Pictures of women doing all types of work need to be screened and shown to both men and women. Though, attitude is changing but it is slow and needs to be accelerated. Face life and its upheavals around you. Be active and tirelessly dynamic. Each exertion undertaken is a shooting spark of "life" from the well of Existence in you. Fearlessly work. With a clear vision, plan and selflessly execute it. Fear not sweat! Hesitate not to face disappointments. Live life, so long as you are alive. Grow through work. Evolve in work. Expand while striving. Make your own life thus rich and sweet. You can. You must. The highest and noblest type of an individual working in the world is known as the "man of achievements" (Yogi).

Such men work, neither for the sake of wages, nor for success; they are not after mere sensual pleasures, nor do they aspire to reform the world; they delicately perform their obligatory duties finding peace and fulfilment in their very activity. Their fulfilment consists of doing their duties to the best of their ability without claiming any rights and they are totally unmindful of whether the society commends or condemns their actions.

Sri K. Anbazhgan, Minister of Education, Government of Tamil Nadu, delivered the Convocation Address at the eighth convocation of Avinashilingam Institute for Home Science and Higher Education for Women (Deemed University). He said, "Women's empowerment is a complex issue having many societal ramifications. It cannot be solved by women alone. Men also should understand the need for women's empowerment and support their cause. Women should learn to articulate their needs and rights in clear terms and work for them, without at the same time upsetting the domestic harmony and family life. They have to work tirelessly in their march towards their empowerment and a life with an identity of their own."

Women's empowerment is a complex issue having many societal ramifications. It cannot be solved by women alone. Men also should understand the need for women's empowerment and support their cause. Women should learn to articulate their needs and rights in clear terms and work for them, without at the same time upsetting the domestic harmony and family life. They have to work tirelessly in their march towards their empowerment and a life with an identity of their own. The great poet

Bharathidasan had laid down categorically that until women became independent, the independence of the nation is meaningless. In the literature, we find several attempts to uphold the dignity of womanhood. Hence, women should use their education to recognize their status in life and to improve by taking up and exercising their rights by themselves. Education is a means of liberation for everyone. But it is more so for women.[24]

5. Women Elected Representatives of PRIs give way to their Men Folk: Need of taking Independent Decisions

Women representatives in PRIs must be trained in the art and science of decision-making so that they are not influenced by extraneous factors. They should discuss among other women and take their opinion. They must develop leadership qualities. K.D. Gangrade in his Article, "Gandhi and Empowerment of Women—Miles to Go" Smt. Savita Singh (International Centre of Gandhian Studies and Research, Gandhi Samiti and Darshan Samiti, New Delhi, "The 74th and 73rd Constitutional Amendments on Panchayati Raj and Nagarpalika with 33 per cent reservation for women has created political space for women. But in most cases they exercise "proxy" power on behalf of men. In reality, women have never been able to get more than ten-percent seats in Parliament or other bodies of decision-making. It is hoped that 81st Constitutional Amendment when passed will give 33 per cent reservation of seats in Parliament and State legislatures. This will go a long way to have their say. We should be ashamed of ourselves that after more than half a century of freedom we have neither been able to clothe our women nor able to provide them something as basic as secure and adequate number of toilets and shelter even in the capital city of Delhi."

6. Lack of Interest and Enthusiasm: Need of Enthusiasm

Women lack interest in PRI on account of lukewarm attitude to PRIs by state and Union Government. To make life worthwhile and fruitful, they must generate enthusiasm within themselves. Generation of enthusiasm will take place when they discover for themselves a goal and attach ourselves to the Altar with a spirit of dedication, reverence and love. Once they have surrendered themselves to it, the ideal itself will provide them with the inspiration and strength. Then nothing can hinder the progress of women's march towards that Goal and the ideal. The love for the ideal will overcome and vanquish all the hurdles from the ideal, and if it comes to that, life itself will be cast off with a smile, a dedication at that Altar. That was how Bhagat Singh could walk to the gallows with a smile on his face. What is important is that one should choose the right ideal an ideal worthwhile even it comes to sacrificing one's own life in the endeavour. The ideal should be inspiring, it should arouse the spring of activity in us. Thus, the discovering of the ideal is the secret of generating in ourselves, dynamism and vitality in its fullness.

Dr. Ela R. Bhatt, Founder, Self Employed Women's Association (SEWA)

Ahmedabad delivered convocation address at the Ninth Convocation of Sri Padmavati Mahila Visvavidyalayam, Tirupati on Monday, the 8th March, 1999 (Women's Day). She said, "Over a period of time, we realized that the right to vote was not enough for the poor and women. They wanted a voice and visibility. It took still more years for us to realize that this was not possible without access to and ownership of economic resources by these poor women. Coming out of their state exploitation by men, society, and the State, the poor women wanted to enjoy what I now call second Freedom: Doosri Azadi." Exerpts.[25]

7. No Forum to Exchange Ideas: Need for All Women Forum

Elected representatives of three tiers should meet once in three months. At present elected representatives rarely meet at one platform to form opinion upon different activities being carried out at various levels. There is a need to have a quarterly meeting of all the elected representatives to exchange their view points. In this way, he would be more participate while deliberating on important issues.

8. Women MLAs and MPs do not take Interest in them

Need for all Women Forum—by their own examples Women MLAs and MPs should visit frequently the elected representatives of PRIs to solve the problems faced by women members.

9. Women do not Struggle for Employment

Need to acquire empowerment Sarojini Vardappan in her Article, "The Challenge of the 21st Century and Role of Indian Women"—"The emphasis now is empowerment, Empowerment is now active process. Power is not a commodity to be transacted. . . . Power cannot be given away as alms. Power has to be acquired, once acquired it needs to be exercised, sustained and preserved. Women have to empower themselves. It is a multidimensional process which should enable individuals or group and individuals to realise their full identity and power in all spheres of life. It consists of greater access to knowledge and resources, greater autonomy in decision-making to enable them to have greater ability to plan their lives or have greater control over the circumstances that influence their lives and freedom from shackles imposed on them by customs, belief and practice. Discrimination of women from womb to tomb is well known, age long traditions and worn out customs are handicaps, woman have to struggle, on their way up."

One of India's greatest poets, Rabindranath Tagore, a pain and inequity of the situation more than half a century ago, thus:

"O Lord Why have you not given
woman the right to conqu'er her destiny?
Why does she have to wait head bowed,

By the roadside,
Waiting with tired patience, I
Hoping for a miracle in the morrow.

10. Mere Legislations do not Keep "Women": Need of Action

Every new legislation has only worsened the position of women. And now her right to property granted by law in a recent judgement by the Supreme Court poses a new threat to her life.

These developments only reinforce the belief that laws alone do not lead to social transformation, unless followed by resolute action and societal awareness of the wrong from time immemorial. And as the eminent jurist V.R. Krishna Iyer rightly says, "The Constitutional provisions are weapons, not victories. Law has to be activated." In short, the struggle for justice—social, economic and political remains to be fought and won. In this scenario, all talk of women Empowerment is nothing more than empty jargon. The situation demands a revolution of consciousness in the minds of women—in the ways they think about themselves. Women must realize that gender deprivation is inconsistent with their basic human rights. They must realize that they have Constitutional rights to quality healthcare, economic security, access to education, employment opportunities, equity and political power.

11. Group Discussions are not Sufficient: Need of Positive Mass Media

Arun K. Gupta, Nisha Jain in their Article, Gender, Mass Media and Social Change: A Case Study of T.V. Commercials in Universal News (August 11, 1997) observe that T.V. commercial also place heavy emphasis on the sexuality of women. In fact, the modernized version of commercials has resulted in a greater emphasis on woman's body and beauty. In the process, woman is reduced to her sexual personality. Whatever else maybe the basis of projection of women, the sexual stereotyping of women continues.

A strong awareness requires to be inculcated among leaders of industry, business and corporate sectors, advertising executives and media directors and personnel to exhibit realistic but emancipated attitude with respect to women. Such an outlook should be in tune with the requirement of increasing consciousness among both men and women about women. As commercials have mass appeal, these can and should be used for generating gender friendly consciousness and for reducing bias against women.[26]

CONCLUSION

The Government of India has declared the year 2001 as Women's Empowerment Year with the three-fold objectives of:

(i) creating a nation-wide awareness about the problems and issues affecting women and their importance for national development;

(ii) initiating and accelerating action to improve access to and control of resources by women;

(iii) creating an enabling environment to enhance the self-confidence and autonomy of women so that they can take their rightful place in the mainstream of the nation's social, political and economic life.

Women empowerment should ensure harmonious existence. Dr. Farncis Soundaraj, Principal, Kodaikanal Christian College, Kodaikanal, delivered the Convocation Address at the annual convocation of the Fatima College (Autonomous), Maduari. He said, "Education has empowered women: they compete better, perform more efficiently and secure values and traditions more carefully than their male counterparts. Are these not reasons and justifications enough for educated women to shake-off pessimism and rise up to meet the challenges which none else but they alone can meet?"

God created human race male and female. He made neither of them superior to the other; on the other hand, he created them for a harmonious existence together. Therefore, the challenges that lie ahead of you cannot be met unless they are approached with a sense of humility and with a sense of togetherness with men. While some of them can be met exclusively by women, they can achieve more by pooling the resources of all.

Notes and References

1. GOI, Deptt. of Social Welfare, Ministry of Education and Social Welfare, Towards Equality, Report on the Committee on the Status of Women in India, 1974, p. 38.
2. Beena Shah, Women and Empowerment in India—The Educational Dimension, in *University News*, Aug. 31, 2000.
3. GOI, Planning Commission, Ninth Five Year Plan, 1997-2000, Vol. II, p. 322.
4. India, 2002, Ministry of Information and Broadcasting, GOI, New Delhi, p. 230.
5. J.P. Singh, Indian Democracy and Empowerment of Women, in *IJPA*, Oct.-Dec., 2000.
6. GOI, Ministry of Rural Development, Annual Report, 1999-2000, p. 66.
7. GOI, Planning Commission Draft Tenth Plan (2002-07), New Delhi, pp. 238-41.
8. Ministry of Environment and Forests, 2002, Empowers People for Sustainable Development, pp. 20-21.
9. Sumitra Sen, Minister of States, Department of Women and Child Development, Ministry of Resource Development, GOI, New Delhi, Message, Deptt. of Women and Child Development, Ministry of HRD, Year of Achievements and New Initiatives.
10. "Towards Equality", Report of the Status of Women, p. 6.
11. Status of Women and Family Planning, C/o No. *6/5fi5* Ref. No. E-75, 1975.
12. Worm, Population and Development, Population Profiles, No. 7, p. 10.

13. Rigveda, *2/17fi1* ; 9/67/10.12.
14. *Shelter*, Vol. III, No. 4, Oct., 2000, XIV.
15. B.K. Chaturvedi, Secretary, Deptt. of Women and Child Development, Ministry of HRD, GOI, New Delhi, Foreword, Year of Achievements and New Initiatives.
16. *Shelter*, Vol. III, No. 4, Oct. 2000, p. IV.
17. Annual Report, Ministry of Rural Development, GOI, New Delhi, 2001-02, p. 60.
18. G.Palanithurai, "The Genere of Women Leaders in Local Bodies Experience from Tamil Nadu", in *IJPA*, January-March, 2001, p. 49.
19. Devki Jain and P. Sujaya, Challenges before Elected Panchayat and Women, in A Round Table on "Financial for District Level Development", 19th May, 2001, United Nations Development Fund for Women, New Delhi, 2002, p. 25.
20. *Ibid.*, p. 24.
21. "Women participation in politics: Hard Choice Workshop" by Research Centre for Women Studies, SNDT University, *Economic and Political Weekly*, September 21, 1991, p. 2191. (17. Roopa Sharma, The Women's Reservation Bill: A Crisis of Identity" in *IJPA*, January-March, 2001, pp. 66.)
22. *University News*, Dec. 6, 1999, p. 27.
23. *University News*, April 6, 1999.
24. *University News*, January 13, 1997.
25. *University News*, January 26, 1999
26. *University News*, April 6, 1998.

CHAPTER 3

HEALTH AND WOMEN DEVELOPMENT

"Happiness, happiness, happiness
It may be of different origin on this earth
But the happiness of being healthy
Is the real happiness."

—*Dashdorjin Natragdorj*

Health and Women Development

Before we discuss about women health, let us discuss about the significance of health in the development of the country.

SIGNIFICANCE OF HEALTH

Good health is a prerequisite to human productivity and the "development" process. It is essential to economic and technological development. A healthy community is the infrastructure upon which to build an economically viable society. The progress of society greatly depends on the quality of its people (both men and women). Unhealthy people can hardly be expected to make any valid contribution towards developmental programmes. Health is man's greatest possession, for it lays a solid foundation for his happiness. Charaka, the renowned Ayurvedic physicians is known to have said: "Health was vital for ethical, artistic, material and spiritual development of human being."

Buddha has said that of all the gains, the gains of health are the highest and the best. Health is not only basic to leading a happy life for an individual but it is also necessary for all productive activities in the society. Who would deny that a soldier who is not keeping good health cannot be expected to defend the frontiers of his country even when he is provided with the latest sophisticated weapons? Similarly, who would deny that an unhealthy farmer with the best possible technological know-how would not succeed in producing the best that can be expected of him? Obviously what is true of an unhealthy soldier or an unhealthy farmer is also true of other categories of workers. Thus, no industry can expect the optimum output if it does not employ healthy workers or does not make and provide adequate facilities for proper maintenance of their health. Undoubtedly, professional efficiency, good health and productivity are inter-related. Yet, health cannot be bestowed upon people if they themselves do not make any effort to maintain a proper balance between their external and internal environments.

Whatever one may say, a disease-stricken society can hardly hope to extricate itself from the clutches of poverty and ignorance that keep it backward and underdeveloped in many areas of life. A nation can become truly healthy only when it succeeds in over-coming all these deficiencies stemming from cultural, social, economic and other causes. A nation that is ill-fed can hardly afford to exhibit efficiency in any field. In fact, an epidemic or endemic disease in any part of the world can pose a potential danger to all mankind and even a challenge to modern science.

Health is fundamental to the national progress in any sphere. In terms of resources for economic development, nothing can be considered of higher importance than the health of the people which is a measure of their energy and capacity as well as of the potential man-hours for productive work in relation to the total number of persons maintained by the nation. For the efficiency of industry and of agriculture, the health of the worker is an essential consideration.

Thus, there can be no two opinions that health is basic to national progress and in terms of resources for economic development nothing could be of greater significance than the health of the people. To quote Herophilas, C., 300 B.C.

"When health is absent
Wisdom cannot reveal itself
Art cannot manifest
Strength cannot fight,
Wealth becomes useless
And Intelligence cannot be applied."

As such, good health must be a primary objective of every development programmes. It is a precursor to improving the quality of life for a major portion of mankind.

Now, let us discuss the special need of women's health in the overall process of health development. A world health organization report rightly submits:

Health conditions in one phase of a woman's life affect other phases of her life as well as the health and well-being of future generations. This concept guided the Technical Discussions on Women, Health and Development at the 45th World Health Assembly in 1992. Since then WHO has advocated strongly for a lifespan approach to women's health—from conception to old-age. It has also called for multicultural action for women's health, particularly in the areas of raising female literacy, creating opportunities for income generation, increasing the participation of women in national development, and in short, empowering women to make decisions on matters that impact their health.[1]

There is a growing realization that investing in women's health is investing in the health of families, communities and societies, in other words—investing in health for all.

"Gender" is used to describe those characteristics of men and women which are socially constructed and therefore can change, in contrast to those that are biologically determined and therefore cannot change. Gender is thus a dynamic concept which looks at the social divisions and the interrelations between men and women.

A "gender approach to health" is based on an analysis of how differences and disparities between women and men determine their differential exposure to risk, their access to technology and healthcare, their rights and responsibilities, and their control over their own lives.[2]

A Report on the status of women in India reports that health of women is directly related to their status and hence status need to be improved as already dealt with in Chapter 1 and Chapter 2. To quote the report:

Health is both an important factor in the achievement of status as well as an indicator of social status, particularly for women, whose health is conditioned to a great extent by social attitudes. The health status of women includes their mental and social condition as affected by prevailing norms and attitudes of society in addition to their biological and physiological problems. Societies delineate women's roles partly according to their biological and physiological problems. Societies delineate women's roles partly according to their biological functions and partly from prevailing attitudes regarding their physical and mental capacity. These social attitudes also influence the provision and use of preventive and curative healthcare, including maternal care. The healthcare facilities offered by a community in the form of medical particularly maternity services for women, is a significant index of the emphasis that community places on the health of its women. Some studies in both the developed and developing countries have shown a definite link between low status of women and deficiencies in the knowledge and utilisation of preventive health services.[3]

Committee on Empowerment of women rightly observes the need of Gender specific approach to health:

There is a growing recognisation that since women also suffer from other disabilities and morbidities, some of which are again very gender specific, there is need to examine the adequacy of our strategies in ensuring that they are appropriately covered. The scanty data available has shown that women in reproductive age groups of 18-45 years, constituting a bulk of the working population, suffer from TB, Malaria, UTI, STDs, Cancer, Leprosy, etc. Women working in cities are also subject to stressful conditions and are seen to suffer from mental health problem as well as heart ailments, blood pressure and other stress induced diseases. Likewise, the National Commission for Women had also brought out the special needs of women working in agriculture and informal sectors where they are exposed to chemicals and pesticides. Besides the longevity of life has resulted in a higher burden of diseases among the older aged women. The women in this age group suffer medical disorders such as Alzheimer's and arthritis, etc.

The various Disease Control Programmes are being implemented without any specific allocation for women. However, it is felt that the sensitisation to women's health is the need of the hour. Certain areas on women's health may require specific interventions especially those disabilities and morbidities which are very gender specific such as cervical and breast cancer. Main constraints are: inadequate funding and inadequate development of gender perspective in programme formulation.[4]

National perspective Plan for Women 1988 spell out the following activities for better health to girls and women:

(i) Change our attitudes to provide prompt and adequate medical care for girls.
(ii) Prepare girls for better motherhood.
(iii) Reduce infant and child mortality of girls.
(iv) Reduce maternal mortality.
(v) Ensure adequate maternal healthcare—pre-natal, natal and post-natal.
(vi) Ensure proper knowledge and services for family planning.
(vii) Provision of basic health and nutrition services for girls and women.
(viii) Raise the level of literacy and education among women.[5]

Beijing UN International Conference emphasized a life span perspective for health of women.

A lifespan approach addresses the health issues of women—at conception and birth, in infancy and childhood, during adolescence, throughout the reproductive years, into old age—within the context of their biological and social vulnerabilities and their status in society. It also takes into account both the specific as well as the cumulative effects of poor health and nutrition.

A lifespan approach to women's health takes into account both the specific as well as the cumulative effects of poor health and nutrition. There is increasing evidence that health problems that begin in childhood and adolescence affect the health status of women during their reproductive years and beyond, as well as the health of their newborns. Discrimination against the girl child as seen in some countries of the Region can also significantly retard her growth and development.[6]

NINTH FIVE YEAR PLAN STRESSES HOLISTIC APPROACH TO HEALTH OF WOMEN

The Ninth Plan recognises the special health needs of women and the girl child and the importance of enhancing easy access to primary

CHART 3.1

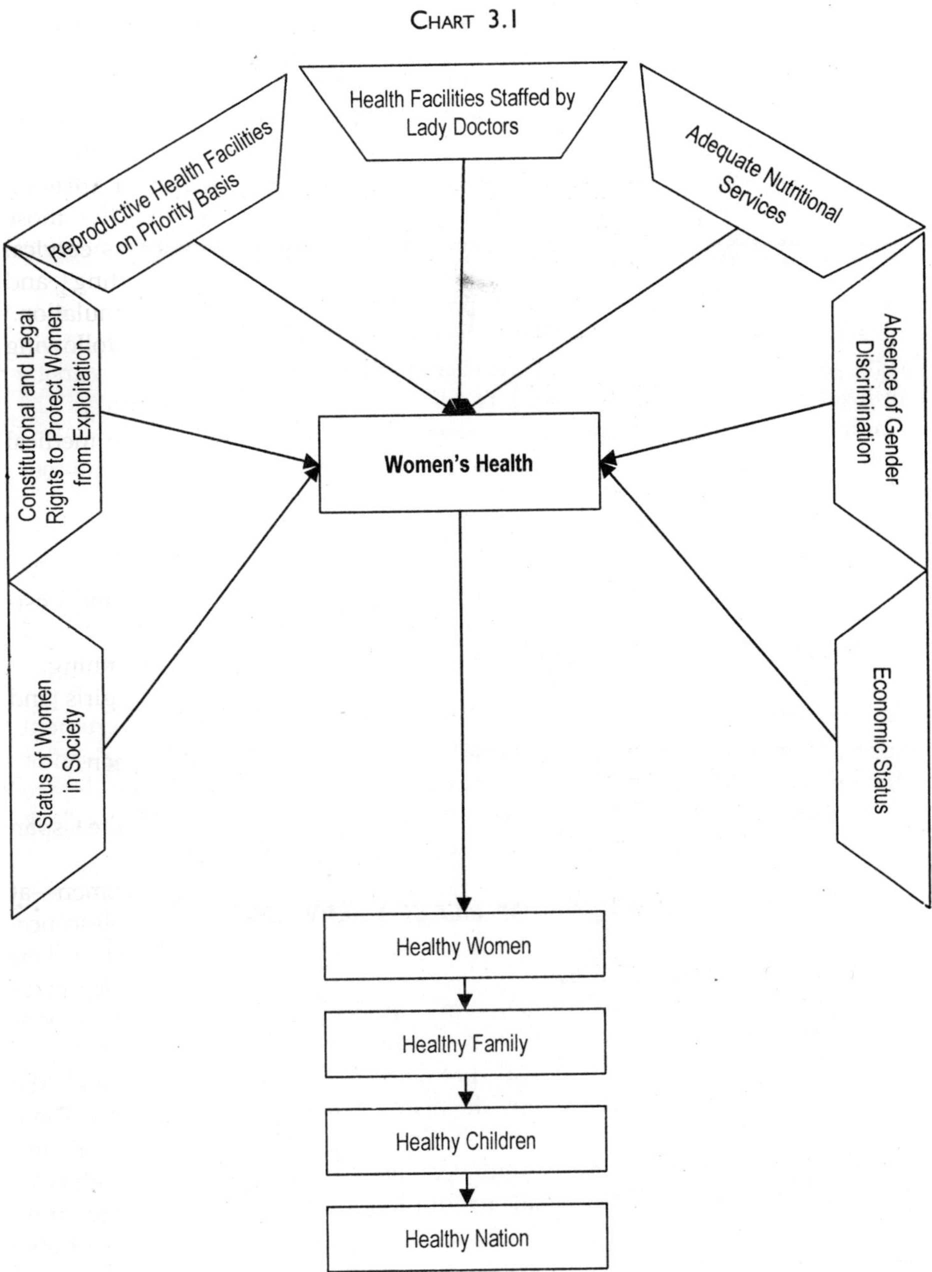

healthcare. There are many indicators to point out that the neglect of health needs of women especially that of the pregnant women, adolescent girls and girl-babies, is responsible for the present high rates of IMR/CMR/MMR. Therefore, a holistic approach with Reproductive Child Health (RCH) measures will be adopted in improving the health status of women by focussing on their age-specific needs.[7]

We may discuss the areas in which women health services need be promoted.

In this context committee on Empowerment has also suggested the following observations which are of great significance.

Since the vast majority of women live in rural areas, where there are hardly any medical facilities available, women become victims of various diseases due to mal-nutrition, lack of clean and safe drinking water, unhygienic conditions, etc. The government ought to integrate various programmes and take a holistic approach to immunization, nutrition, healthcare, drinking water, cleanliness, health infrastructure, trained personnel, etc. so as to improve the health of the rural women. As 33 per cent women are now in panchayats and other local bodies they can be utilized for improving the condition of women all over the country. The Committee desire that the government should coordinate with various concerned Departments in this regard to draw up appropriate programmes and schemes along these lines.

The demand and supply of health facilities is highly skewed. There is urgent need to improve the conditions of the Government hospitals by making available doctors, para-medical staff, requisite medicines and necessary medical equipments. Not only is there need for more doctors and nurses but the norms for doctor-patient ratio and nurse patient ratio needs to be reviewed and appropriate steps taken to provide medical staff as per those norms. It is known fact that the emergency wards of Government hospitals in major cities are managed by junior doctors while the senior doctors have to be called, if need arises. The Government should take appropriate steps to ensure the presence of senior doctors round the clock in each discipline in the emergency wards of major hospitals.[8]

PROVISION OF HEALTH SERVICES

I. Adequate Health Facilities

Health facilities are undoubtedly inadequate, especially in rural areas. The women services have four components: care of general medical problems; care of gynaecological problems; obstetric care and family problems. The purpose is to provide planned maternal and child health services to ensure that expectant and nursing mothers maintain good health, have a normal delivery and bear healthy children. It is a service planned for the promotion and restoration of health of mothers and children and provision of safe confinement. The following suggestions may be considered to improve the health services for women:

(a) Since a major part of our population stay in villages, where dais play a significant role, we should accelerate the training programme for them. This would reduce greatly the maternal and infant mortality rates.

(b) Arrangements may be made for special identifiable services for women in all types of institutions, especially in the PHCs.
(c) At present, one PHC is provided for 30,000 population. It is suggested that one PHC be provided for not more than 25,000 population.
(d) Cooperation of the private practitioners of the indigenous system of medicine should be sought for identification and referral of high risk pregnancies and for delivery and expansion of family-welfare services.
(e) Blood transfusion services may be streamlined to provide blood to women, who are likely to lose their lives due to haemorrhage.

There is a need of increasing women's access to appropriate, affordable and quality healthcare throughout their lifespan and strengthening preventive programmes that promote women's health.

A gender perspective to health must also take into account the differences between men and women relative to their access to health services and the quality of care they receive. This can only be done, through an analysis of health service utilization statistics obtained, from facilities along with community-based statistics, which include population groups not using health facilities.

2. Provision of Nutritional Services

The nutritional status of women especially that of the rural poor is far from what is desired. Inspite of the prophylactic programmes against nutritional anaemia targeted at the expectant and lactating mothers, these women continue to suffer from acute anaemia. It has been pointed out that much wasting and stunting of growth takes place during young age. With early and multiple pregnancies, women miss the opportunity of attaining full bodily growth. The low nutritional status of women in India applies to all the age groups but is more acute in the cases of young girls, pregnant and aged women. While in the lowest socio-economic groups, the low nutritional status of women is mainly due to poverty and the burden of family responsibilities, in the lower middle income groups, it is aggravated by general neglect and is the indirect result of stronger gender discrimination.

Women in developing countries are generally more malnourished than men. The additional biological demands due to menstruation, pregnancy and lactation have made nutritional deficiencies the most widespread and disabling health problem among women. For example, low birth weight in newborns is partly a reflection of poor maternal nutrition. In 1990-94, the proportion of newborns weighing less than 2500 grams ranged from 13% to 50% in countries of the South-East Asia.

Iron deficiency anaemia is more common in women than in men. About 55% of pregnant women and 44% of all women suffer from anaemia in developing countries. At ages between 15-44 years, the burden of iron deficiency anaemia in developing countries in 1990 in terms of thousands of DALYs per year was 4898 for men and 7135 for women. Anaemia lowers the physical work capacity of women and their ability to cope with various infections. It also has serious repercussions on their reproductive health, with maternal mortality being significantly higher in anaemic women.[9]

The most serious problem afflicting women is lack of adequate nutrition. Girls and women generally get the leftovers because of the social customs, poverty and their poor social status. A pleasant and healthy diet, not necessarily an expensive one, is one of the most satisfying and stimulating activities of family life. It contributes to the physical, the mental and social well-being of all the members of the family. Man does not always instinctively choose the right nutrition for maintaining his health. He is influenced in his food habits by religion, culture, social status, traditions and beliefs.

Nature abounds in good nutritious foods within reach of the economically under-privileged families. A balanced diet does not mean an expensive diet. With proper education, families with limited financial resources can take better care of their nutritional needs. It is, therefore, essential for the health department and voluntary organisations to impart this type of education as this can go a long way in promoting the health and well-being of family members. Health institutions do not provide, at present, any special nutritional services. There is a need to plan well-equipped and staffed nutrition clinics attached to all hospitals and PHCs. There may be arrangements to educate the women about the nutritive value of locally available foods and also teach methods of cooking that would retain food value. The properties of medical herbs and medicines and traditional cures can be analysed and popularized among mothers.

The Prime Minister, in his Independence Day speech on 15th August, 2001 announced the setting up of a National Nutrition Mission. Under this Mission, subsidized food grains would be made available to adolescent girls and expectant and nursing mothers, belonging to below-poverty-line families.

A two-tier structure is envisaged for the Mission. The National Nutrition Mission would be headed by the Prime Minister and its Executive Committee would be under the Human Resource Development Minister.[10]

3. Planning and Development of Health Personnel for Women's Health

We have already discussed the various aspects of health manpower planning. We may suggest here some methods which can help in making more women health personnel available to cater to the health needs of women:

(a) More reservation of seats for women in medical colleges till a sufficient number of qualified lady doctors are available.

(b) More women may be encouraged to undergo training in ISM through the reservation in service as well.

(c) In order to encourage self-employment among women doctors, financial assistance may be provided to set-up clinics, etc.
(d) Community Health Workers' Scheme must include at least fifty per cent women to deal effectively with the women health problems.

4. Planning Adequate Facilities for Reproductive Health

The greatest burden of reproductive health problems, however, falls on women. It is they who face the risks from complications of pregnancy and childbirth, from unwanted pregnancies and from unsafe abortions. Over one-third of all healthy life lost in adult women in the developing world is due to reproductive health problems, as compared to only 12% in men. And yet large number of women remain ill-informed about basic facts related to their reproductive health.[11]

Women must be encouraged to adopt family planning in rural areas. Women start their reproductive life when they are barely out of adolescence and may have four or five children by the time they are thirty. This adversely affects their health and well-being.

Women in the rural and urban areas have hardly any say in family planning. It is men who decide matters, but among the educated women, some mutual understanding is evident. The education of women, population change and overall development are closely inter-related. Women have a crucial role to play in all these areas still uncovered. A study of the inter-relationship between the status of women and family planning was conducted in accordance with the Economic and Social Council Resolution. The report affirmed—

(a) The right to decide freely and responsibly on the number and spacing of their children is a fundamental right of individuals which facilitates the exercise of other human rights especially by women;
(b) Adequate information, education and services enabling individuals to exercise this right are essential pre-requisites for the promotion of the status of women, and for ensuring their complete integration in social and economic development at all levels; and
(c) Family planning which should constitute an integrated and essential part of development plan and programmes, in countries suffering from over-population can only succeed in concert with other measures which also improve the status of women."

The establishment of a close doctor-patient relationship is an absolutely essential requirement for the success of the programme. Careful follow-up by doctors of vasectomy and tubectomy cases is as necessary as the operation itself, for the psychological rehabilitation of the patient, as well as for the assurance of potential acceptors.

A maternal death is defined as the death of a woman while pregnant or within 42 days of the termination of pregnancy, irrespective of the duration and site of the pregnancy, from any cause related to or aggravated by the pregnancy or its management but not from accidental or incidental causes.

Most maternal deaths are preventable. The medical interventions necessary to prevent them are trained assistance at delivery, a well established primary healthcare infrastructure with a good referral system, and referral facilities (e.g. at district level) for managing complications. Most women do not receive the services of a skilled attendant (midwife, nurse or doctor) at the time of delivery.

For example, the report of a three-year study covering a population of 686,000 in a rural area of India showed that "delay in seeking care and too many and inappropriate referrals through lower levels of the health system not capable of dealing with the problem, significantly increased the risk of dying. Similarly, residence in the village proper (which has better transport facilities) as compared to the hamlets had a protective effect. A trained attendant at delivery, presence of an ANM (Auxiliary Nurse Midwife) in the village, an educated husband (the usual decision-maker) and the social custom of migrating to the natal home for delivery all had a protective effect."[12]

5. Planning Women Education for Family Health

Healthy families make healthy people. The family is the primary unit of healthy care, a front line in the sequence of education, prevention, diagnosis, treatment and rehabilitation of its constituents. "Health begins at Home" was the theme chosen for World Health Day (1973) on 25th Anniversary of WHO in recognition of the important role of the family in promoting and protecting the health of its members. Women occupy an important place in shaping the lives of its family members. The mother is still the best teacher on life and health. The education imparted by her remains with children as long as they live. Government should provide health education to women as notions of health and hygiene given at home to children would help them to be good citizens. Women, if properly educated, can really help in the socio-economic development of the country. This would release the potential energy of the women and help in channelizing it for the welfare of the family and ultimately national development.

6. Planning for HIV/AIDS and STDs, Infertility and Gynaecological Disorders

Acquired immune deficiency syndrome (AIDS), unknown even 15 years ago, has now become a major challenge to public health. It is important to educate women about STDs and HIV infection. It is even more important to empower them to say "NO" to unsafe-sex. STDs in women are not easily identified or cured because over 50% of STDs in women are a symptomatic, diagnosis is difficult, and women's access to services for STD treatment is poor. STDs in pregnant women cause complications such as seplis, spontaneous abortion, premature birth, still-birth and congential infection. Almost two-thirds of cases of infertility among women and 35% of cases of post-partum morbidity are attributable to STDs.

Worldwide, the disease burden of STDs in women is more than five times that in men.[13]

During the Ninth Plan, attempts are being made to provide for screening for syphiliis, gonorrhoea and HIV infection at PHC/CHC level wherever possible. Utilising the microscope and laboratory technician available at PHCs vaginal/cervical smears in women with symptoms of RTI are to be screened for identifying organisms responsible and appropriate treatment provided.

Infertility

It is estimated that between 5 to 10% of couples are infertile. While provision of contraceptive advice and care to all couples in reproductive age group is important, it is equally essential that couples who do not have children have access to essential clinical examination, investigation, management and counselling. The focus at the CHC level will be to identify infertile couples and undertake clinical examination to detect the obvious causes of infertility, carry out preliminary investigations such as sperm count, diagnostic curettage and tubal potency testing. Depending upon the findings, the couples may then be referred to centres with appropriate facilities for diagnosis and management. By carrying out simple diagnostic procedures available at the primary healthcare institutions it is possible to reduce the number of couples requiring referral. Initial screening at primary healthcare level and subsequent referral is a cost-effective method for management of infertility both for the healthcare system and those requiring such services.

Gynaecological Disorders

Women suffers from a variety of common gynaecological problems including menstrual dysfunctions at peri-menarchal and peri-menopausal age. Facilities for diagnosis of these are at the moment available at district hospitals or tertiary care centres. During the Ninth Plan period the CHCs, with a gynaecologist, have started providing requisite diagnostic and curative services. Yet another major problem in women is prolapse uterus of varying degrees. The PHCs and CHCs refer women requiring surgery to district hospitals or tertiary care centres.

Cancer Cervix is one of the most common malignancies in India and accounts for over a third of all malignancies in women. Cancer Cervix can readily be diagnosed at the PHCs and CHCs. Early diagnosis of Stage I and Stage II and referral to places where radiography is available will result in rapid decline in mortality due to cancer cervix in the country in the near future.

7. Environment and Work Related Health Problems

Health problems that are work-related or those arising out of averse environment conamons, cover a broad range or Illnesses disabilities. Such problems arise out of injuries, infections, exposure to dust, chemicals and gases, from psychological stresses, and from the harmful effects of a degrading environment.

Women often work long hours, increasing their exposure to illness and injuries. A large proportion of women are engaged in agricultural work. This can expose them to worm infestations, which aggravate anaemia, to injuries, snake bites and insecticide poisoning on as well as to disorders resulting from extreme climatic conditions. Exposure to pesticides and chemical fertilizers can also result in abortion and stillbirth. The health department must provide facilities against such risks.[14]

8. Violence against Women

Many women face violence throughout their lives, like rape and domestic violence. Although national statistics on violence against women are not readily available, the problem is serious.

Domestic violence is relatively common. Available evidence suggests that thousands of cases of domestic violence are reported directly to police stations each year like dowry deaths are regularly reported by the media. However, domestic violence is often regarded as a private family matter and many cases may therefore go unreported. Fear and shame also contribute to the non-reporting of domestic violence.

9. Increasing General and Functional Literary for Good Health

Education is the most potent factor for changing women's position in society. We must correct the imbalances by encouraging the education of girls. We can use the adult education or non-formal education system. What can be the future of a country where general illiteracy, especially among women, is very high? Besides, the women have also to handle the new generation, i.e.. the child who is the future hope.

All this would remain a dream unless women are themselves enlightened. Education is the key factor in elevating the status of women. It equips them to contribute in different fields more meaningfully. Dr. (Mrs.) P.K. Devi, Professor of Gynaecology, in PGI, Chandigarh, has rightly stated on the basis of her critical examination of the various states of the Indian Union, that "Literacy, especially of women seems to be a significant factor in differences in the mortality and morbidity rates between various Indian states and infant mortality rates coincide with a very low female literacy rate."

In India, planners, statesmen, educationists and administrators have come to realise that the pace of development cannot accelerate unless women are also properly qualified. So to improve the education of women quantitatively and qualitatively, the following steps are submitted for consideration:

(a) Expansion of the facilities of women education including adult and vocational education tremendously so that the literacy in respect of this group may be increased.

(b) Removal of disparity between rural and urban literacy by: (i) provision of good institutions in villages to avoid the attraction for cities; (ii) to bring awareness towards hygiene among women through community development programmes; (iii) preference in employment to rural people; (iv) setting up of professional and other training institutions in the villages; (v) setting up of rural-based industries in village; (vi) training of women in modern methods of agriculture; (vii) encouraging the formation of mahila mandals to exchange information on various problems facing the nation; and (viii) setting up of model villages.

(c) The contents of women education may be somewhat; different from men as women have to devote a lot of their time in homes as well. Jobs in the country are limited and hence the women education (general) can create more frustration rather than prove an asset. Hence along with general education, some course like Home Science, Agriculture, Music, etc. may also be imparted.

(d) Involvement of women at the policy-making, planning and implementation of all the programmes aimed at national reconstruction, e.g. Family Planning, Rural Planning, Rural Development, etc. This would give the impetus to women education.

(e) The share of the women in the Government jobs is very limited at present as the men presume without any justification that women cannot be effective in good administration. The State must employ more and more women if eligible and even, I would suggest that preference may be given till they are properly represented. Strangely, when one sees the University results, the girls are surpassing the boys but the same is not true in Government jobs. More and more women may also be assigned gazetted jobs of responsibility. Women may be encouraged even to take up part-time jobs.

(f) Women may be imparted education in the fields like management, marketing, etc. so that they can actively participate in cooperative organisations. They can make the cooperative movement a success.

(g) Incentive like mid-day meals, scholarships, free school uniforms, free books and study material, stipends, awards, etc., should be extended to all girls in the rural areas and urban slums.

(h) Scheme to activate the reduction of dropouts may be planned.

It may be concluded that women education can help in nation-building. Napoleon once said, "Give me good mothers, I will give you a good nation."

Illiteracy is a great obstruction in the path of development and education is the backbone of democracy. The Director-General of UNESCO has described illiteracy as "the most monstrous of all the many instances of wasted human potential which still at the present time keeps more than one-third of the human race in a state of hopelessness—below the level of modern civilisation." Therefore, in order to translate the essence of the Preamble and the Directive Principles of the State Policy enshrined in the Constitution of India into practical life, it is imperative for us to increase the literacy rate in general and of women in particular.

10. Collecting Accurate Data for Improving Health Status of Women

A lot of difficulty has been experienced with regard to data pertaining to the status of women. Lack of data in quantity and quality would impede effective planning. The action plan suggested that there is a need to augment the information available in the field of health, family planning and nutrition through the following research studies:

1. The data available at present regarding maternal morbidity and mortality are based on hospital statistics and hence are of limited value. The system of registration of vital events is also incomplete. It is suggested that periodic special surveys be undertaken to study the pattern and causes of mortality and morbidity among women and female children. The studies should cover different communities and different regions. Such studies would also provide information on the relative value of age-structure, parity and other "High Risk" factors in the delivery of maternity services.
2. Practical service-oriented field studies should be undertaken to assess the felt needs of the community and their attitudes towards the services offered, with a view to providing guidelines for framing health policy decision relating to the delivery of maternal care and family planning services.
3. Studies be conducted on the inter-relationship between pattern of family formation, nutrition, health and causes and incidence of sterility.
4. Studies of attitudes, beliefs and practice of traditional birth attendants (dais) should be made, to improve upon the training programme now designed for them and to obtain their greater participation in maternity and family planning services.
5. The base-line data will have to be established first against which the impact of this plan of action would be measured.

The World Plan of Action has also emphasised that "A scientific and reliable data base should be established and suitable economic and social indicators urgently developed which are sensitive to the particular situation and needs of women as an integral part of the national and international programme of statistics."[15]

11. Planning Women's Participation in their own Welfare

Women should themselves exert pressure to get the due benefits for their welfare. They should unite to form voluntary organizations to help themselves and ultimately the nation. It was rightly stated in the National Plan of action for women that:

> "Women voluntary organisations are best suited for motivation in the field of health, family planning and nutrition. There is therefore, every need for creating a conducive climate, so that they can render the needed service effectively."[16]

The women's voluntary organisation in the form of Mother's Club in the Republic of Korea has been quite useful in raising the status of women. By mid-1997, nearly 70,000 such clubs had been organised. The clubs provide opportunities for village women to get together to talk about health, education of children and improvement of environment. The club helps in family planning, vaccination and treatment of emergency cases. The mother's clubs are a genuinely grass-root community network, which owes little to outside administrators or planners. I.C. Abacde, in his article on "Women Power in Korea" observes that mother's clubs are helping to change age-old social attitudes towards women. He says: "The growth of women's clubs in Korea has coincided with considerable changes in social attitudes towards women. The trend is towards greater recognition between husband and wife, and more open discussion of family planning matters. It seems clear that the enhanced status of women and the growth of mothers' clubs have gone hand-in-hand and are contributing significantly to the development of rural communities in Korea."[17]

Such clubs should be set-up in other countries as well. These would help mobilise voluntary resources lying idle and if not used can be a source of destruction. In the developing countries like India, voluntary organisations are urban-based and serve the urban area. These organisations must create a strong base by setting up such clubs and diffuse information to them to be passed on to the members of the community. This would bring about a socio-economic revolution and contribute substantially to modernisation and development.

The planners, policy-makers and administrators responsible for the improvement of the status of women should not be satisfied only with effective planning and policy-making, but should think of the vehicle or administrative structure through which plans and policies are to be implemented. Myron Weiner has rightly pointed out:

> "India's forte is one of the crisis management. Instincts of leadership are to cope, rather than innovate, and to work within an existing framework not only of institutions but of ideas as well."[18]

Thus, with the help of well designed administrative machinery using modern management methods we should try to put the policy into action.

In this implementation process, women themselves will have to be the most forceful agents for change and active participants in the development effort, wherever they have the opportunity to play a dynamic role. The contemporary social situation of women in India should not be frustrating and disheartening but should be rather challenging and it is the men and women of India, particularly the women who have to face the challenge. It has been demonstrated by the women in the field that they are as capable and efficient as men in carrying out various kinds of work and have even much more endurance for hardships than is commonly believed. All of us who are associated with the development of the country in any capacity, must renew our dedication to the cause of women which would eventually lead to national development and modernisation.

The National Health Policy, 2001 (Draft) promises to ensure increased access to women to basic healthcare and commits highest priority to the funding of the identified programmes relating to women's health. During the Ninth Plan period, several new initiatives were taken as part of the Reproductive and Child Health (RCH) Programme (1997), in order to make it broad-based and client-friendly. All the interventions of the erstwhile programme of Child Survival and Safe Motherhood (CSSM) became part of RCH. During this period, the focus shifted from the individualised vertical interventions to a more holistic integrated life-cycle approach with more attention to reproductive healthcare. This includes access to essential obstetric care during the entire period of pregnancy, provision of emergency obstetric care as close to the community as possible, improving and expanding early and safe abortion services and provision for treatment of Reproductive Tract Infections/Sexually Transmitted Infections (RTI/STI) cases at the sub-district level.

Under the Universal Immunisation Programme, launched in 1985-86, which became part of the RCH Programme in 1997, the coverage of Tetanus Toxoid Vaccination of pregnant women increased from 40 per cent in 1985-86 to 76.4 per cent in 1996-97 and to 83.4 per cent in 2000-01. The scheme of Training of Dais was initiated in 2000-01 in 142 districts in 17 states. An extensive network of 2,935 Community Health Centres (CHCs), 22,975 Primary Health Centres (PHCs) and 1,37,271 village level Sub-Centres was put into operation by the end of the Ninth Plan. The Ninth Plan also envisaged to promote institutional deliveries, both in urban and rural areas. A comparison of National Family Health Survey (NFHS) I and II shows that the institutional deliveries has risen from 26 per cent in 1992-93 to 34 per cent in 1998-99. As a result of the above initiatives, the Crude Birth Rate fell from 29.5 to 26.1 and the Crude Death Rate from 9.8 to 8.7 between 1991 and 1999.

The National Nutrition Policy (1993) advocates a comprehensive inter-sectoral strategy for alleviating all the multi-faceted problems of under malnutrition and its related deficiencies and diseases so as to achieve an optimal state of nutrition for all sections of society but with a special priority for women, mothers and children who are vulnerable as well as 'at-risk'. Of the two major problems of macro and micro-nutritional deficiencies that the women, mothers and children suffer from, while the former are manifested through chronic energy deficiency (CED), the latter are reflected in Vitamin A, Iron and Iodine deficiencies. The strategies adopted in the Ninth Plan include—screening of all pregnant women and lactating mothers for CED; identifying women with weight below 40 kg and providing adequate ante-natal, intra-partum and neo-natal care under the RCH programme and ensuring they receive food supplementation through the Integrated Child Development Services (ICDS) Scheme. The ICDS, launched in 1975, provides supplementary feeding to bridge the nutritional gaps that exist in respect of children below 6 years and expectant and nursing mothers.

Besides this, since 2000-01, the Government of India has been providing Additional Central Assistance to the states under the nutrition component of Pradhan Mantri Gramodaya Yojana (PMGY) in an effort to prevent the onset of under-nutrition in the age-group 6-24 months. Supplementary nutrition is also provided to 105 million school-going children under the National Programme of Nutritional Support to Primary Education (also popularly known as Mid-Day Meals Programme).[19]

Inspite of these singular policies, programmes and achievements, there are certain critical areas, which call for immediate attention, as following:

- Inadequacy of institutional mechanisms for the advancement of women.
- Persistent and institutionalised discrimination against the girl child.
- Feminisation of poverty.
- Gender blindness in macro-economic policies.
- Invisibility of women's contribution to the economy and environmental sustenance.
- Poor participation by women in decision-making structures and processes.
- Gender gaps in literacy, education and health.
- Growing trend of violence against women.
- Barriers encountered by women in accessing legal entitlements.
- Gender biased societal norms.
- Negative portrayals and perpetuation of gender stereotypes by mass media.

Prevailing ill-health among women is a major concern. These are being addressed through several programmes, such as nutrition, RH, MCH and WHD. Inspite of realisation that it is women who die in the process of reproduction, who pay the highest toll for untreated sexually transmitted disease, who bear the largest brunt of poverty, and yet who are conditioned to remain silent. Accordingly, investment in women's health has been one of the actions identified in the Declaration for Health Development in the South-East Asia Region in the 21st Century. It has been recognised in the Declaration that since women's health is integral to development, a multi-sectoral approach would be needed through the development of partnerships with other relevant sectors.[20]

There is a need of increasing women's access to appropriate, affordable and quality healthcare throughout their lifespan and strengthening preventive programmes that promote women's health. Investing in women's health has strong synergistic effects on other dimensions.

PROBLEMS AND SUGGESTIONS

The Members of the National Commission For Women briefed the Committee about the various problems being faced by women with regard to Health and Family Welfare and spelt out certain areas to which the commission had restricted its activities. These were stated to be as under:

(i) Need to look at health for women in a holistic and integrated way including physical, mental and social health.

(ii) Lack of primary healthcare facilities, viz. primary health centres and sub-centres to cater to women at the district and block level.

(iii) Inaccessibility of healthcare facilities by women in remote areas like hilly and tribal regions and need for mobile health clinics.

(iv) Inadequate budget allocation for women's health and need for specific allocation in the budget allocation for women's health especially in hospital treatment.

(v) Ignorance about beneficial aspects of other alternate systems of medicine (Ayurveda, Homoeopathy, etc.) for health and family welfare and need to rejuvenate the Ayurveda and other Indian systems of Medicine.

(vi) Malnutrition among women and lack of gender specific data in this regard.

(vii) Female Foeticide and infanticide leading to a falling female-male ratio.

(viii) Misuse of pre-natal diagnostic techniques for promoting sex-related abortion.

(ix) Unmet need for contraceptives both for birth control and prevention of AIDS.

(x) Lack of proper survey in the field of family welfare and gender specification.

(xi) Increasing prevalence of Sexually Transmitted Diseases and HIV/AIDS among sex workers.

(xii) High rate of prevalence of Urinary Tract Infection (UTI) among women.

The Members shared with the commission their views and experience on the lack of basic health facilities specially among the rural women and sex workers and the problems being faced by them. They asked the members of the commission to concentrate in this direction with the help of NGOs, etc. so as to highlight their problems and impress upon the State and Central Government to act speedily for their welfare. Members wanted that more Hospitals are opened in rural and semi-rural areas, making it compulsory for all doctors to serve in rural areas for a specified period and ensuring that sufficient number of lady doctors posted there.

We may conclude in the words of Pt. Jawaharlal Nehru: "To awaken people; it is the women who must be educated. Once she is on the move, the family moves, the village moves, the nation moves."

We may also in this chapter briefly discuss about the (A) girl child health, (B) Adolescent girl, and (C) elderly women health.

(A) Health of The Girl Child

I Eliminate all forms of discrimination against
the girl-child.
Eliminate negative cultural attitudes and
practices against girls.
Promote and protect the rights of the girl-child and
increase awareness of her needs and potential.
Eliminate discrimination against girls in
education, skills development and training.
Eliminate discrimination against girls in health
and nutrition.
Eliminate the economic exploitation of child
labour and protect young girls at work.
Eradicate violence against the girl-child
Promote the girl child's awareness of and
participation in social, economic and political life.
Strengthen the role of the family in improving the
status of the girl-child.

—*Strategic Objectives,* L.1-L.9. Platform for Action I

Child development is integral to over all socio-economic, development of a nation. "Children's health-tomorrow's wealth" the theme affords an occasion to convey to a world-wide audience the message that children are a priceless resource, and that any nation which neglects them would do so at its peril. World Health Day, 1984 thus highlighted the basic truth that we must all safeguard the healthy minds and bodies of the world's children, not only as a key factor in attaining health for all by the year 2000, but also as a major part of each nations health in the twenty-first century

There is an old saying, attributed to Jesuit teachers: "Give me the child for seven years and I will give you the man for life"

Regarding the welfare of the children—Mahatma Gandhi said very rightly that Prayer of the Nation is child's smile and fortune. Pt. Jawaharlal Nehru said: "Nation marches on the tiny feet of the children." IYC slogan of India was Happy Child is Nation's Pride.

Children's health is linked to many inter-sectoral factors, e.g. health, environmental and nutritional needs, social and psychological needs, educational needs and special attention of girl child. (see Chart 3.2)

Mounting evidence of the special needs of girl children is increasingly focusing world attention on this very vulnerable group of the young. Exploring the problems of the girl child in the Region has raised several important issues.

It is a common fact that girl children are less desired, largely for economic reasons and the roles they will play in adult life. Tradition does not consider them as future bread winners. In fact, they become an economic liability at the time of marriage, with large dowries expected from their families.

Such discrimination begins in intrauterine life. Selective abortions of female foetuses have been reported in some countries. A study in an urban area of one country in the South East-Asia Region showed that, out of 8000 abortions performed after parents learned the sex of the foetus, only one was a male. Female infanticide has also been reported in some countries.

There are also gender differences in childhood mortality, with under-five mortality rates higher in girl children in a few countries of the Region. Since female mortality is typically lower than male mortality during childhood, this suggests some gender-related differences in child-rearing practices, and possibly in feeding patterns and use of healthcare services.

Under-nturition is also more prevalent in girls. Inadequate feeding in childhood has serious health consequences. It can lead to impaired intellectual capacity, delayed puberty, possible impaired fertility and stunted growth, resulting in higher risks of complications during childbirth.

Child prostitution and sexual abuse of young girls include rape and incest are also issues of serious concern. Education is less accessible to girls in some countries of the Region. Even in countries where primary and secondary school enrolment is relatively equal, dropout rates in girls are higher and enrolment at higher educational and vocational training courses is lower. Young girls, particularly in rural areas, contribute substantially to domestic chores and caring for smaller children in the family, and hence are often unable to attend school. We have to take care of Girl Child in 21st Century through positive discrimination.[21]

Ninth Five Year Plan lays down the strategy as:

- To arrest the declining sex ratio and curb its related problems of female foeticide and female infanticide and thus ensure 'Survival, Protection and Development of Children'.

CHART 3.2

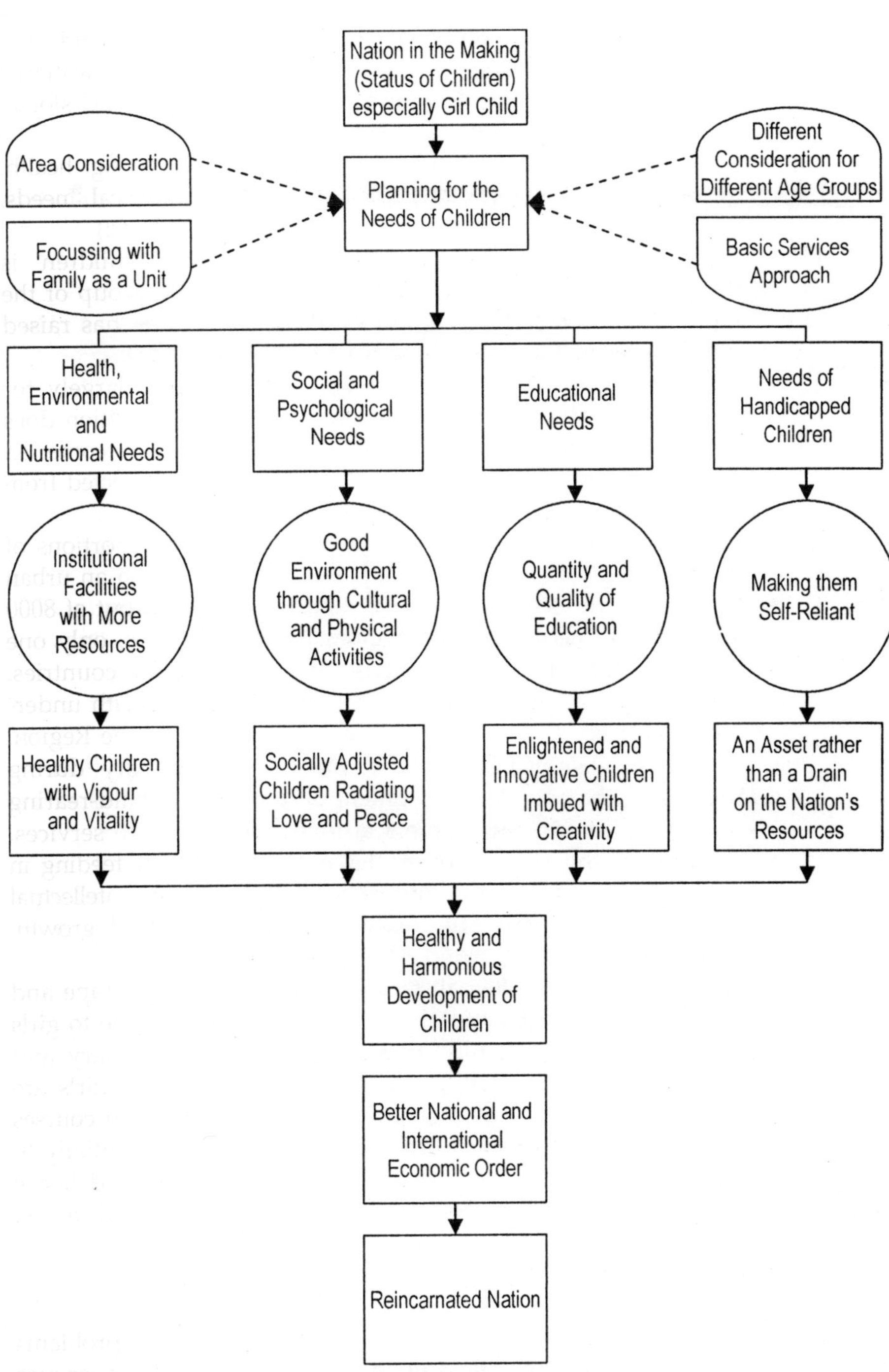
Nation in the Making (Status of Children) especially Girl Child
Area Consideration
Focussing with Family as a Unit
Planning for the Needs of Children
Different Consideration for Different Age Groups
Basic Services Approach
Health, Environmental and Nutritional Needs
Social and Psychological Needs
Educational Needs
Needs of Handicapped Children
Institutional Facilities with More Resources
Good Environment through Cultural and Physical Activities
Quantity and Quality of Education
Making them Self-Reliant
Healthy Children with Vigour and Vitality
Socially Adjusted Children Radiating Love and Peace
Enlightened and Innovative Children Imbued with Creativity
An Asset rather than a Drain on the Nation's Resources
Healthy and Harmonious Development of Children
Better National and International Economic Order
Reincarnated Nation

- To ensure Survival, Protection and Development through effective implementation of the two National Plans of Action one for children and the other for the Girl Child.
- To continue to lay a special thrust on the three major areas of child development: health, nutrition and education.
- To bring down the IMR to less than 60 and the CMR to below 10 by 2002 through providing easy access to healthcare services including RCH services and 100% coverage of immunization in respect of all vaccine-preventable diseases.
- To universalise the Nutrition Supplementary Feeding Programmes to fill the existing gaps in respect of both pre-school and school children and expectant and nursing mothers with a special focus on the girl child and the adolescent girl.
- To view girl's education as a major intervention for breaking down the vicious inter-generational cycle of gender and socio-economic disadvantages.
- To expand the support services of creche/day care services and to develop the linkages between the primary schools and the child care services to promote educational opportunities for the girl child.
- To widen the scope and the spectrum of child development services with necessary interventions related to empowerment of women and children, families and communities through effective convergence and coordination of various sectoral efforts and services.
- To universalise ICDS as the main-stay of the 9th Plan for promoting the overall development of young children especially the girl child and the mothers all over the country.
- To expand the scheme of adolescent girls in preparation for their productive and re-productive roles as confident individuals not only in family building but also in nation building.
- To promote the nutritional status of the mother and the child by improving the dietary intake through a change in the feeding practices and intra-family food distribution.
- To strengthen the early joyful period of play and learning in the young child's life and to ensure a harmonious transition from the family environment to the primary school.

(a) Special Programmes for the Girl Child

SAARC declared 1990 "The Year of the Girl Child" and 1991-2000 as the "Decade of the Girl Child." During this period programmes are proposed to:

- Increase public awareness of the value of the girl child;
- Reach girls with basic services for their survival and development;

- Ensure their participation in programmes of child development, health, nutrition and education;
- Increase the age of marriage; and
- Create a positive environment to allow girls to develop into productive and confident young women.

A National Plan of action for the Girl Child for 1991-2000 A.D. has been drawn up by the Government. The Plan recognises the rights of the girl child to equal opportunity, to be free from hunger, illiteracy, ignorance and exploitation.

Towards ensuring survival of the girl child, the objectives are to:

- Prevent cases of female foeticide and infacticide and ban the practice of amniocentesis for sex determination;
- End gender disparity in infant mortality rate;
- Eliminate gender disparities in feeding practices, expand nutritional interventions to reduce severe malnourishment by half and provide supplementary nutrition to adolescent girls in need;
- Reduce deaths due to diarrhoea by 50% among girl children under 5 years and ensure immunization against all forms of serious illnesses; and
- Provide safe drinking water and ensure access to fodder and drinking water nearer home.

Protection of the girl child is to be ensured through the following:

- Relief for those girls who are economically and socially deprived and belong to special groups;
- Intervention to sensitize various agencies on the need to protect the girl child and adolescent girls from exploitation, assault and physical abuse;
- Education and sensitization of male members of the family to the special needs of the girl child;
- Equal treatment, dignity and respect for girl children in the family and community as well as providing support and help in their day-to-day work so that they get time to avail of the opportunities for self-development;
- Rehabilitation services to reduce the growing instances of exploitation of girl-children and adolescent girls; and
- Protection of girl-children and adolescent girls from prevalent social evils such as dowry, child marriage, prostitution, rape, incest, molestation, etc. through appropriate legislation and proper enforcement.

(b) Youth Girl Health (see Chart 3.3)

One may be tempted to call this period as that of extended childhood. But the interests, attitudes, characteristics or worries of the youth do not resemble those of children. Youths even have some illnesses which are peculiar to those years or which demand special consideration at this time of life. One immediately thinks of such conditions as acne, epiphysitis, athletic injuries, growth and development disorders, the psychologic conflicts, dysmenorrhea, amenorrhea, and menorrhagia, hypertension, obesity, duodenal ulcer, cerebral palsy, epilepsy and ulcerative colitis (which are absent during childhood).

It has been defined as the period between the onset of puberty, i.e. when the person enters the gateway of manhood or womanhood; with the appearance of secondary sex characters to the completion of 24 years of age. This is the period when the young person girls completes his/her physical growth (adolescence) as well as social and cultural growth (early adulthood). This is the period when he/she attains maturity, gets employed, may get married, develops financial and psychological autonomy, stability, wisdom, reliability, integrity and compassion (Craig, 1980). WHO considers the period between 15-24 years age as youthhood.

Adolescents between 10 and 19 years of age are often considered as young people with special needs. Rapid physical, emotional and social change are taking place in their bodies and lives. With the onset of puberty with learning new ways of behaving that may lead to experimentation with sex drugs and alocohal, adolescents finds themselves exposed to a host of factors which can adversely affect their health.

It is estimated that each year across the world about 15 million girls aged 15 to 19 years give birth, and that about 11% all children are born to adolescents. Adolescent fertility rates in the least developed countries are twice as high as the overall rates in developing countries and four times higher than in developed Countries. In many countries of the Region, girls are marrying at very young ages and getting pregnant—nearly 40-50% of girls in some countries of South Asia. Adolescent fertility rates, conventionally measured as the number of births per 1000 women aged 15-19 years, exceed 100 in Bangladesh and India. Early pregnancy can set into motion an intergenerational cycle of ill-health and growth failure.

Maternal mortality is estimated to be three to four times higher in adolescent women than in adult, and pregnancy-related complications are the leading cause of mortality among adolescent girls in many countries. In addition infacts born to adolescent are more likely to have low birth weight.

Adolescent girls are both biologically and socially more vulnerable to sexually transmitted diseases (STDs) including HIV infection. In Thailand an estimated 800,000 commercial sex workers (CSWs) are under 20 years of age. Of these, one-quarter are below 14 years and approximately 3 in every 10 are HIV infected. In Myanmar, 17.3% of adolescent females between 15 and 19 years of age treated for STDs are infected with HIV. Among CSWs in the same age group, the proportion is even higher (25%).

CHART 3.3

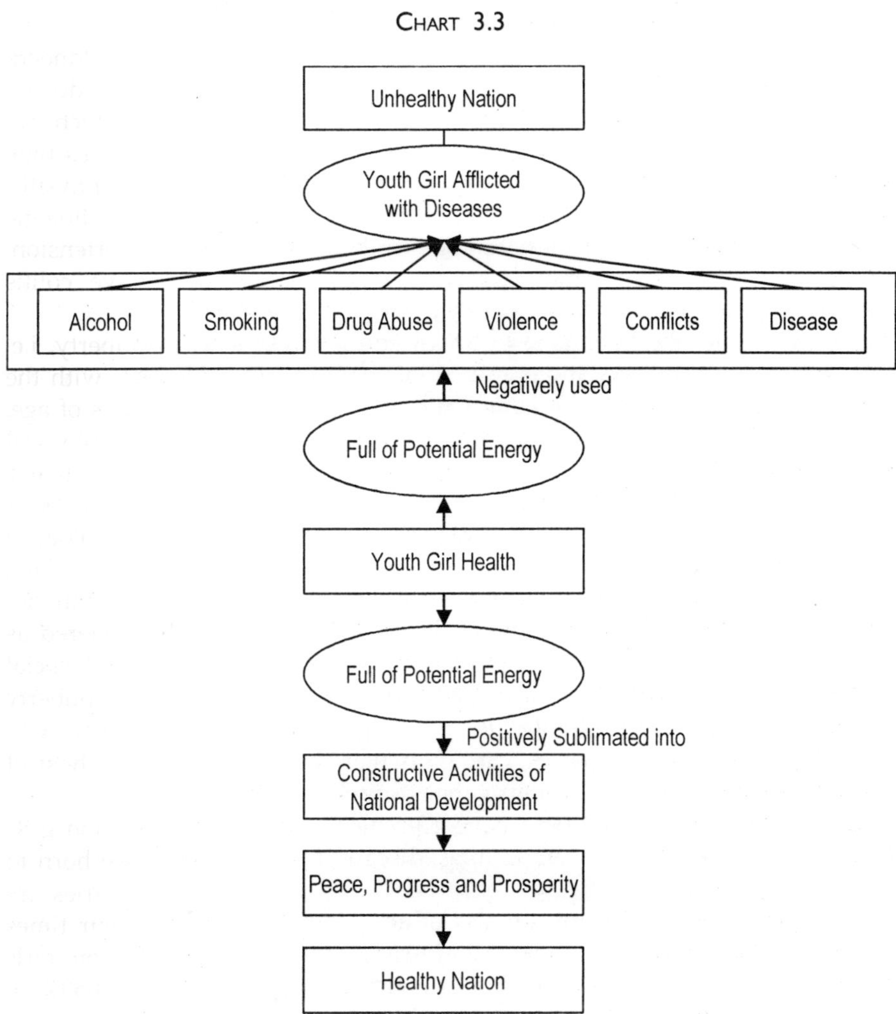

Unwanted pregnancies in single adolescents are of increasing concern and could lead adolescent girls to seek abortions. Often such abortions are sought from illegal and unsafe sources, and may lead to serious complications and even death. We should provide them right education and guidance.[22]

(c) Health of Elderly Women

For many people, living longer is not living better. Adding years to life is important. But adding life to the added years is even more important. "Active ageing makes the difference" was the World Health Day Theme for 1999. By the year 2020 more than 1000 million of the world's population will be over 60 years old. To help promote a global response to this major societal concern. WHO, in 1995, restructured its programme of health of the elderly and gave it as a new name—Ageing and Health. This area of healthcare is becoming a dominant concern as the next millennium approaches.[23]

As life expectancies in women increase, so do the numbers of elderly females in the population. Longer life can be both a penalty and a prize. In the case of women it may be more of the former. As The World Health Report 1998 states, "Many millions of women are made old before their time by the daily harshness and inequalities of their earlier lives, beginning in childhood. They experience poor nutrition, reproductive ill-health, dangerous working conditions, violence and lifestyle-related diseases, all of which exacerbate the likelihood of breast and cervical cancers, osteoporosis and other chronic conditions after menopause. In old age poverty, loneliness and alienation are common."

In the South-East Asia Region, the number of women 60 years and above increased from 37.5 million in 1985 to almost 51 million in 1995, and is projected to surpass 68 million by 2005. The health and other social needs of ageing women in the Region, however, have not yet been adequately studied.

"Although women in the world today live longer than men, their longevity is offset by a higher rate of illness. Elderly women face a number of significant medical problems. Depletion of hormones at menopause may influence cause-specific morbidity and mortality, including cardiovascular diseases and malignant neoplasms.

Musculoskeletal diseases, cardiovascular disorders, diabetes, cancers and injuries seem to be the common health problems of older women in the Region. For example, the most frequent problems seen in elderly women in Myanmar are arthritis (35.9%), lung disease (24.7%) and hypertension (17.7%).

Psychological problems are also of great importance to the health and welfare of the elderly. With increasing urbanization, and the pressure that go with it, disintegration of the extended family structure, economic hardships and the like, the elderly may become disadvantaged. Already in some countries, old people's home have appeared where there were none before.

For older persons to continue to be a resource for their families, their communities and the economy, it is essential that they be active physically, socially and mentally. The best possible foundations on which to build a long and fulfiling life is good health. In many developed countries, large number of older persons are already enjoying a healthy prolonged life and seeking ways to continue to contribute to their society. In developing countries, healthy ageing is even more important. In the absence of universal social security and within severe socio-economic constraints, a longer and more productive life will depend on vigour, vitality and health throughout childhood, youth and middle age.[24]

CONCLUSION

India has built up a vast health infrastructure and manpower at primary, secondary and tertiary care in government, voluntary and private sectors. Technological advances and improvement in access to healthcare technologies have resulted in a substantial improvement in health indices of the population and a steep decline in mortality. However, the extent of access to and utilization of healthcare has varied substantially between States, districts and different segments of society.[25]

- SC/PHC/CHC has increased from 725 in 1951 to 57,363 in 1981 to 1,63,181 (99-RHS) in 2000.
- Dispensaries and Hospitals (all) have increased to 9209 in 1951 to 23,555 in 1981 to 43,322 (95-96-CBHI) in 2000.
- Beds (Pvt. and Public) has increased 117,198 in 1951 to 569,495 in 1981 to 8,70,161 (95-96-CBHI) in 2000.
- Nursing Personnel—18,054 in 1951 to 1,43,887 in 1981 to 7,37,000 (99-INC) in 2000.
- Doctors (Modern System)—61,800 in 1951 to 2,68,700 in 1981 to 5,03,900 (98-99-MCI) in 2002.

Source: National Health Policy, 2002.

The Department of Health has formulated the National Health Policy (NHP) 2002 which was approved by the Cabinet in 2002. The National Health Policy-2002 aims at achieving an acceptable standard of good health amongst the general population of the country and has set the goals for the next two decades.

Areas of attention in the Tenth Plan include the reorganization and restructuring of existing healthcare infrastructure at primary, secondary and tertiary levels so that they have the capacity to render healthcare services to the population residing in well defined geographical areas and have appropriate referral linkages with each other. Appropriate delegation of powers to Panchayati Raj Institutions to ensure local accountability of public healthcare providers, horizontal integration of all aspects of the current vertical disease control programmes, including supplies monitoring, IEC, training and administrative arrangements, development of appropriate two-way referral system utilizing; information technology, exploring alternative systems of healthcare financing, and defining the role of various stakeholders—Government, private and voluntary sectors—are the other focus areas.

NOTES AND REFERENCES

1. WHO: SEARO: Regional Health Report, 1998, Focus on Women, New Delhi; 1998, p. 1.

2. *Ibid.*, p. 2.
3. Government of India, Department of Social Welfare Ministry of Education and Social Welfare, Towards Equality, Report of the Committee on the Status of Women in India, December, 1974, New Delhi, p. 310.
4. Lok Sabha Secretariat, Committee on Empowerment of Women (2001-02), Fourth Report, Thirteenth Lok Sabha, Health and Family Welfare Programmes for Women, New Delhi, Aug. 2001, pp. 13-16.
5. Department of Social Welfare, GOI, Blue Print of Action Points and National Plan of Action for Women, New Delhi, 1988.
6. WHO: SEARO, Regional Health Report, 1998, Focus on Women, New Delhi, 1998, p. 7.
7. GOI, Planning Commission Ninth Five Year Plan, 1997-2002, Vol. II, New Delhi, p. 322.
8. Lok Sabha Secretariat, Committee on Empowerment of Women (2001-02), Fourth Report, 13th Lok Sabha, p. 21.
9. WHO: SEARO Regional Health Report, 1998, Focus on Women, New Delhi, 1998, p. 8.
10. GOI, Economic Survey, 2002-03, p. 233.
11. Regional health Report 1998, *op. cit.*, p. 610.
12. WHO, SEARO: Regional Health Report, 1998, Focus on Women, New Delhi, 1998, p. 13.
13. *Ibid.*, pp. 21-23.
14. *Ibid.*, p. 26.
15. World Plan of Action, Para 166.
16. National Plan of Action for Women, p. 71.
17. WHO: *World Health*, May 1979, p. 19.
18. ICSSSR: Programme of Women's Studies, New Delhi; 1977, p. 10.
19. GOI, Planning Commission, Xth Five Year Draft Plan, 2002-07, pp. 217-23.
20. WHO: SEARO: Highlights of the World of WHO in the South-East Asia Region, 1 July, 1997-30 June, 1998, New Delhi, SEARO, 1998, p. 37.
21. Regional Health Report, 1998, *op. cit.*, p. 9.
22. *Ibid.*, p. 15.
23. WHO: SEARO: Fifty Years of WHO in South-East Asia, New Delhi, 1999, p. 90.
24. Regional Health Report, 1988, *op. cit.*, p. 24.
25. Economic Survey 2002-03, GOI, pp. 226-27.

CHAPTER 4

POPULATION EDUCATION VALUES, SOCIETY AND DEVELOPMENT

> "The ultimate goal of the word's population policy must be to achieve an equilibrium based on low birth and death rates that can be sustained throughout a distant future for the world and its several parts."
>
> —*F.W. Notestein*

Population Education Values, Society and Development*

"The programme of family welfare and family planning is in the interest of peace and humanity in order to improve the quality of life for families in developing countries particularly in rural areas and in urban disadvantaged poor."

—Tokyo Declaration of Parliamentarians
issued in March, 1978

IMPLICATION OF POPULATION EXPLOSION (See Chart 4.1)

The growth rate in population absorbs the national income and lowers the standard of living. The world population conference indicated in the population plan of action that population growth and population policy must be viewed not in isolation, but in the context of development. It was mentioned by the Secretary-General that current and potential world-wide population trends evidently cannot continue for as long as even one century without causing serious dislocations and crises in many areas.[1]

Myrdal in his book "Asian Drama" gave a stern warning to the world in regard to population explosion when he said, "Demographers are of the view that if fertility does not decrease, a time will come when mortality will lose its relative independence of levels of living and begin to rise again.[2]

Thus, there is a great need of stabilizing population. According to Frank W. Notestein:

* See Appendix 4.1 National Population Policy, 2000, Action Plan (Operational Strategies).

CHART 4.1

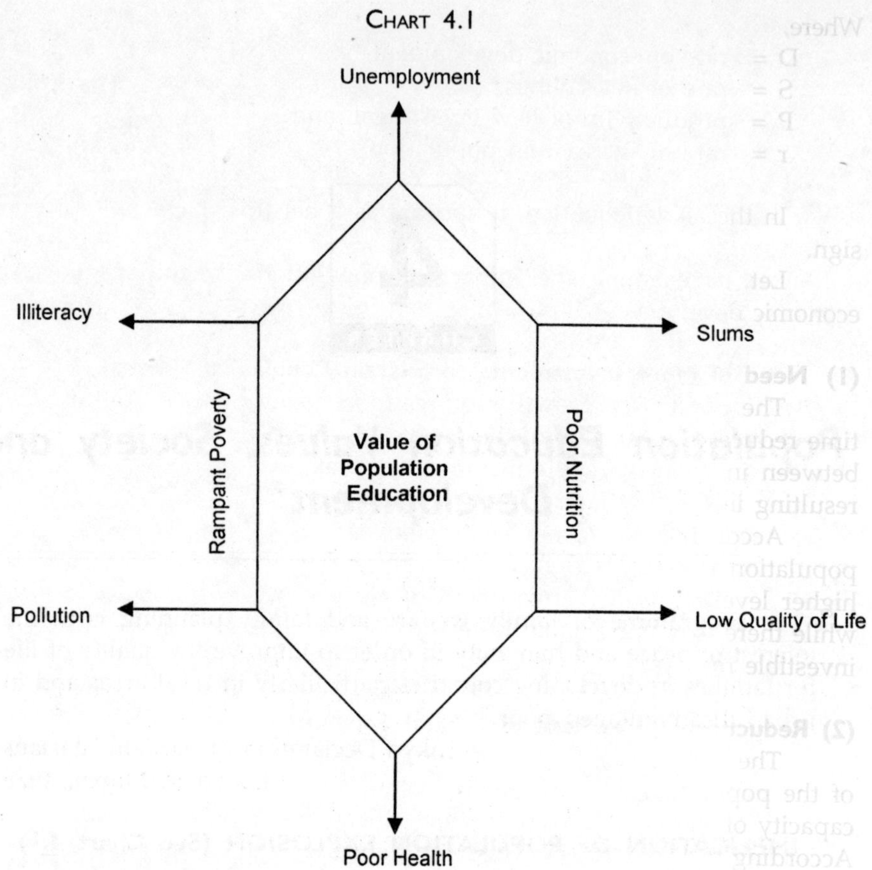

"The ultimate goal of the world population policy must be to achieve an equilibrium based on low birth and death rates that can be sustained throughout a distant future for the world and its several parts."[3]

As long as the birth rate is not restricted in these countries, it would not be possible to bring about improvements in the living standard of the people.

In a 'capital poor' and technologically backward country, growth of population diminishes the rate of capital accumulation, increases the amount of disguised unemployment and lowers the standards of living of the people, i.e., resources go to the formation to population, not capital. According to Prof. A.W. Singir, population growth has a negative effect on the rate of economic development. According to him:

$$D = SP - r$$

Where,

D = rate of economic development,
S = rate of net savings,
P = productivity of new investment, and
r = rate of increase in population.

In the above equation, it appears as a negative factor with a minus sign.

Let us examine the impact of population growth on the socio-economic development.

(1) Need of More Investments to Sustain Population Growth

The population growth requires more investment while at the same time reduces the capacity of the people to save. This creates a serious gap between investment requirements and the availability of investible funds resulting in the low rate of growth of an economy.

According to Coale and Hoover, "The significant feature of population as such is that a higher rate of population growth implies a higher level of needed investment to achieve a given per capita output, while there is nothing about faster growth that generates a great supply of investible resources."[4]

(2) Reduction in the Rate of Capital Formation

The composition of the people in underdeveloped countries (40-50% of the population in unproductive age-group) is such that it reduces the capacity of the people to save which affects the rate of capital formation. According to Prof. Meier, "This high dependency requires the economy to divert a considerable part of its resources, that might otherwise go into capital formation, to the maintenance of high percentage of dependence who may never become producers or, if so, only for relatively short working life."[5]

Recoginsing this, the Third Plan States:

> "In an underdeveloped economy with very little capital per person, a high rate of population growth makes it even more difficult to step up the rate of saving which, in turn, largely determines the possibility of achieving higher productivity and incomes. Moreover, for a given investment, a larger proportion will need to be devoted to the production of essential consumer goods at the expense of investment goods industries thereby still further slowing down the potential rate of growth."[6]

(3) Food Problem

The demand of food is rising faster than the production of food.[7] In a study carried out by Food and Agricultural Organization, it was found that the failure of food production to keep up with population growth was especially pronounced in the case of the developing countries. Out of the total of 106 countries studied, 72 were classified as developing; but in 24 of these (or one-third) food production lagged behind the growth of population. In the more recent period, it was mentioned, the situation was even less favourable.

(4) Unemployment and Underemployment

The impact of more population would affect the employment situation as there is already a back-log of unemployment and under-employment in these countries. The growing unemployment of these countries is not only an economic but it is also a social evil.

(5) Poor Health Standards

Family planning and health are intimately related. Family planning can promote women's health through the prevention of unwanted pregnancies, limiting number of births, and proper spacing, timing of births and foetal health. Family planning also promotes the health of the child through the reduction of child mortality, and promotion of the child development. Maryellen Fullam stresses the importance of family planning as instrument for the promotion of health. He says:

> "Uncontrolled fertility directly threatens the health of mothers and infants and many undermine the health of other family members. Today, no health programme can be considered complete unless it offers ready access to the appropriate family planning measures for all potential parents."[8]

(6) Social and Psychological Tensions

Rapid population growth leads to social and psychological tensions, and breakdown of a distribution system. Civil amenities such as water and power supply, housing, transport and social utilities like schooling, educational, health and medical services fall much short of demand in spite of their constant expansion. Besides, it leads to political and social corruption and accentuates economic disparities.

Thus, we can say that the problem of growing population has reached such menacing proportions that it has become a real threat to the socio-economic stability of the country. The excessive growth in population does not affect the stability of the national economy alone, it disturbs the stability of the entire body politic. It poses a colossal threat to our social structure. In our fight against poverty, disease, hunger, malnutrition and unemployment, checking the rapid growth of population is as important as raising production in the farms and factories and provision of social services. Population control is one of the chief issues which the country has to resolve and accord top priority in its march towards social and economic development. The programme of family planning is of vital importance for our country. It is a positive and constructive approach to the betterment of the quality of life of the community. Thus, it is evident that the key to India's economic future based on social justice lies in the immediate and effective implementation of a nationwide population programme.

J.P. Singh has rightly analysed the impact of population growth. He states that according to the provisional results of the 2001 census, India's population stood at 1,027 million on March 1, 2001, comprising 531 million males and 496 million females. From 361 million at the time of Independence, the population reached one billion in 2001, registering an increase of nearly three times. All this had happened when the country is not in a position to guarantee adequate nutrition, healthcare and education to the burgeoning population. At the same time, it is also true that all this has happened because of mass poverty in the country. Indifferent governance is also partly responsible for the current demographic and health scenario. Every year about 18 million people were added to India's population during 1991-2001 as against 16 million annually during 1981-91 (see Table 4.1). In other words, each year India's population increases by the equivalents of the number of inhabitants of Ghana, Australia, Mozambique or Saudi Arabia.[9]

TABLE 4.1

Decadal Variations in Population Growth in India: 1901-2001

*Census Year**	*Total population in million*	*Average annual exponential growth rate*	*Progressive growth rate over 1901 in per cent*
1901	238.4	—	—
1911	252.1	0.56	5.8
1921	251.3	-0.03	5.4
1931	279.0	1.04	17.0
1941	318.7	1.33	33.7
1951	361.1	1.25	51.5
1961	439.2	1.96	84.3
1971	548.2	2.20	129.9
1981	683.3	2.22	186.6
1991	846.3	2.14	255.0
2001	1027.0	1.93	330.8

* Including Assam and Jammu and Kashmir. The 1981 Census was not held in Assam and the 1991 Census was not held in Jammu and Kashmir due to disturbances. The 1981 and 1991 census data include estimated figures for these two states.

Source: Census of India, 1971, General Population Tables, Series 1, India, Part II-A (i), pp. 33,50, 536-37; Census of India, 1991, Final Population Totals: Brief Analysis of Primary Census Abstract, Series 1, India, Part 2 of 1992, p. 86; Census of India, 2001, Provisional Population Totals, Series 1, India, Paper 1 of 2001, p. 34.

If the country puts for a natural course of demographic transition, then it will have to pay a heavy price in the form of unmanageable unemployment, rampant poverty, political chaos leading to ethnic violence and even dismemberment of the country in the long run. In fact, the whole South Asia would have to encounter a similar experience and would take the shape of Africa and Europe in terms of number of independent nations fighting among themselves. Here the process have already set in, as the population bomb has already exploded. It is altogether a different matter that some of us at the helm of affairs deliverately tend to camouflage the reality or do not want to recognize it. Some of them even ignore the description of dismal demographic scenario scientists seem blissfully unaware of how rising population of India threatens its future, while the population issues have already started dominating India's future. One simply wonders whether new advancements in science and technology will really do any magic to save India from impending disaster following population explosion.

The Government of India in the year 1976-77 announced a National Population Policy. The policy covered a broad range of individual policies including such vital matters as raising the age of marriage, freezing representation of States in Parliament, linking the distribution of federal resources to the performance in family planning, promoting female literacy, increasing the monetary compensation for sterilization operations. The policy statement emphasized the urgent need for a direct attack on the population problem as a national commitment. It suggested a series of measures which, it was hoped, would reduce the birth rate to 25 per thousand of population by the end of the Sixth Plan.

Some of the important measures of this policy are:

1. Age of marriage to be raised to 21 for boys and 18 for girls. Offences under the new law have been made cognizable.
2. Representation in the Lok Sabha and State Legislatures to be frozen till the year 2001 A.D. at the level determined after 1971 Census.
3. Eight per cent of Central assistance to State Plans to be specifically earmarked against performance in family planning.
4. Monetary compensation for both male and female sterilization to be raised so as to provide a motivation to couples to have lesser number of children.
5. No Central legislation is proposed for the time being on the question of compulsory sterilization. States were left free to introduce compulsory sterilization if they were well equipped to meet its demands.
6. Group incentives to be introduced for panchayats, teachers and the labour.
7. Scheme for aiding voluntary organizations to be expanded to make family planning a mass movement.

8. Special measures to be undertaken to raise the level of female education.
9. High priority to be accorded to child nutrition programme to secure appreciable decline in infant mortality.
10. Population values to be introduced in the educational system to sensitize younger generations.
11. Change to be made in the Service and Conduct Rules of Central Government employees to ensure that they adopt small family norm.

The Family Planning Programme became a major political issue and the opposition coalition or Janta Party used it in the election campaigns against the ruling party. This gathered momentum and the Congress lost the election at the hands of the Janta Party. The new party changed the name of the Family Planning Programme to the Family Welfare Programme. The Janta announced the revised policy on the Family Welfare Programme on 29 June 1977.

The new approach towards family planning by the Janta Government is known as the 'Cafetaria Approach'. Under this approach, the people can choose any method suitable to them. There is no undue emphasis on sterilization. It is available only to those who desire it. The main features of this policy are:

(a) Ruling out compulsion or coercion of any sort in the field of family welfare for all times to come; while all methods of contraception will be promoted with equal emphasis, it will be left to each family to make its own choice of the method for maintaining the small family norm.
(b) Assigning a vital role to maternal and child healthcare by providing maternity services to all those who many need them and expanding the immunization programme further.
(c) Raising the age of marriage for girls and boys, although the statement envisaged raising the minimum age of marriage for girls to 16 years, it was decided subsequently that the minimum age for girls would be raised to 18 for the time being while that for boys would remain 21 years.
(d) Giving higher priority to the improvement of women's educational level through formal and non-formal channels.
(e) Using the population figures of 1971 as a base till the year 2001 in all cases where population is a factor as the allocation of Central assistance to State plans, devolution of taxes and duties and grants-in-aid.
(f) Linking of 80 per cent of Central assistance to the State Plans with their performance and success in the Family Welfare Programme.
(g) Giving population education the attention it deserves, specially

in the courses for schools and colleges aimed at influencing that segment of population which would soon be entering reproductive age and marital life.

(h) Emphasizing a multimedia motivational approach in which all media units of the various departments in the Centre and the State would be fully associated.

(i) Involving actively all voluntary bodies and the organized sector as agents of change.

(j) Allowing full rebates in the income tax assessment for amounts given as donations for family welfare purposes.

(k) Paying special attention to the necessary research inputs in the field of reproductive biology and contraception.

(l) Soliciting active cooperation and involvement of all ministries and departments of the government of India as well as the States in the programme.

(m) Monitoring of the programme intensively and carefully. Annual review of the situation in depth is to be made by the Union Cabinet.

(n) All restrictions aimed at limiting the size of the family in the case of government employees through conduct rules and the disincentives introduced by the Ministry of Finance in respect of those who violated the small family norm have been withdrawn.

The Family Welfare Programme was included in the New 20 Point Programme of the Prime Minister announced in January 1982. It envisages promotion of family planning on a voluntary basis as people's movement.

A well-defined long-term strategy has been evolved to ensure that the adoption of the 'small family norms' is done entirely on a voluntary basis. The salient features of this strategy consist of intensified efforts to spread awareness and information through imaginative use of multimedia and interpersonal communication strategies, providing services and supplies as close to the doorsteps of the acceptors as possible, developing facilities for rapid increase in female literacy, extending population education to youth in schools and colleges as well as those out of schools, assisting and supporting the association of elected representatives of the people at all levels with the programme, developing linkages with other concerned ministries and departments, ensuring effective observance of the law relating to minimum age for marriage of girls and boys and ensuring close monitoring and follow-up of the programme at all levels.

A critical examination of the existing and past population policies indicate that the family planning programme has become more political rather than technical. Well-designed and articulated public policy can keep the structural components and their elements integrated. We should not change the population policy too often. There are no two different opinions regarding the need for control of population and reducing the growth rate to zero. The views differ regarding the methodology and strategy. We must try to evolve the strategy in cooperation with the people.

Although many dedicated and wise people have been working on the Indian population problem for several years, there are few ideas, and less agreement, about what needs to be done to recruit significantly large numbers of acceptors.[10]

The creation of awareness is integral to the process of social development. The possibility for the power of communication to liberate the minds and potential of people to critical awareness is real in every field linked to human development, and the generation of public will hinges on effective communication of information and ideas that relate to people's needs, aspirations and capacities for progress in thought and action. In this sense, getting the development process started is largely the task of information, education and communication.

The communication aspect of a national family planning programme is generally termed as IEC-Information, Education Communication. The Year Book (1986-87) of Family Welfare Programme in India has rightly mentioned that the success of the Family Welfare Programme depends primarily upon the voluntary and widespread acceptance of the concept of small family and delayed marriages and well spaced and properly linked births are an effective way of achieving this objective. Mass education and Media activities, accordingly, were given multi-dimensional and integrated thrust through Information-Education-Communication activities in the form of a comprehensive package of social transformation to bring behavioural and attitudinal changes in the people so as to enable them to adopt family planning as a way of life. In brief, we can simplify it, and can call it simply as communication function. Sometimes, the activities under IEC are also referred to as "Mass Communication", "Mass Education" and "Mass Education and Media."

Donald J. Bogue has rightly said that IEC is a term widely used to identify the activities of family planning programme to inform the public and stimulate them to adopt contraception.[11] In every technical component of the Family Planning Programme provided by family planning workers, there exists a corresponding educational aspect, which has to be imparted more or less simultaneously, so as to enhance the continuing usefulness of the services provided at the time of need. This would have permanent value.

An added importance of communication in family planning resulted from the experience and studies which indicated that pure clinical approach did not bear fruit. A. Govindachari has mentioned some of the findings of the studies, which have brought to notice the limited impact of clinical approach. These are:

(i) The population reached by the clinics was very limited;
(ii) Education on family planning in the clinics was mostly through individual contacts. There was no organized community education;
(iii) The educational efforts were mostly directed towards women,

since the clinics normally have female social workers. Husbands, who are important from the point of view of decision-making in family planning, especially in an Indian cultural context, were not given due attention;

(iv) Couples felt shy to visit clinics for fear of identification by their friends and neighbours;

(v) The working hours of the clinics were found to be inconvenient, especially for the low income groups;

(vi) There was a lack of social support for the programme due to inadequate involvement of the community;

(vii) People generally prefer to obtain contraceptives in an informal way which does not involve formal recording procedures and publicity. This was not possible in a clinic situation; and

(viii) There was very little involvement of other supporting staff, like the village level workers, extension officers, etc. in the family planning programme.[12]

Today, Family planning programmes around the world are applying a broad range of service delivery and communication strategies. To make family planning services and supplies more accessible, conventional clinic-based programmes have been supplemented by innovative approaches to services delivery. These include community-based outreach, social marketing through commercial outlets at subsidized prices, and employment-based programmes organized or supported by employees or Unions. Extensive communication campaigns, combining a variety of modern and traditional mass-media are spreading family planning awareness and encouraging more people to seek out family planning services.[13]

The Information, Education, Communication (IEC) component of National Family Welfare programme is mainly to create an effective communication strategy, to inform the masses about the means and measures of Family Welfare Programme, educate them about the perils of over-population and motivate and persuade them to adopt small family norm, using all possible channels of media.[14]

In a Family Planning organisation, external communication is very important in the implementation of its programme, as information about the utility and means of planned parenthood through appropriate choice and correct use of contraceptives by the eligible married couples is important. Moreover, communication being two-way process brings to the attention of the management the needs, reactions and complaints of the people concerned for necessary initiative or remedial actions. The external communication process needs to be guided by considerations of relevance of information, the choice of communication channels and the existing understanding capacity (education, etc.) of the people concerned outside the organisation. Moreover, it should not by any means be only one sided, i.e., from the organisation to the people. The reverse flow of information from the people to the organisation would make the latter to judge the impact of the programme as well as provide the basis for any changes in the strategies of the Programme. Here again, barriers and disruptions in the two-way communication process have to be dealt with appropriately.[15]

Broadly speaking, communication is the means by which intentions of the programme are classified to ensure fruitful results. It may even be looked upon as the means by which special information inputs are fed into social systems. It is the means by which behaviour of the personnel engaged in the programme is modified; change is effected, information is made productive and goals are achieved. Barnard has aptly viewed it as the means by which people can be linked together in an organisation to achieve the objectives of the programmes. Communication is a universal phenomenon among living beings. Newman and Summer have viewed communication as an exchange of facts, ideas, opinion, or emotions by two or more persons.[16]

Family Planning Communication implies a number of actions starting with identifying the audience, assessing needs and channels for response, identifying specific messages especially in areas of resistance to change in attitude and behaviour, selecting complementary media for optimal combination, producing communication materials and refining messages and techniques after pre-testing, revision and re-testing, dissemination of communication, continuous support through stages of programmes implementation mainly to ensure community involvement and participatory monitoring and evaluation. Since, Family Planning is a challenging and arduous task, communication technology must be well planned. A successful communication effort blends the use of traditional communication media with the modern, brings together the channels of government communication with those of the community and of voluntary organisations and a variety of other groups. Family Planning ideology can be registered in the minds of the people not simply by providing the information on Family Planning, but because people can be told that they exist, shown that they work and encouraged (and empowered) to try them and make them work for themselves. This is the nature of the support which communication lends to a family planning programme.

ESSENTIALS AND ASPECTS OF MASS MOTIVATION CAMPAIGN

Essentials

Dr. John Hubley quoted by Gloria Gorden in his Article, "Let's Communicate" in *World Health* (January-Feb. 1989) has rightly described the essentials of Communication—

- Promote actions which are realistic and feasible within the constraints faced by the community.
- Build on ideas, concepts and practices that people already have.
- Repeat and reinforce information overtime, using different methods.

- Use existing channels of Communication such as songs, drama and story-telling, and be adaptable.
- Entertain and attract the attention of the Community.
- Use clear, simple language with local expressions and emphasize short-term benefits of action.
- Provide opportunities for dialogue and discussion to allow learner participation and feedback on understanding and implementation.
- Use demonstrations to show the benefits of adopting practices.[17]

E.M. Rogers mentions the following essentials:

(i) Family Planning Communication campaigns should be preceded by extensive planning of the strategies to be followed.

(ii) A Consumer Orientation in family planning communication activities will be more effective in achieving the objectives of the National Family Planning Programme.

(iii) A new family planning communication approach should be launched on a small scale pilot project basis.

(iv) Social research can perform an important function in more effective family planning communication, (a) by providing feedback for the design of communication messages through pre-testing, and (b) by yielding, evaluative data about the efforts of communication activities.[18]

MEANING AND GENESIS OF POPULATION EDUCATION

The National Seminar on Population Education organized by the NCERT at Bombay in 1969 observed, "The objectives of population should be to enable the students to understand that family size is controllable, that population limitation can facilitate the development of a higher equality of life in nation and that a small size family can contribute to the quality of living for the individual family. It should also enable the students to appreciate the fact that for preserving the health and welfare of members of the family, to ensure the economic stability of the family and to assure good prospects for the younger generation, that the Indian families of today and tomorrow should be small and compact."

The Seminar giving a comprehensive definition of population education emphasized knowledge about the quantity and quality of population and the need to control them for happy human existence. Population education has been regarded as a strategy for human resource development. It aims at developing desired awareness, values and attitudes both for quality and quantity of population. It must enable students to make rational decisions on population. It must enable students to make rational decisions on population matters for themselves for others by acquiring knowledge about cause and effect relationship.

The Asian Regional Seminar organized by the UNESCO at Bangkok in 1970 defined population education as "an educational programme which provided for a study of the population situation in the family, community, nation and world for the purpose of developing in the students national and responsible attitudes and behaviour towards that situation." According to Stephen Viedeeman population education is "an educational process which assists persons (a) to learn the probable causes and consequences of population phenomena for themselves and their community (including the world), (b) to define for themselves and their communities, the nature of the problems associated with population processes and characteristics, and (c) to assess the possible effective means by which society as a whole and as an individual can respond to and influence these processes in order to enhance the quality of life now as in future.

The NCERT document (1987) has aptly enunciated, "By doing so they are expected to develop national attitude towards the desirable size and structure of our population and the quality of life in their respective family. They are also expected to appreciate and promote the development of small family norms in the society. The acceptance of observance of small family norms depends a great deal on inculcation of commitment on the part of students." (p. 68) Proper education is, therefore, felt essential to develop right attitudes amongst the vast population which is to enter the fertility age-group after a few years. Such education can enable the young people to know the actual facts and position of our country in particular and of the world in general which will motivate them with a desire to adopt small family norms.

ROLE OF HIGHER EDUCATION (See Chart 4.2)

As stated in the UGC guidelines for the Development of Population Education Resource Centres in the Indian Universities (1995). In 1983, the concept of population education was introduced in some universities by setting up population education clubs as a co-curricular activity. The main objective of the programme was to provide opportunities to the University/ College youth and through them to the people in the community, on the relationship to the people in the community, on the relationship between population and quality of life.

The UGC-UNFPA projects on Population Education in Higher Education was launched in 1986. The commitment of the University Grants Commission to population education at the University and college levels go back to 1983 when about 92 universities and 1300 colleges were provided financial support to organize population education activities both for college youth on campus and through them in the communities through Population Education Clubs. The launching of the population education programmes in 1986 with the financial support of UNFPA and technical assistance of UNESCO, provided further impetus to the programme to cover

CHART 4.2

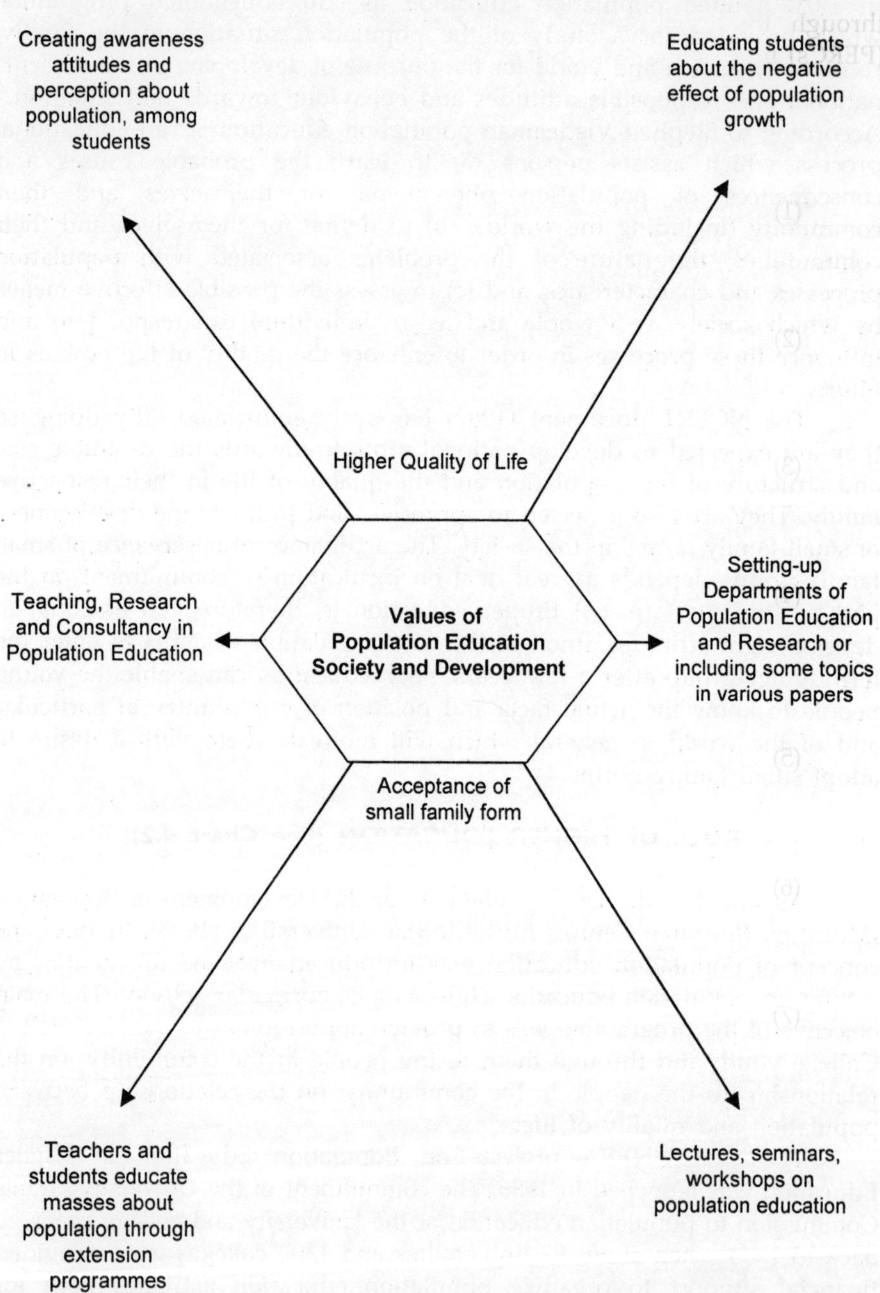

the three functional areas of the universities, viz. development of population education contents for introduction into courses of study at the under-graduate and post-graduate levels, research, and extension education.

Since 1985 the programme has been implemented in 12 universities through the establishment of Population Education Resource Centres (PERCs) in the Department of Adult, continuing Education and Extension.

AIMS AND OBJECTIVES

(1) Change the present attitudes/values in society regarding gender's roles and rights, to one of equal participation in all social, economic and political processes and national and international development;

(2) To counter the reactionary forces emanating from certain sections of the media, economic, social and political institutions, that uncovering the demotion of superstitious from productive to more reproductive roles;

(3) To revitalize university education, bringing it closer to population related issued to work towards their solution, and to produce sensitive persons able to play more committed and meaningful roles in development activities for the country;

(4) To fulfil a special responsibility—to produce for all levels of the educational system, teachers who are aware of the need for a non-formal education, and who would actively pick up the challenge to promote, values, of social equality, including gender equality, secularisms, socialism and democracy;

(5) To update university curricula by incorporating the results of new research and the issues related to population as they challenge some of the established theories, analytical concepts and methodologies of various disciplines;

(6) To promote increased collaboration between different disciplines in teaching, curriculum designing, research and extension activities since population studies are interdisciplinary by nature;

(7) To generate new and organic knowledge through intensive field work. This would help generation of data essential for evaluation and correction of development policies and programmes and in extending the areas to academic analysis into hertherto neglected sectors. For better understanding and investigation of problems being experienced at the grassroots, a closer contact between institution of higher education and groups directly involved in action, to assist men and women to enjoy their rights within the family, the community and at work) would be very valuable. Such contact would also help universities and colleges to design their extension activities in a more meaningful manner; and

(8) To contribute to be global debate on the population problems throughout development of material, training, teaching, research and extension activities.

ACTIVITIES

Teaching

The Population Education Resource Centres would be responsible for the integration of population education in the curriculum at UG/PG/B.Ed. and M.Ed. levels. Efforts will also be made to incorporate Population Education through distance education mode—

(a) A Foundation course for all undergraduates students in all universities, professional and teaching institutions.

(b) curriculum Development; to incorporate population dimension into courses in different disciplines.

(c) Review of existing text books and to integrate the population issues in the curriculum.

(d) Workshops to plan restructuring of courses and syllabus formation.

Development of Learning Materials (Print and Audio-Visual)

The PERCs would be responsible for the procurement, preparation of learning materials depending upon the local needs of the area. Learning materials would be in printed form as well as Audio-Visual cassettes. The PERC will duplicate the audio-visual cassettes to be used in their university and also in the service area.

Training (Functionaries/College Principals? Public Leaders/Medical Officers/ Students/Others)

(a) Workshop for the functionaries of the (Vice-chancellors, Principals, Medical Officers, Project Officers, etc.) Universities and colleges to generate better understanding and interest in Population-related issues.

(b) Summer/Winter institutes for orientation training of teachers/ researchers, etc. to handle population-related topics.

(c) Workshops for research methodology and syllabus/curriculum restructuring at the UG/PG levels in different disciplines.

(d) Orientation of Vice-chancellors and Public leaders related to the Population Education issues.

Extension Activities

Greatest importance needs to be attached to extension work, as a learning and developmental instrument, for the benefit of the community through students and teachers. A few such extension activities are exhibitions, posters, films, songs, plays, etc. on issues pertaining to the population:

- (i) to organize debates, essays competitions, elocution competitions, group discussions, symposia, drawing painting competitions, quises.
- (ii) To arrange lectures by experts on population-related issues.
- (iii) To organize and monitor the programme of population Education Clubs in the Service area.
- (iv) To enact demands/rallies on the themes on Population problems on important occasions such as World Population Day, World's Aid Day, University Day, etc.
- (v) Working closely with NGOs, NSS, etc. collaboration with other departments of audit and continuing education and extension will enrich such activities

Universities and colleges through their departments of Adult and continuing education and population research centers can help the students to understand the dynamics of population control. It can as well support the government. Universities and colleges in India are living in Ivory towers as they do not take much interest in social and economic issues found in the community. It is the duty of higher education system in the country to take interest in such issues by incorporating these into undergraduate and postgraduate syllabus or setting up individual departments to support community and government so that these issues can be solved. This is also known as extension function of the University. Faculty in the University possess immense potentially and they can take keen interest in these extension activities provided they are supported by the system of higher education with financial and material support. They can take up following activities for population education:

- (a) Educating the youth about population growth so that they understand the implications of small family norms in their life.
- (b) Creating understanding and a spirit in the youth about population education so that they spread the message to people.
- (c) Students after getting education can work in the community to remove doubts among the people about population control.
- (d) Students can convince families about quality of life, which can be possible only with small family.
- (e) Prepare charts, video films, etc. for educating students and people about population education.
- (f) Arrange debates and discussions on various issues of population education.
- (g) Dissemination of information about population education.
- (h) Prepare groups of students to visit villages on holidays to promote population education.
- (i) Promote the teaching of population education as an independent subject at all educational levels or as part of the regular curricula to meet the needs of each age group.

(j) Create a better understanding of population education by organizing population education workshops for family planning administrators at various levels.
(k) Support research studies and evaluation so that the findings can be applied to further the development of population education.
(l) Encourage educational institutions and relevant agencies to carry out studies and research in order to develop appropriate techniques for implementing information, education and communication services on population activities.

Educational approach is a healthy method and will motivate people to accept family welfare voluntarily. Any other scheme without educational base will miserably fail as it will generate reaction. We must encourage population education through formal and informal education to imbibe the confidence of the people in the family welfare programme. Population education is an educational programme to develop in young men rational and responsible attitude and behaviour towards population problem. NCERT suggested the following curriculum:

(1) The population growth.
(2) Economic development and population.
(3) Social development and population.
(4) Health, nutrition and population.
(5) Family life and population.

Wayland suggests six basic topics for study:

(1) Basic instructions in population dynamics.
(2) Development of basic understanding of the process of human reproduction.
(3) Understanding of health problem concerned with bringing up of children.
(4) Appreciation of relationship between quality of life and family size.
(5) Government policies regarding population growth and economic development.
(6) Familiarity with the family planning programme of one's own country.

J.P. Singh feels, "What has happened elsewhere can happen in India too provided there is a massive campaign to educate eligible couples, particularly in villages, about the benefits of limiting the size of the family. This point has of course been emphasized innumerable times and at different places but it has never been sincerely implemented. Rural people, steeped in ignorance and obsolete religious belief, still do not know the harm that big family size brings to them and consider every child as a gift of God. This notion must be altered if family planning is to succeed. However, the education campaign must always be backed by easy availability of modern contraceptive measures that can enable people to plan their families. One of the reasons why family planning measures have not yielded the desired results is that it has not been honestly implemented. The unmet need for family planning has been reported to be quite high. According to the National Family Health Survey the current unmet need for family planning is 16 percent and it is higher in rural areas than in urban areas.[19]

National Population Policy, 2000

Government of India has enunciated the new Population Policy in February 2000. Commenting on the New Population Policy, *Business Standard* Editorial "Sense on Population" dated February 17, 2000 remarked that the new national population policy, 2000, however may have a greater chance of acceptance as it incorporates some of the lessons learnt from recent successes in curbing population growth. While the earlier attempts merely emphasized physical targets and ignored the vital aspects of health and education, especially that of the girl child, which are vitally linked to birth rates, the latest policy seeks to squarely address these issues. Besides, it also makes the right kind of noises about investment in social infrastructure as an essential prerequisite for promoting small family norms.

Success of the new policy will depend largely on the way it is implemented by the laggard states and the pace of socio-economic development (including in the field of health and education) that accompanies. It measures like freezing the number of seats in the Lok Sabha at the current level are essentially facilitators, dispelling states fears that population control will reduce their quota of MPs. There has to be an adequate political will to achieve the twin, veritably inseparable, objectives of reducing family size and improving the quality of life.

However, *The Tribune* Editorial, "Gaps in Population Policy" dated February 17, 2000, suggested the gaps in new policy and stressed the need to make up these gaps. Increasing population packs a greater destructive power than what Pakistan can cause by hurling a few nuclear bomb blasts. That is because it is concentrated at the bottom of the social and economic pyramid covering three-fourth of the population. The failure to control the exploding numbers is the most damaging of all failures. What the country needed was a radical review of the old policies, alertness to deploy all available instruments and establish enduring contacts with the target segment in rural India. Sadly these are missing in the new National Population Policy unveiled. The document still pins its hopes on a few tried incentives and shapeless promises to run in population growth. Such sops will be available only after the event—that is, after individuals or couples take themselves out of the reproduction cycle. Actually, the concentration should have been on goading people to enter the charmed circle.

CONCLUSION

Without evaluating the impact of FP education programmes on the bulk of the people, one cannot possible identify positive as well as negative aspects of the programme. An objective evaluation of the FP education programme alone can help one improve guidelines for future action. Cost benefit analysis should be an integral part of this evaluation, so that one may assess how available resources have been utilized. Through objective evaluation, one may also be able to curtail mass production of ritualistic FP education material as produced by various FP education bureaus. The amount thus saved can be effectively utilized for a more purposeful and meaningful health education programme.

FP education is the most difficult task as habits, usages and customs are deeply entrenched. But, FP administration would fail in its purpose, if it could not produce social change, as it is easier to destroy our villages than to change our customs. Professional training helps the FP experts to deal with the health changes effectively. Their pharamcopoeia in both fields must be strong in order to translate the findings of biological investigations into social application. So over and above each technical act, there is a corresponding education function which doubles the value of the act, increases its efficiency and endows it with real human and social value.[20]

Noel David Burleson has rightly said, "The history of the twentieth century becomes more and more a race between numbers and the quality of life. If we are to utilize our intelligence in our present population dilemma, we must make our educational systems relevant. Participants and those who are about to become participants in the vital revolution will require an education that includes population education. It is felt that through education students, the future participants of population explosion will be able to understand the relationship between the increasing numbers and socio-economic development of our country. The coming generations can be made aware of the impact of population on our environment, on our resources, and on all aspects of our life and society. It is hoped that the future citizens should be involved right from their student life in understanding this major concern formation.

The NCERT document (1987) has aptly enunciated, "By doing so they are expected to develop national attitude towards the desirable size and structure of our population and the quality of life in their respective family. They are also expected to appreciate and promote the development of small family norms in the society. The acceptance of observance of small family norms depends a great deal on inculcation of commitment on the part of students." (p. 68) Proper education is, therefore, felt essential to develop right attitudes amongst the vast population, which is to enter the fertility age-group after a few years. Such education can enable the young propel to know the actual acts and position of our country in particular and of the world in general which will motivate them with a desire to adopt small family norms.

Notes and References

1. UN: E.F.S. 75, XIII, 4, p. 76.
2. Gunnar, Myrdal, "Asian Drama: An Inquiry into the Poverty of Nations", Vol. III, London, 1968, p. 154.
3. Frank, Notestein, W., "Population Policy and Development, a Summary View", *Population Debate*, Vol. I, Part Four, Para 5).
4. Coale and Hoover, Population Growth and Economic Development in Low Income Countries, 1958, p. 19.
5. Geral Meier, Leading Issues in Economic Development,1975, p. 591.
6. GOI Planning Commission, Third Five Year Plan, p. 22.
7. FAO: Population, Food Supply and Agricultural Development, *Population Debate*, Vol. I, Part Four, Para 8.
8. Maryellen Fullan in *People*—A Journal of the International Planned Parenthood Federation, Vol. 5, Number 4, 1978, p. 27.
9. J.P. Singh, Problems of Population and Sustainable Development in India, in *IJPA*, January-March 2003, pp. 85-86, 94.
10. World Bank, "Management Problems in National Family Planning Programe", in UN: E/F/S, 75, XIII, 5, p. 511.
11. Donald J. Bogue, "A Five Year Information—Education Communication Perspective to meet the Population, Health, Food Crisis, 1975-80" in *Family Planning Resumed*, p. 117, 1977, No. 1.
12. A. Govindachari, "The Role of Extension Education in Family Planning", in *Aspects of Population Policy in India*, New Delhi, 1969, pp. 124-25.
13. Population Reports, Series, Number 35, November 1987, p. 2.
14. Annual Report of the Ministry of Health and Family Welfare, 1998-99, p. 73
15. H. Koontz and C. O'Donnell, "Principles of Management: An Anlysis of Managerial Functions", London: McGraw Hill, Kogakusha Ltd., 1972, pp. 538-40.
16. W.H. Newman and C.E. Summer, "The Process of Management Concepts: Behaviour and Practice", Anglewood, Cliffs, N.J. Prentice Hall, 1961, p. 59.
17. *World Health*, Jan.-Feb. 1989.
18. E.M. Rogers in Joung Whang, ed. pp. 130-31.
19. J.P. Singh, *op. cit.*, p. 93.
20. WHO, Technical Report Series, 1954, No. 89, p. 4.

APPENDIX 4.1

NATIONAL POPULATION POLICY, 2000 ACTION PLAN

OPERATIONAL STRATEGIES

(i) and (ii) Converge Service Delivery at Village Levels

1. Utilise village self-help groups to organise and provide basic services for reproductive and child healthcare, combined with the ongoing Integrated Child Development Scheme (ICDS). Village self-help groups are in existence through centrally sponsored schemes of: (a) Department of Women and Child Development, Ministry of HRD, (b) Ministry of Rural Development, and (c) Ministry of Environment and Forests. Organise neighbourhood acceptor groups, and provide them with a revolving fund that may be accessed for income generation activities. The groups may establish rules of eligibility, interest rates, and accountability for which capital may be advanced, usually to be repaid in instalments within two years. The repayments may be used to fund another acceptor group in a nearby community, who would exert pressure to ensure timely repayments. Two trained birth attendants and the Anganwadi Worker (AWW) should be members of this group.

2. Implement at village levels a one-stop integrated and coordinated service delivery package for basic healthcare, family planning and maternal and child health-related services, provided by the community and for the community. Train and motivate the village self-help acceptor groups to become the primary contact at household levels. Once every fortnight, these acceptor groups will meet, and provide at one place 6 different services for: (i) registration of births, deaths, marriage and pregnancy; (ii) weighing of children under 5 years, and recording the weight on a standard growth chart; (iii) counselling and advocacy for contraception, plus free supply of contraceptives; (iv) preventive care, with availability of basic medicines for common ailments; antipyretics for fevers, antibiotic ointments for infections, ORTIORSI for childhood diarrhoeas, together with standardised indigenous medication and homeopathic cures; (v) nutrition supplements; and (vi) advocacy and encouragement for the continued enrolment of children in school up to age 14. One health staff, appointed by the panchayat, will be suitably trained to provide guidance. Clustering services for women and children at one place and time at village levels will promote positive interactions in health benefits and reduce service delivery costs.

3. Wherever these village self-help groups have not developed for any reason, community midwives, practitioners of ISMH, retired school teachers and ex-defence personnel may be organised into neighbourhood groups to perform similar functions.

4. At village levels, the Anganwadi Centre may become the pivot of basic healthcare activities, contraceptive counselling and supply, nutrition education and supplementation, as well as pre-school activities. The

Aanganwadi Centres can also function as depots for ORS/basic medicines and contraceptives.

5. A maternity hut should be established in each village to be used as the village delivery room, with storage space for supplies and medicines. It should be adequately equipped with kits for midwifery, ante-natal care, and delivery; basic medication for obstetric emergency aid; contraceptives, drugs and medicines for common ailments; and indigenous medicines/ supplies for maternal and new-born care. The panchayat may appoint a competent and mature mid-wife, to look after this village maternity hut. She may be assisted by volunteers.

6. Trained birth attendants as well as the vast pool of traditional dais should be made familiar with emergency and referral procedures. This will greatly assist the Auxiliary Nurse Midwife (ANM) at the sub-centres to monitor and respond to maternal morbidity/emergencies at village levels.

7. Each village may maintain a list of community mid-wives, village health guides, panchayat sewa sahayaks, trained birth attendants, practitioners of indigenous systems of medicine, primary school teachers and other relevant persons, as well as the nearest institutional healthcare facilities that may be accessed for integrated service delivery. These persons may also be helpful in involving civil society in monitoring availability, quality and accessibility of reproductive and child health services; in disseminating education and communication on the benefits of smaller and healthier families, with emphasis on education of the girl child; and female participation in the work force.

8. Provide a wider basket of choices in contraception, through innovative social marketing schemes to reach household levels. *Comment*: Meaningful decentralisation will result only if the convergence of the national family welfare programme with the ICDS programme is strengthened. The focus of the ICDS programme on nutrition improvement at village levels and on pre-school activities must be widened to include maternal and child healthcare services. Convergence of several related activities at service delivery levels with, in particular, the ICDS programme, is critical for extending outreach and increasing access to services. Intersectoral coordination with appropriate training and sensitisation among field functionaries will facilitate dissemination of integrated reproductive and child health services to village and household levels. People will willingly cooperate in the registration of births, deaths, marriages and pregnancies if they perceive some benefit. At the village level, this community meeting every fortnight, may become their most convenient access to basic healthcare, both for maternal and child health, as well as for common ailments. Households may participate to receive integrated service delivery, alongwith information about ongoing micro-credit and thrift schemes. Government and non-government functionaries will be expected to function in harmony to ensure integrated service delivery. The panchayat will promote this coordination and exercise effective supervision.

(iii) Empowering Women for Improved Health and Nutrition

1. Create an enabling environment for women and children to benefit from products and services disseminated under the reproductive and child health programme. Cluster services for women and children at the same place and time. This promotes positive interactions in health benefits and reduces service delivery costs.

2. As a measure to empower women, open more child care centres in rural areas and in urban slums, where a woman worker may leave her children in responsible hands. This will encourage female participation in paid employment, reduce school dropout rates, particularly for the girl child, and promote school enrolment as well. The Anganwadis provide a partial solution.

3. To empower women, pursue programmes of social afforestation to facilitate access to fuel wood and fodder. Similarly, pursue drinking water schemes for increasing access to portable water. This will reduce long absences from home, and the need for large number of children to perform such tasks.

4. In any reward scheme intended for household levels' priority may be given to energy saving devices such as solar cookers, or provision of sanitation facilities, or extension of telephone lines. This will empower households, in particular women.

5. Improve district, sub-district and panchayat-level health management with coordination and collaboration between district health officer, sub-district health officer and the panchayat for planning and implementation activities. There is need to:

- Strengthen the referral network between the district health office, district hospital and the community health centres, the primary health centres and the sub-centres in management of obstetric and neo-natal complications.
- Strengthen community health centres to provide comprehensive emergency obstetric and neo-natal care. These may function as clinical training centres as well. Strengthen primary health centres to provide essential obstetric and neo-natal care. Strengthen sub-centres to provide a comprehensive range of services, with delivery rooms, counselling for contraception, supplies of free contraceptives, ORS and basic medicines, together with facilities for immunisation.
- Establish rigorous problem identification mechanisms through maternal and peri-natal audit, from village level upwards.

6. Ensure adequate transportation at village level, sub-centre levels, zila parishads, primary health centres and at community health centres. Identifying women at risk is meaningful only if women with complications can reach emergency care in time.

7. Improve the accessibility and quality of maternal and child health

services through:

- Deployment of community mid-wives and additional health providers at village levels; cluster services for women and children at the same place and time, from village level upwards, e.g. ante-natal and post-partum care, monitoring infant growth, availability of contraceptives and medicine kits; and routinised immunisations at sub-centre levels.
- Strengthen the capacity of primary health centres to provide basic emergency obstetric and neo-natal healthcare.
- Involve professional agencies in developing and disseminating training modules for standard procedures in the management of obstetric and neo-natal cases. The aim should be to routinise these procedures at all appropriate levels.
- Improve supervision by developing guidance and supervision checklists.

8. Monitor performance of maternal and child health services at each level by using the maternal and child health local area monitoring system, which includes monitoring the incidence and coverage of ante-natal visits, deliveries assisted by trained healthcare personnel and post-natal visits, among other indicators. The ANM at the sub-centre should be responsible and accountable for registering every pregnancy and child birth in her jurisdiction, and for providing universal ante-natal and post-natal services.

9. Improve technical skills of maternal and child healthcare providers by:

- Strengthening skills of health personnel and health providers through classroom and on-the-job training in the management of obstetric and neo-natal emergencies. This should include training of birth attendants and midwives at district-level hospitals in life-saving skills, such as management of asphyxia and hypothermia.
- Training on integrated management of childhood illnesses for infants (1 week-2 months).

10. Support community activities such as dissemination of IEC material, including leaflets and posters, and promotion of folk jatras, songs and dances to promote healthy mother and healthy baby messages, along with good management practices to ensure safe motherhood, including early recognition of danger signs.

11. Programme development comprising:

- Partnership in family health and nutrition. The Anganwadi worker will identify women and children in the villages who suffer from malnutrition and/or micro-nutritional deficiencies,

including iron, vitamin A, and iodine deficiency; provide nutritional supplements and monitor nutritional status.
- Convergence, strengthening and universalisation of the nutritional programmes of the Department of Family Welfare and the ICDS run by the Department of Women and Child Development, ensuring training and timely supply of food supplements and medicines.
- Include STD/RTI and HIV/AIDS prevention, screening and management, in maternal and child health services.
- Provide quality care in family planning, including information, increased contraceptive choices for both spacing and terminal methods, increase access to good quality and affordable contraceptive supplies and services at diverse delivery points, counselling about the safety, efficacy and possible side effects of each method, and appropriate follow-up. Develop a health package for adolescents.

13. Expand the availability of safe abortion care. Abortion is legal, but there are barriers limiting women's access to safe abortion services. Some operational strategies are:

- Community-level education campaigns should target women, household decision-makers and adolescents about the availability of safe abortion services and the dangers of unsafe abortion.
- Make safe and legal abortion services more attractive to women and household decision-makers by: (i) increasing geographic spread; (ii) enhancing affordability; (iii) ensuring confidentiality; and (iv) providing compassionate abortion care, including post-abortion counselling.
- Adopt updated and simple technologies that are safe and easy, e.g. manual vacuum extraction not necessarily dependant upon anaesthesia, or non-surgical techniques which are non-invasive.
- Promote collaborative arrangements with private sector health professionals, NGOs and the public sector, to increase the availability and coverage of safe abortion services, including training of mid-level providers.
- Eliminate the current cumbersome procedures for registration of abortion clinics. Simplify and facilitate the establishment of additional training centres for safe abortions in the public, private, and NGO sectors. Train these healthcare providers in provision of clinical services for safe abortions.
- Formulate and notify standards for abortion services. Strengthen enforcement mechanisms at district and sub-district levels to ensure that these norms are followed.
- Follow norms-based registration of service provision centres,

and thereby switch the onus of meticulous observance of standards onto the provider.

- Provide competent post-abortion care, including management of complications and identification of other health needs of post-abortion patients, and linking with appropriate services. As part of post-abortion care, physicians may be trained to provide family planning counselling and services such as sterilisation and reversible modern methods such as IUDs, as well as oral contraceptives and condones.
- Modify syllabus and curricula for medical graduates, as well as for continuing education and in-house learning, to provide for practical training in the newer procedures.
- Ensure services for termination of pregnancy at primary health centers and at community health centres.

14. Develop maternity hospitals at sub-district levels and at community health centres to function as FRUs for complicated and life-threatening deliveries.

15. Formulate and enforce standards for clinical services in the public, private, and NGO sectors.

16. Focus on distribution of non-clinical methods of contraception (condoms and oral contraceptive pills) through free supply, social marketing as well as commercial sales.

17. Create a national network consisting of public, private and NGO centres, identified by a common logo, for delivering reproductive and child health services free to any client. The provider will be compensated for the service provided, on the basis of a coupon, duly counter-signed by the beneficiary, and paid for by a system to be devised. The compensation will be identical to providers across all sectors. The end-user will choose the provider of the service. A group of management experts will devise checks and balances to prevent misuse.

(iv) Child Health and Survival

1. Support community activities, from village level upwards to monitor early and adequate ante-natal, natal and post-natal care. Focus attention on neo-natal healthcare and nutrition.

2. Set-up a National Technical Committee on neo-natal care, to align programme and project interventions with newly emerging technologies in neo-natal and peri-natal care.

3. Pursue compulsory registration of births in coordination with the ICDS Programme.

4. After the birth of a child, provide counselling and advocacy about contraception, to encourage adoption of a reversible or a terminal method. This will also contribute to the health and well-being of both mother and child.

5. Improve capacities at health centres in basic midwifery services,

essential neo-natal care, including the management of sick neo-nates outside the hospital.

6. Sensitise and train health personnel in the integrated management of childhood illnesses. Standard case management of diarrhoea and acute respiratory infections must be provided at sub-centres and primary health centres, with appropriate training, and adequate equipment. Besides, training in this sector may be imparted to healthcare providers at village levels, especially in indigenous systems.

7. Strengthen critical interventions aimed at bringing about reductions in maternal malnutrition, morbidity and mortality, by ensuring availability of supplies and equipment at village levels, and at sub-centres.

8. Pursue rigorously the pulse polio campaign to eradicate polio.

9. Ensure 100 per cent routine immunisation for all vaccine preventable diseases, in particular tetanus and measles.

10. As a child survival initiative, explore promotional and motivational measures for couples below the poverty line who marry after the legal age of marriage, to have the first child after the mother reaches the age of 21, and adopt a terminal method of contraception after the birth of the second child.

11. Children form a vulnerable group and certain sub-groups merit focused attention and intervention, such as street children and child labourers. Encourage voluntary groups as well as NGOs to formulate and implement special schemes for these groups of children.

12. Explore the feasibility of a national health insurance covering hospitalisation costs for children below 5 years, whose parents have adopted the small norm, and opted for a terminal method of contraception after the birth of the second child.

13. Expand the ICDS to include children between 6-9 years of age, specifically to promote and ensure 100 per cent school enrolment, particularly for girls. Promote primary education with the help of Anganwadi workers, and encourage retention in .school till age 14. Education promotes awareness, late marriages, small family size and higher child survival rates.

14. Provide vocational training for girls. This will enhance perception of the immediate utility of educating girls, and gradually raise the average age of marriage. It will also increase enrolment and retention of girls at primary school, and likely also at secondary school levels. Involve NGOs, the voluntary sector and the private sector, as necessary, to target employment opportunities.

(v) Meeting the Unmet Needs for Family Welfare Services

1. Strengthen, energise and make publicly accountable the cutting edge of health infrastructure at the village, sub-centre and primary health centre levels.

2. Address on priority the different unmet needs detailed in Appendix 4.1, in particular, an increase in rural infrastructure, deployment

of sanctioned and appropriately trained health personnel, and provisioning of essential equipment and drugs.

3. Formulate and implement innovative social marketing schemes to provide subsidised products and services in areas where the existing coverage of the public, private and NGO sectors is insufficient in order to increase outreach and coverage.

4. Improve facilities for referral transportation at panchayat, zilla parishad and primary health centre levels. At sub-centres, provide ANMs with soft loans for purchase of mopeds, to enhance their mobility. This will increase coverage of ante-natal and post-natal check-ups, which, in turn, and will bring about reductions in maternal and infant mortality.

5. Encourage local entrepreneurs at village and block levels to start ambulance services through special schemes, with appropriate vehicles to facilitate transportation of persons requiring emergency as well as essential medical attention.

6. Provide special loan schemes and make site allotments at village levels to facilitate the starting of chemist shops for basic medicines and provision for medical first aid.

(vi) Under-Served Population Groups

(a) Urban Slums

1. Finalise a comprehensive urban healthcare strategy.

2. Facilitate service delivery centres in urban slums to provide comprehensive basic health, reproductive and child health services by NGOs and private sector organisations, including Corporate houses.

3. Promote networks of retired government doctors and para-medical and non-medical personnel who may function as healthcare providers for clinical and non-clinical services on remunerative terms.

4. Strengthen social marketing programmes for non-clinical family planning products and services in urban slums.

5. Initiate specially targeted information, education and communication campaigns for urban slums on family planning, immunization, ante-natal, natal and post-natal check-ups and other reproductive healthcare services. Integrate aggressive health education programmes with health and medical care programmes, with emphasis on environmental health, personal hygiene and healthy habits, nutrition education and population education.

6. Promote inter-sectoral coordination between departments/ municipal bodies dealing with water and sanitation, industry and pollution, housing, transport, education and nutrition, and women and child development, to deal with unplanned and uncoordinated settlements.

7. Streamline the referral systems and linkages between the primary, secondary and tertiary levels of healthcare in the urban areas.

8. Link the provision of continued facilities to urban slum-dwellers with their observance of the small family norm.

(b) Tribal Communities, Hill Area Populations and Displaced and Migrant Populations

1. Many tribal communities are dwindling in numbers, and may not need fertility regulation. Instead, they may need information and counselling in respect of infertility.

2. The NGO sector may be encouraged to formulate and implement a system of preventive and curative healthcare that responds to seasonal variations in the availability of work. income and food for tribal and hill area communities and migrant and displaced populations. To begin with, mobile clinics may provide some degree of regular coverage and outreach.

3. Many tribal communities are dependent upon indigenous systems of medicine which necessitates a regular supply of local flora, fauna and minerals, or of standardised medication derived from these. Husbandry of such local resources and of preparation and distribution of standardised formulations should be encouraged.

4. Healthcare providers in the public, private and NGO sectors should be sensitised to adopt a "burden of disease" approach to meet the special needs of tribal and hill area communities.

(c) Adolescents

I. Ensure for adolescents access to information, counselling and services, including reproductive health services, that are affordable and accessible. Strengthen primary health centres and sub-centres, to provide counselling, both to adolescents and also to newly weds (who may also be adolescents). Emphasise proper spacing of children.

2. Provide for adolescents the package of nutritional services available under the ICDS programme.

Comment: Improvement in health status of adolescent girls has an inter-generational impact. It reduces the risk of low birth weight and minimizes neo-natal mortality. Malnutrition is a problem that seriously impairs the health of adolescent and adult women and has its roots in early childhood. The causal linkages between anemia and low birth weight, prematurity, pre-natal mortality, and maternal mortality has been extensively studied and established.

3. Enforce the Child Marriage Restraint Act, 1976, to reduce the incidence of teenage pregnancies. Preventing the age of girls below the legally permissible age of 18 should become a national concern.

Comment: It will promote higher retention of girls at schools, and is also likely to encourage their participation in the paid work force.

4. Provide integrated intervention in pockets with unmet needs in the urban slums, remote rural areas, border districts and among tribal populations.

(d) Increased Participation of Men in Planned Parenthood

I. Focus attention on men in the information and education campaigns to promote the small family norm, and to raise awareness by emphasising the significant benefits of fewer children, better spacing, better heath and nutrition, and better education.

2. Currently, over 97 per cent of the sterilisations are tubectomies. Repopularise vasectomies, in particular the no-scalpel vasectomy, as a safe, simple, painless procedure, more convenient and acceptable to men.

3. In the continuing education and training at all levels, there is need to ensure that the no-scalpel vasectomy, and all such emerging techniques and skills are included in the syllabi, together with abundant practical training. Medical graduates, and all those participating in "in-service" continuing education and training, will be equipped to handle this intervention.

(vii) Diverse Healthcare Providers

1. At district and sub-district levels, maintain block-wise data base of private medical practitioners whose credentials may be certified by the Indian Medical Association (IMA). Explore the possibility of accrediting these private practitioners for a year at a time, and assign to each a satellite population, not exceeding 5,000 (depending upon distances and spread), for whom they may provide reproductive and child health services. The private practitioners would be compensated for the services rendered through designated agencies. Renewal of contracts after one year may be guided by client satisfaction. This will serve as an incentive to expand the coverage and outreach of high quality healthcare. Appropriate checks and balances will safeguard misuse.

2. Revive the earlier system of the licensed medical practitioners who, after appropriate certification from the IMA, may participate in the provision of clinical services.

3. Involve the non-medical fraternity in counselling and advocacy so as to demystify the national family welfare effort, such as retired defence personnel, retired school teachers and other persons who are active and willing to get involved.

4. Modify the under/post-graduate medical, nursing, and paramedical professional course syllabi and curricula, in consultation with the Medical Council of India, the Councils of ISMH, and the Indian Nursing Council, in order to reflect the concepts and implementation strategies of the reproductive and child health programme and the national population policy. This will also be applied to all in-service training and educational curricula.

5. Ensure the efficient functioning of the First Referral Units, i.e. 30 bed hospitals at block levels which provide emergency obstetric and child healthcare, to bring about reductions in Maternal Mortality Ratio (MMR) and Infant Mortality Rate (IMR). In many states, these FRUs are not operational on account of an acute shortage of specialists, i.e. gynaecologist obstetrician, anaesthetist and pediatrician. Augment the availability of specialists in these three disciplines, by increasing seats in medical institutions, and simultaneously enable and facilitate the acquisition of in-service post-graduate qualifications through the National Board of Medical Examination and open universities like IGNOU in larger numbers. As an

incentive, seats will be reserved for those in-service medical graduates who are willing to abide by a bond to serve for 5 years at First Referral Units after completion of the course. States would need to sanction posts of Specialists at the FRUs. Further, these specialists should be provided with clear promotion channels.

(viii) (a) Collaboration with and Commitments from the Non-Government Sector

1. There remain innumerable hurdles that inhibit genuine long-term collaboration between the government and non-government sectors. A forum of representatives from government, the non-government organisations and the private sector may identify these hurdles and prepare guidelines that will facilitate and promote collaborative arrangements.

2. Collaboration with and commitments from NGOs to augment advocacy, counselling and clinical services, while accessing village levels. This will require increased clinic outlets as well as mobile clinics.

3. Collaboration between the voluntary sector and the NGOs will facilitate dissemination of efficient service delivery to village levels. The guidelines could articulate the role and responsibility of each sector.

4. Encourage the voluntary sector to motivate village-level self-help groups to participate in community activities.

5. Specific collaboration with the non-government sector in the social marketing of contraceptives to reach village levels will be encouraged.

(viii) (b) Collaboration with the Commitments from Industry

1. The corporate sector and industry could, for instance, take on the challenge of strengthening the management information systems in the seven most deficient states, at primary health centre and sub-centre levels. Introduce electronic data entry machines to lighten the tedious work load of ANMs and the multi-purpose workers at sub-centres and the doctors at the primary health centres, while enabling wider coverage and outreach.

2. Collaborate with non-government sectors in running professionally sound advertisement and marketing campaigns for products and services, targeting all segments of the population, from village level upwards, in other words, strengthen advocacy and IEC, including social marketing of contraceptives.

3. Provide markets to sustain the income-generating activities from village levels upwards. In turn, this will ensure consistent motivation among the community for pursuing health and education-related community activities.

4. Help promote transportation to remote and inaccessible areas up to village levels. This will greatly assist the coverage and outreach of social marketing of products and services.

5. The social responsibility of the corporate sector in industry must, at the very minimum, extend to providing preventive reproductive and child healthcare for its own employees (100 workers are engaged).

6. Create a national network consisting of voluntary, public, private and non-government health centres, identified by a common logo, for delivering reproductive and child health services, free to any client. The provider will be compensated for the service provided, on the basis of a coupon system duly counter-signed by the beneficiary and paid for by a system that will be fully articulated. The compensation will be identical to providers, across all sectors. The end user exercises choices in the source of service delivery. A committee of management experts will be set-up to devise ways of ensuring that this system is not abused.

7. Form a consortium of the voluntary sector, the non-government sector and the private corporate sector to aid government in the provision and outreach of basic reproductive and child healthcare and basic education.

8. In the area of basic education, set-up privately run/managed primary schools for children up to age 14-15. Alternately, if the schools are set-up/managed by the panchayat, the private corporate sector could provide the mid-day meals, the text-books and/or the uniforms.

(ix) Mainstreaming Indian Systems of Medicine and Homeopathy

I. Provide appropriate training and orientation in respect of the RCH programme for the institutionally qualified ISMH medical practitioners (already educated in midwifery, obstetrics and gynaecology (over 5½ years), and utilise their services to fill in gaps in manpower at appropriate levels in the health infrastructure, and at sub-centres and primary health centres, as necessary.

2. Utilise the ISMH institutions, dispensaries and hospitals for health and population-related programmes.

3. Disseminate the tried and tested concepts and practices of the indigenous systems of medicine, together with ISMH medication at village maternity huts and at household levels for ante-natal and post-natal care, besides nurture of the newborn.

4. Utilise the services of ISMH 'barefoot doctors' after appropriate training and orientation towards providing advocacy and counselling for disseminating supplies and equipment, and as depot-holders at village levels.

(x) Contraceptive Technology and Research on RCH

1. Government will encourage, support and advance the pursuit of medical and social science research on reproductive and child health, in consultation with ICMR and the network of academic and research institutions.

2. The international Institute of Population Sciences and the Population Research Centres will continue to review programme and monitoring indicators to ensure their continued relevance to strategic goals.

3. Government will restructure the Population Research Centres, if necessary.

4. Standards for clinical and non-clinical interventions will be issued and regularly reviewed.

5. A constant review and evaluation of the community needs assessment approach will be pursued to align programme delivery with good management practices and with newly emerging technologies.

6. A committee of international and Indian experts, voluntary and non-government organisations and government may be set-up to regularly review and recommend specific incorporation of the advances in contraceptive technology and, in particular, the newly emerging techniques, into programme development.

(xi) Providing for the Older Population

1. Sensitize, train and equip rural and urban health centres and hospitals towards providing geriatric healthcare.

2. Encourage NGOs and voluntary organizations to formulate and strengthen a series of formal and informal avenues that make the elderly economically self-reliant.

3. Tax benefits could be explored as an encouragement for children to look after their aged parents.

(xii) Information Education and Communication

1. Converge IEC efforts across the social sectors. The two sectors of Family Welfare and Education have coordinated a mutually supportive IEC strategy. The Zila Saksharta Samitis design and deliver joint IEC campaigns in the local idiom, promoting the cause of literacy as well as family welfare. Optimal use of folk media has served to successfully mobilize local populations. The state of Tamil Nadu made exemplary use of the IEC strategy by spreading the message through every possible media, including public transport, on milestones on national highways as well as through advertisement and hoardings on roadsides, along city/rural roads, on billboards, and through processions, films, school dramas, public meetings, local theatre and folk songs.

2. Involve departments of rural development, social welfare, transport, cooperatives, education with special reference to schools, to improve clarity and focus of the IEC effort, and to extend coverage and outreach. Health and population education must be inculcated from the school levels.

3. Fund the nagarpalikas, panchayats, NGOs and community organizations for interactive and participatory IEC activities.

4. Demonstration of support by elected leaders, opinion-makers, and religious leaders with close involvement in the reproductive and child health programme greatly influences the behaviour and response patterns of individuals and communities. This serves to enthuse communities to be attentive towards the quality and coverage of maternal and child health services, including referral care. Public leaders and film stars could spread widely the messages of the small family norm, female literacy, delayed

marriages for women, fewer babies, healthier babies, child immunization and so on. The involvement and enthusiastic participation of elected leaders will ensure dedicated involvement of administrators at district and sub-district levels. Demonstration of strong support to the small family norm, as well as personal example, by political, community, business, professional, and religious leaders, media and film stars, sports personalities and opinion-makers, will enhance its acceptance throughout society.

5. Utilise radio and television as the most powerful media for disseminating relevant socio-demographic messages. Government could explore the feasibility of appropriate regulations, and even legislation, if necessary, to mandate the broadcast of social messages during prime time.

6. Utilise dairy cooperatives, the public distribution systems, other established networks like the LIC at district and sub-district levels for IEC and for distribution of contraceptives and basic medicines to target infant/ childhood diarrhoeas, anaemia and malnutrition among adolescent girls and pregnant mothers. This will widen outreach and coverage.

7. Sensitise the field level functionaries across diverse sectors (education, rural development, forest and environment, women and child development, drinking water mission, cooperatives) to the strategies, goals and objectives of the population stabilisation programmes.

8. Involve civil society for disseminating information, counselling and spreading education about the small family norm, the need for fewer but healthier babies, higher female literacy and later marriages for women. Civil society could also be of assistance in monitoring the availability of contraceptives, vaccines and drugs in rural areas and in urban slums.

MILESTONES IN THE EVOLUTION OF THE POPULATION POLICY OF INDIA

1946

Bhore Committee Report.

1952

Launching of Family Planning Programme.

1976

Statement of National Population Policy.

1977

Policy Statement on Family Welfare Programme.

Both statements were laid on the Table of the House in Parliament, but never discussed or adopted.

1983

The National Health Policy of 1983 emphasized the need for

"securing the small family norm, through voluntary efforts and moving towards the goal of population stabilisation." While adopting the Health Policy, Parliament emphasized the need for a separate National Population Policy.

1991

The National Development Council appointed a Committee on Population with Shri Karunakaran as Chairman. The Karunakaran Report (Report of the National Development Council (NDC) Committee on Population) endorsed by NDC in 1993 proposed the formulation of a National Population Policy to take "a long-term holistic view of development, population growth and environmental protection" and to "suggest policies and guidelines (for) formulation of programmes" and "a monitoring mechanism with short, maritime and long-term perspectives and goals" (Planning Commission, 1992). It was argued that the earlier policy statements of 1976 and 1977 were placed on the table, however, Parliament never really discussed or adopted them. Specifically, it was recommended that "a National Policy of Population should be formulated by the Government and adopted by Parliament."

1993

An Expert Group headed by Dr. M.S. Swaminathan was asked to prepare a draft of a national population policy that would be discussed by the Cabinet and then by Parliament.

1994

Report on a National Population Policy by the Expert Group headed by Dr. Swaminathan. This report was circulated among Members of Parliament, and comments requested from central and state agencies. It was anticipated that a national population policy approved by the National Development Council and the Parliament would help produce a broad political consensus.

1997

On the 50th anniversary of India's Independence, Prime Minister Gujral promised to announce a National Population Policy in the near future. During 11/97 Cabinet approved the draft National Population Policy with the direction that this be placed before Parliament. However, this document could not be placed in either House of Parliament as the respective Houses stood adjourned followed by dissolution of the Lok Sabha.

1999

Another round of consultations was held during 1998, and another draft National Population Policy was finalised and placed before the Cabinet in March 1999. Cabinet appointed a Group of Ministers (headed by

Dy Chairman, Planning Commission) to examine the draft Policy. The GOM met several times and delivered over the nuances of the Population Policy. In order to finalise a view about the inclusion/exclusion of incentives and disincentives, the Group of Ministers invited a cross-section of experts from among academia, public health professionals, demographs, social scientists, and women's representatives. The GOM finalised a draft population policy, and placed the same before Cabinet. This was discussed in Cabinet on 19 November, 1999. Several suggestions were made during the deliberations. On that basis, a fresh draft was submitted to cabinet.

CHAPTER 5

REPRODUCTIVE AND CHILD HEALTH PROGRAMME

> "It is the flagship programme of family welfare which combines the trinity of objectives, viz. reproductive health, child survival and fertility regulations with a policy and programme orientation markedly different from previous programmes."
>
> —*India, 2004*

Reproductive and Child Health Programme

I. GENESIS

The Universal Immunisation Programme (UIP) aimed at reduction in mortality and morbidity among infants and younger children due to Vaccine Preventable Diseases, was started in 1985-86. The Oral Dehydration Therapy (ORT) was also started in view of the fact that diarrhoea was a leading cause of deaths among children. Various other programmes under Maternal and Child Health (MCH) were also implemented during the Seventh Plan. The objectives of all these programmes were convergent and aimed at improving the health of the mothers and young children and to provide them facilities for prevention and treatment of major disease conditions. While these programmes did have a beneficial impact, but the separate identity for each programme was causing problems in its effective management and this was also reducing somewhat the outcomes. Therefore, in the Eighth Plan, these programmes were integrated under Child Survival and Safe Motherhood (CSSM) Programme which was implemented from 1992-93.

The process of integration of related programmes initiated with the implementation of the CSSM Programme was taken a step further in 1994, when the International Conference on Population and Development in Cairo recommended that the participant countries should implement unified programmes for Reproductive and Child Health (RCH). The RCH approach has been defined as "People have the ability to reproduce and regulate their fertility, women are able to go through pregnancy and child birth safely, the outcome of pregnancies is successful in terms of maternal and infant survival and well-being and couples are able to have sexual relations free of fear of pregnancy and of contacting diseases." This concept is in keeping with the evolution of an integrated approach to the programmes aimed at improving the health status of young women and children, which has been going on in the country. It is obviously sensible that the integrated RCH Programme would help in reducing the cost of inputs to some extent because overlapping of expenditure would no longer be necessary and integrated implementation would optimise outcomes at the field level. During the Ninth Plan, the RCH Programme, accordingly, has integrated all the related programmes of the Eighth Plan. The concept of RCH is to provide to the beneficiaries need-based, client-centred, demand driven, high quality and integrated RCH services. The RCH Programme is a composite programme incorporating the inputs of the Government of India as well as funding support from external donor agencies including the World Bank and the European Commission.

The RCH programme incorporates the components covered under the Child Survival and Safe Motherhood Programme and includes two additional components, one relating to sexually transmitted diseases (STD) and the other relating to reproductive tract infection (RTI). The main highlights of the RCH Programme are:

(i) The Programme integrates all interventions of fertility regulation, maternal and child health with reproductive health of both men and women.

(ii) The services to be provided will be client-centred, demand-driven, high quality and based on the needs of the community arrived at, through decentralised participatory planning and a target free approach.

(iii) The programme envisages upgradation of the level of facilities for providing various interventions and quality of care. The First Referral Units (FRUs) being set-up at sub-district level will provide comprehensive emergency obstetric and new born care. Similarly, RCH facilities in PHCs will be substantially upgraded.

(iv) The Programme will improve access of the community to various services which are commonly required. It is proposed to provide facilities for MTP at the PHCs, counselling and IUD insertion at SCs in a phased manner.

(v) The Programme aims at improving the outreach of services, particularly for the vulnerable groups of population who have till now substantially been let out of the planning process:

- Special programmes will be taken up for urban slums, tribal population and adolescents.
- Non-Governmental Organisations will be involved in a much larger way to improve out-reach and make it people's programme.
- Skills of practitioners of ISM will be upgraded by training and research and development in ISM will be supported to improve the range of the RCH services.

- Panchayati Raj system will have a greater role in planning, implementation and assessment of client satisfaction.[1]

Ninth Five Year Plan (Draft) has mentioned the following features of RCH Programme:

- Effective maternal and child healthcare,
- Increased access to contraceptive care,
- Safe management of unwanted preganancies,
- Nutritional services to vulnerable groups,
- Prevention and treatment of RTI/STD,
- Reproductive health services for adolescents,
- Prevention and treatment of gynaecological problems, and
- Screening and treatment of cancers, especially that of uterine cervix and breast.

For over 30 years Family Welfare Programme was known for its rigid, target-based approach in contraceptives. The performance was measured by the reported numbers of the four contraceptive methods—Sterilisation, Intrauterine device, Oral pills and Condoms. This was widely criticised for being a coercive approach.

The 1994 Cairo International Conference on Population and Development (ICPD) formulated a growing International consensus that improving reproductive health and family planning is essential to human welfare and development.

A growing body of evidence and the Cairo consensus suggest "Numerical method specific contraceptive target and monetary incentives" for providers to be replaced by a broader system of "programme performance goals" and measures focussed on a range of reproductive health services.

We can say in brief that reproductive and Child Health Services which is equivalent to:

- Family Planning, to focus on fertility regulation,
- Child Survival and Safe Motherhood Programme, and
- Treatment of Reproductive Tract Infections and Sexually Transmitted Infections and prevention of AIDS,

Through

1. Client-Oriented/Mother-Friendly/user-specific, family welfare services, and
2. High quality services.

The specific programmes under Reproductive and Child Health Services are:

1. Prevention and management of unwanted pregnancies,
2. Maternal care:
   (a) Ante-natal services,
   (b) Natal services,
   (c) Post-natal services,
3. Child Survival, and
4. Treatment of Reproductive Tract Infections (RTI) and Sexually Transmitted Infections (STI).[2]

The following definition of reproductive health was approved in April 1994, by the WHO Global Policy Council, provides the basis for action in this field:

"Reproductive health implies that people are able to have a responsible, satisfying and safe sex life and that they have the capability to reproduce and the freedom to decide if, when and how often to do so. Implicit in this last condition are the right of men and women to be informed of and to have access to safe, effective, affordable and acceptable methods of fertility regulation of their choice, and the right of access to appropriate healthcare services that will enable women to go safely through pregnancy and childbirth and provide couples with the best chance of having a healthy infant."

Reproductive health must address, as its basic elements, sexual behaviour, family planning, maternal care and safe motherhood, abortion, reproductive tract infections (including sexually transmitted diseases and HIV/AIDS, and certain reproductive tract malignancies such as cervical cancer.[3]

II. THE PACKAGE OF REPRODUCTIVE AND CHILD HEALTH SERVICES

The different services provided under RCH programme are:

I. For the Mothers

- TT Immunization,
- Prevention and treatment of anaemia,
- Ante-natal care and early-identification of maternal complications,
- Deliveries by trained personnel,
- Promotion of institutional deliveries,
- Management of Obstetric emergencies, and
- Birth spacing.

2. For the Children

- Essential newborn care,
- Exclusive breast feeding and weaning,
- Immunization,
- Appropriate management of diarrhoea,
- Appropriate management of ARI,
- Vitamin A prophylaxis, and
- Treatment of Anaemia.

3. For Eligible Couples

- Prevention of pregnancy, and
- Safe abortion.

4. RTI/STD

- Prevention and treatment of reproductive tract and sexually transmitted diseases.[4]

Principles and Approach

The guiding principles and approach of reproductive healthcare are to a great extent different than those of the existing dominant approach of MCH and FP programme.[5] A glimpse of the shift in approach and principle can be studied from the Table 6.1.

The guiding principles of reproductive healthcare are those of human rights, ethics, equity, quality of care, universal access, participation, partnership, integration, optimal use of resources and sustainability. Partnerships and sharing of responsibilities between government, governmental organizations and the private sector are important in stimulating new ideas and approaches and ensuring service coverage and quality of care. These principles are the same as the principles of primary healthcare.

We must keep in mind that reproductive health is a crucial part of general health and is central to human development. It affects everybody; it involves intimate and highly valued aspects of life. Not only is it a reflection of health in infancy, childhood and adolescence, it also sets the stage for health beyond the reproductive years, for both men and women, and has effects from one generation to another. Reproductive health includes sexual healthcare, for maintaining and enhancing the functions of the reproductive system, and the prevention and management of RTIs, HIV/AIDS and infertility. Reproductive healthcare is an integral part of primary healthcare. The guiding principles and the approaches of reproductive healthcare are similar to the delivery of primary healthcare. These are:

TABLE 6.1

Principles and Approach of Existing MCH/FP Programme and of RHC Programme

Existing MCH/FP Programmes	*Reproductive Health Programmes*
Target population is primarily women	Target population is both women and men
Vertical programmes	Integrated and inter-sectoral programmes
Top-down planning and implementation	Bottom-up planning respoding to local reprodutive health needs within socio-cultural and economic milieu and decentralised implementation
Focus on individual cases	Public health approach with familiy and community focus
Pregnancy-based approach	Life cycle approach
Medical approach: health needs identified by providers; reliance on medical solutions	Community-based approach: respect women's knowledge and definition of their health needs; reliance on holistic solutions that take into account the social, biological and psychological factors determining health
Provider centred: prescribe fertility control methods	Client centred: provide inforamtion and enable women to choose the methods they wish to adopt
Method specific information provided	Apart from information on all methods of fertility regulation, provide knowledge on sexuality and reproduction
Emphasis on achieving output targets	Emphasis on coverage and quality of services
Services provided in a clinical atmosphere	Provide services in a humane and caring setting
Vague general health rights	Respect specific reproductive health rights

Source: WHO: SEARO, Managing Essential Reproductive Healthcare, New Delhi, p. 5.

- education concerning prevailing health problems and the methods of preventing and controlling them;
- promotion of food supply and proper nutrition;
- an adequate supply of safe water and basic sanitation;
- maternal and child healthcare, including family planning;
- immunisation against the major infectious diseases;
- appropriate treatment of common diseases and injuries; and
- provision of essential drugs.

Let us new mention the health interventions required for different services at different levels. (See Table 6.2).

Advantages of the Scheme

RCH can avoid the problems prevalent in earlier family planning programme and can improve the coverage and quality of services provided the RCH programme is implemented as scheduled.

1. Target-free Approach can make the Programme Flexible

The achievements of family planning programmes were judged simply on the completion of targets fixed from above. It was found that the top down approach is not realistic and based on field situations. Thus, the users preference is not reflected in the targets. A major feature of the target-free approach in its emphasis on the promotion of modern spacing methods. The approach intends also to achieve a greater participation of males in the family welfare programme. Moreover, in the absence of method-specific targets, the grass-root level workers including the ANM and the Multi-purpose Health Workers (both male and female) are expected to work closely with the community and arrive at an estimate of the various family welfare activities required in the area/population covered by them. The male health workers, in particular, are made responsible for motivation for vasectomy and condoms. These activities are expected to result in an improvement in the knowledge of modern temporary methods as well as male methods of contraception; and an improvement in the proportion of spacing as well as male methods in the contraceptive method-mix.

2. Target-free Approach can make the Reporting Honest and Reliable

Field Staff used to do false reporting in order to prove the progress to avoid disciplinary action. This approach has made the reporting realistic and thus can help in effective policy-making and planning.

Earlier, we had malpractices of performing sterilisation/vasecotomy upon ineligible persons. All such cases and practices would be avoided.

3. New Programme can Infect Forward and Backward Linkages

The RCH programme can promote linkages to make it effective forwards positive health. Since it is not merely a family planning programme, it is a total package covering the total health of women and children, a very positive view.

4. Over-head Cost can be Reduced

Costs incurred in managing programmes in an integrated way can reduce a lot of cost as overhead cost can be reduced.

5. Effective Maternal and Child Health

At the village level, the Auxiliary Nurse Midwife is responsible for rendering maternal and child health services alongwith family welfare

TABLE 6.2

Essential Reproductive and Child Health Services at Different Levels of the Health Services System

Health Intervention	*Community Level*	*Sub-centre Level*	*Primary Health Centre Level*	*First Referral Unit/ District Hospital Level*
1. Prevention and management of unwanted pregnancy	1. Sexuality and gender information education and counselling 2. Community mobilization and education for adolescents, newly married youth, men and women* 3. Community-based contraceptive distribution** (through panchayats, Village Health Guides, Mahila Swasthya Sanghas, etc. with follow-up) 4. Motivating referral for sterilization 5. Social marketing of condoms and oral pills through community sources and G.P. (Oral pills to be distributed through health personnel including GPS to women who are starting pills for the first time) 6. Free supplies to health services * to be piloted ** Panchayats to distribute only condoms	No. 1. as in community level 2. Providing* oral contraceptives (OCS) and condoms 3. Providing IUD after screening for contraindications 4. Counselling and early referral for medical termination of pregnancy 5. Counselling/ management/ referral for side effects, method-related problems, change of method where indicated 6. Add other methods to expand choice 7. Providing treatment for minor ailments and referral for problems * Social marketing of pills and condoms through HW (M & F) may be explored by permitting her to retain the money.	Nos. 1-6 and 7. Performing tubal ligation by minilap on fixed dates* 8. Performing vasectomy 9. Providing first trimester medical termination of pregnancy upto 8 weeks (includes MR) 10. Facilities for Copper 'T' insertion to post-natal cases 11. Treatment facilities for all types of referrals * PHCs should have facilities for tubal ligation and mini-lap including OTs and equipments	Nos. 1-11 and 12. Providing services for medical termination of pregnancy in the first and second trimester (upto 20 weeks) where indicated

TABLE 6.2 *(Contd.)*

Health Intervention	*Community Level*	*Sub-centre Level*	*Primary Health Centre Level*	*First Referral Unit/ District Hospital Level*
2. Maternity Care Prenatal Services	1. Early registration of all pregnant women 2. Awareness raising for importance of appropriate care during pregnancy and identification of danger signs 3. To mobilise community support for transport, referral and blood donation 4. Counselling education for breast feeding nutrition, family planning, rest, exercise and personal hygiene, etc. 5. Early detection and referral of high risk pregnancies 6. Observing five cleans or through social marketing of disposal delivery kits. Delivery planning as to where? when and from whom? * The need of IC support and establishment of first referral facilities.	No. 1-4 and 5. Three ante-natal contacts with women either at the sub-centre or at the outreach village sites during immunisation/ MCH sessions 6. Early detection of high risk factors and maternal complications and prompt referral 7. Referral of high risk women for institutional delivery 8. Treatment of malaria (facilities including drugs to be made available at sub-centres) 9. Treatment for TB and follow-up 10. Preventive measure against all communicable disease	Nos. 1-10 and 11. Treatment of TB 12. Testing of syphilis for high risk group and treatment where necessary including for RTI's * training of laboratory technicians, equipment and reagents required.	Nos. 1-12 and 13. Diagnosis and treatment of RTIs/STIs 14. Weekly clinics for High risk pregnancies

TABLE 6.2 *(Contd.)*

Health Intervention	*Community Level*	*Sub-centre Level*	*Primary Health Centre Level*	*First Referral Unit/ District Hospital Level*
3. Delivery Services	1. Early recognition of pregnancy and its danger signals (rupture of membranes of more than 12 hours duration, prolapse of the cord, hemorrhage) 2. Conducting clean deliveries with delivery kits by trained personnel 3. Detection of complications referral for hospital delivery 4. Providing transport for referral 5. Referral of new born having difficulty in respiration 6. Management of Neonatal hypothermia	No. 1-4 and 5. Supervising home delivery 6. Prophylaxis and treatment for infection (except sepsis) 7. Routine prophylaxis for gonococi eye infection	Nos. 1-7 and 8. Modified partograph 9. Delivery services 10. Repair of episiotomy and perennial tears	Nos. 1-9 and 10. Treatment of severe sepsis 11. Delivery of referred cases 12. Treatment of high risk cases 13. Services for obstetrical emergencies anesthesia, cesarean section, blood transfusion through close relatives linkages with blood banks and mobile services
4. Post-partum Services	1. Breast-feeding support 2. Family Planning counselling 3. Nutrition counselling 4. Resuscitation for asphyxia of the newborn 5. Management of neonatal hypothermia 6. Early recognition of post-partum sepsis and referral	Nos. 1-6 and 7. Referral for complications 8. Giving inj. Ergometrine after delivery of placenta	Nos. 1-8 and 9. Referral of FRUs for complications after starting an I.V. line and giving initial dose of antibiotics and oxytocin when indicated 10. Management of asphyxiated new born (equipment to be provided)	Nos. 1-10 and 11. Management of referred cases PHCs and FRUs would require additional equipment and training for management of asphyxiated new borns and hypothermia. These include a resuscitation bag and mask and radiant warmers
5. Child Survival	1. Health education for breast feeding nutrition immunization, utilisation of services, etc.	Nos. 1-6 and 7. Treatment of dehydration and pneumonia and referral of severe cases	Nos. 1-9 and 10. Management of referred cases	Nos. 1-10 and 11. Handling of all paediatric cases including encephalopathy

TABLE 6.2 *(Contd.)*

Health Intervention	*Community Level*	*Sub-centre Level*	*Primary Health Centre Level*	*First Referral Unit/ District Hospital Level*
	2. Detection and referral of high risk cases such as low birth weight, premature babies, babies with asphyxis, infections, severe dehydration acute respiratory infections (ARI), etc. 3. Help during Immunization by ANM 4. Help during Vitamin 'A' supplementation by ANM 5. Detection of pneumonia and seeking early medical care by community and treatment by ANM 6. Treatment of diarrhoea cases and ARI cases	8. First-aid for injuries, etc. 9. Closing watching on the development of child and creating awarness of cheap and nutritious food		12. Identification of certain FRU's to provide specialist services and training
6. Management of RTIs/STIs	1. IEC, counselling and awareness and prevention 2. Condom distribution 3. Creating awareness about usage of sanitary pads by women of reproductive period 4. Creating awareness of about RTI's and personal hygiene	Nos. 1-4 and 5. Identification and referral for vaginal discharge, lower abdominal pain, genital ulcers in women, and urethra discharge, genital ulcers, swelling in scrotum or groin in men 6. Diagnosis of RTI's and STI's by Syndrome approach 7. Referral of cases not responding to suavely treatment 8. Partner notification/ referral	Nos. 1-8 and 9. Treatment of RTIs/STIs 10. Syphilis testing in ante-natal women	Nos. 1-9 and 10. Laboratory diagnosis and treatment of RTIs/STIs 11. Syndromic approach to detect and treat STD in ante-natal, post-natal and at risk groups

Source: Department of Family Welfare, GOI, Reproductive and Child Health, Vol. I, March 1997, pp. 42-45.

services. She is supposed to register pregnant women as assess their health throughout pregnancy, by at least three visits. Regular height and weight checkup, blood pressure test, urine test as well as providing tetanus toxoid injections and iron and folic acid tablets constitute important aspects of any antenatal check-up. Another responsibility of the ANM is to refer pregnant women who have symptoms of abnormal pregnancy or labour, or who have gynaecological problems that are beyond her level of competence, to the Primary Health Centre.

At the instance of the Ministry of Health and Family Welfare, Government of India, New Delhi and as a part of monitoring and evaluation of the performance of the family welfare programme under the new target-free approach, the Population Research Centre, J.S.S. Institute of Economic Research, Dharwad, undertook a rapid survey in the rural areas of Belgaum District, Karnataka state during the last two weeks of December 1997 and first two weeks of January 1998. Using a simple and short questionnaire, the survey interviewed a total of 1,000 currently married women age 15-44, from 50 villages, at the rate of 20 women per village. Apart from several background characteristics of women, the survey collected information on utilization of ante-natal care, place of delivery, and assistance during delivery, child immunizations, knowledge and practice of family planning, visits by the ANM and services received from her; health problems of the women including side-effects of family planning methods, and respondents ratings on various aspects of quality of care provided by the nearest PHC, sub-centre or the ANM.

(a) While the provision of tetanus toxoid injections and iron/folic tablets is better, other components of ante-natal care such as monitoring the weight and blood pressure, and urine tests were not carried out for the majority of women during their pregnancy by multi-member females.

(b) Overall, 51 percent of the deliveries which occurred during the five years preceding the survey took place at home, 30 percent in private hospitals or nursing homes, and little less than one-fifth in government health facilities. Of the births that took place at home, the majority (62 percent) were attended by untrained persons including relatives, friends and neighbours.

(c) Little less than one-quarter of women in the rural areas of Belgaum District have an unmet need for family planning, that is, they are not using contraception even though they do not want any more children or want to wait at least two years before having their next child. The unmet need for spacing (11 percent) is almost the same as that for limiting births (12 percent). If all the women with an unmet need were to use family planning, the contraceptive prevalence rate would increase from 62 percent to 85 percent.

(d) Among the three registers (Eligible Couple register, ANC register, and immunization register) examined, the EB register was found to be relatively more complete and accurate than the other two registers.[6]

In another study a rapid research survey was conducted in rural areas of Dharwad district in Karnataka during February-April 1997 to check the coverage, quality of services and client satisfaction under the new strategy of 'target-free' approach. The analysis of service statistics for the district showed that removal of targets appears to have made no significant impact on the total number of annual acceptors. However, it had a favourable impact on method mix as sterilizations have come down slightly while acceptors of IUD and Pill have gone up from that of the previous year.

The unmet need for contraception was estimated to be 10 percent, 6 percent for limiting and 4 percent for spacing.

It was found that immunization levels are yet to become universal. About 70 percent of pregnant women had two doses of Tetanus toxoid vaccination and only half of the children were fully immunized.

Measurement of weight and blood pressure, as well as urine tests were reported rarely. Only 40 percent of deliveries were attended by trained persons. On record maintenance, it was observed that EC register was better maintained than ANC and immunization registers. Some of the important policy recommendations emerging from the study are:

1. Improve ANM services, especially make them visit women with unmet need for contraception, and past acceptors of sterilization.
2. As a large number of sterilization acceptors complain about method side effects, a special health campaign for sterilized men and women should be launched by multi-purpose workers female. In order to safeguard future levels of acceptance, past acceptors should be made to feel that they are looked after well by programme functionaries.
3. It should be ensured that sub-centres have adequate supply of drugs, and attempts should be made to reduce waiting time and provide free services at primary health centres. The guilty should be punished.
4. A television set could be placed in PHC waiting room and also a VCP to disseminate information and messages on health and family welfare and facilities in sub-centres.
5. Concerted attempts should be made to raise immunization levels by workers as they appear to have reached a point of stagnation before acquiring universality.[7]

National Institute of Health and Family Welfare (Role in RCH)

History and Need

The National Institute of Health and Family Welfare came into being with effect from 9 March, 1977, by the amalgamation of the erstwhile institutes, namely, the National Institute of Family Planning and the National Institute of Health Administration and Education. It has been established as an autonomous body (registered under the Societies Registration Act, 1860) and its object is to act as an apex technical institute for promoting the Health and Family Welfare Planning Programme in the country through education, training, services, research and evaluation. The overall objective of the Institute has been to play a leading role in orienting training and research in health administration and education to the newer concepts of administration and education and thereby strengthen and accelerate India's health and family welfare programmes.

Organisation

The Institute is governed by a General Executive Council with the Union Minister for Health and Family Welfare as the President/Chairman. The day-to-day activities are administered by the Director. The Institute is supported in its activities by International Agencies such as WHO/SEARO and UNICEF. Closer contacts and collaboration exist between the Institute and numerous other organisations in the country. The finances for the functioning of the Institute are provided by the Government of India through grants-in-aid.

Structure

As health administration is based on the concept of 'multi-disciplinary' approach, the Institute has departments embracing various disciplines. These are the departments of Public Health Administration, Hospital Administration, Family Welfare, Maternal and Child Health Programme Planning, Evaluation, Social Sciences, Epidemiology, Health Education, Public Administration, Biostatistics, Education and Training, Field Training, Public Health Nursing and Field Services. A field practice area in the Rohtak district of Haryana State exists for experimentation and field training exercises of the participants of the institute. Research in the field of Health Administration is reckoned to be a key factor for the development of the activities of the Institute and is therefore, an integral part of the functioning of all departments of the Institute. The new Institute has been renamed as the National Institute of Health and Family Welfare.

Activities

The main activities of the Institute are:

(a) Education and Training.
(b) Research.

(c) Evaluation of Health Programmes.
(d) Consultation Services.
(e) Clearing House Functions.
(f) Publications and Documents.

Objectives in the Context of RCH

(i) To organise, co-ordinate and monitor training in the country.
(ii) To upgrade the competence of family welfare personnel and managers to provide technically sound client centred and gender sensitive RCH services.
(iii) To create mass awareness of RCH and population stabilization issues by holding orientation training programme.
(iv) To involve other government departments in promotion of RCH programme by team training for convergence of services.

III. SPECIFIC OBJECTIVES

(a) *To coordinate*: (i) Training financed by the Family Welfare Department in RCH management, clinical and interpersonal counselling skills and communications (IEC), and (ii) Awareness generation and community mobilization (including convergence of related programmes such as ICDS) as requested by MOHFW.
(b) To coordinate the development and or adaptation, as necessary, of model training curricula, facilitators, guides, and prototype manuals/materials, and provide such materials to collaborating centres and training centres for local adaptation and use.
(c) To assist MOHFW in the development of clinical management protocols for safe motherhood, fertility regulation methods, reproductive tract infections and sexually transmitted diseases and child survival as specified in the essential package of RCH services and ensure that such protocols are integrated into training.
(d) To assist MOHFW and national procurement support agency for appointment of suitable collaborating institutions from Government, NGO and private/corporate sector in accordance with World Bank Guidelines and to organise training of trainers of these institutions.
(e) To review the work of the collaborative institutions annually and to assist the MOHFW in determining suitability of the institution to continue as a collaborating institution.
(f) To assist states, districts through collaborating institutions, in formulation of integrated training plans at State and District levels so as to: (i) avoid unnecessary duplication; (ii) ensure here are no critical gaps in the training plans; and (iii) coordinate

scheduling of training with other programme inputs such as equipment, civil works, IEC and NGO activities.

(g) To assist States in the establishment of system of proficiency certificate award to trainees and monitor and report on state specific achievements on the project performance.

The RCH programme should take care of following factors before formulation, implementation and evaluation strategy:

(a) according to the topography of the District,
(b) according to the priority needs of the people,
(c) linked properly with the objectives and goals of District planning,
(d) fitted into the overall economic and social development of the country,
(e) properly linked with projects in the allied area, and
(f) able to achieve useful and permanent results.

Let us now analysis the factors which impede the effective functioning of RCH programme. It is based on authors' study in Punjab and Karnataka. We have also given suggestions to improve RCH programme.

Let us mention the schedule of operation of RCH programme in Punjab and Karnataka (See Tables 6.3 and 6.4). We may also mention the facilities required in A, B and C categories of Districts. The project has not so far been implemented fully. However, we discuss our observations and findings on the basis of the experiments done so far.

Though it is desirable that the entire package of services indicated above is made available to all those who need it, it will not be possible to immediately implement such a comprehensive package on a nation-wide basis. Hence, it is envisaged that improvement in quality and coverage of services over and above the existing level will be attempted in all states in an incremental manner so that maternal and child health indices improve.

After consultation with experts a package of essential reproductive health services for nation-wide implementation at various levels of healthcare has been identified. Essential components recommended for nation-wide implementation include:

- Prevention and management of unwanted pregnancy.
- Services to promote safe motherhood.
- Services to promote child survival.
- Prevention and treatment of RTI/STD.

Most of the services are already included in the Family Welfare Programme. However, there are wide variations in the quality and coverage of services not only between states but also between various districts in the

TABLE 6.3

Punjab—Year-wise Category of Districts

Category	Year-I	Year-II	Year-III
A			
B	Hoshiarpur Patiala Moga	Jalandhar Ludhiana Kapurthala Gurdaspur Amritsar Sangrur	Faridkot Rupnagar Bathinda Muktsar Nawanshahar
C	Firozepur Fatehgarh Sahib	Mansa	

TABLE 6.4

Karnataka—Year-wise Category of Districts

Category	Year-I	Year-II	Year-III
A	Dakshin Kannada Kadagu (Coorg) Mandya		
B	Uttar Kannada Chikmaglur Dharwad	Hassan Bangalore (R) Tumkur Mysore Belgaum	Shimoga Chitradurga
C	Bijapur Bidar Gulbarga Bangalore	Bellary Raichur	

same state. The focus is therefore on the improvement in the quality and coverage of the services. A project preparation workshop held in September 1995 discussed the issues and problems in implementation of essential RCH package and recommended reproductive and child health services that should be made available at community, sub-centre, PHC and FRU/ District Hospital.

Implementation schedule of Punjab and Karnataka is given in Tables 6.3 and 6.4.

The Ministry of Health and Family Welfare has got the research conducted on the impact of RCH programme in the districts. Analysis of the reports indicate that:

(a) Infrastructure facilities non-existent.
(b) Personnel responsible for RCH lack motivation.
(c) Lack of effective supervision.

(d) Slackness in work.
(e) Non-availability of funds.
(f) Lack of team work.
(g) Not following the work as schedules.

The study in Punjab in some districts revealed not impact of the new RCH programme. The personnel responsible lack motivation and interest. Because of financial crisis, normal functioning of the health department is at a stand still. Besides, there is no supervision, resulting into a absentism and irregulately.

1. Lack of Adequate Facilities in the Institutions Responsible for the Provision of RCH Services

After the project is formulated, the project manager must ensure the availability of necessary inputs. It has been generally observed that the projects are delayed because of the absence of timely availability of all the inputs simultaneously. In one of the projects, the health personnel had no work to do because of the non-availability of vaccine. Obtaining resources is a process that takes place periodically throughout the life of the project. It was revealed that failure to obtain resources simultaneously in time is the most common cause of delay in implementation. The project manager must begin the process of procuring resources immediately after the formulation stage. Sometimes, the process may be started quite early if the resources are scarce and not easily available. The absence of one resource would inflate the cost of the project as the other resources would remain idle. The project manager must take the following steps:

(a) Working with the relative administrative units in preparing a time-table of administrative steps to be taken to obtain the planned resources.
(b) Monitoring this time-table to ensure that the administrative steps are being completed in time.
(c) Taking corrective action as and when necessary.

Inspite of all these precautions, there is a possibility of not reaching the resources in time. What can be done under such critical situation? Most of the experts indicated that the whole project staff remains idle for months together. This is very serious in big projects. It is suggested that project officers may be delegated powers to purchase the inputs locally or employ persons, if not available from the agency as planned. This would ensure that the project is one schedule.

2. Lack of Clarity among the Person Responsible for Implementation of RCH Programme

There is a dichotomy between the personnel responsible for the formulation and the personnel responsible for the implementation of the

RCH project. The latter are not clear about the implications of the project. Because of lack of identity, they develop low morale resulting into the poor management. It was mentioned by a number of persons working on some projects that, "they are thrown into the fields to operate the RCH project without proper briefing about the project and its rationale in the total system. Besides, the supervisors, at the head-quarters, never guide them about their role in the projects."

3. Poor Linkages Among the Allied Projects

In a particular geographical or functional area, a number of projects are being implemented to improve the standard of living of the people. Most of the projects are complementary and supplementary. Because of the poor co-ordination among the various departments, at the state level, the projects are implemented in the area without developing linkages with each other. For example, a project for the agriculture development to grow more food can be beautifully linked with the health projects on nutrition. Population control has many dimensions and needs the co-operation of many agencies. Thus, there is a need of area planning and developing an integrated area approach where different projects may develop linkages to have optimum benefit.

4. Absence of the Full Involvement of the Beneficiaries in the Formulation and Implementation of Projects

The success or failure of the RCH project ultimately depends upon the acceptance of these projects by the people. If the people are not taken into confidence during the formulation and implementation of RCH projects, these would be less successful. People's participation would provide extra nuclear energy to the success of the RCH projects. Most of the beneficiaries contacted by the writer were of the view that they are not treated as equal partners in the process of formulation and implementation of projects. The failure of the scheme is because of the absence of identity of the people with the programmes. It is essential for the experts to motivate and encourage the people to participate in the formulation and implementation of projects. Although people's participation in affairs governing their lives dates back to the beginning of human society, the concept has taken a new dimension as societies have grown in size and complexity. This is partly because the management has become more and more a specialized enterprise, an area for technocrats and trained general administrators and political leaders. Although they officially advocate and preach people's involvement, in practice, they bring them into picture only after the major decisions have been made. Hence, they often leave the ordinary citizens to follow their pre-determined paths. Peter Druker agrees with this contention when he says that "the overwhelming majority of these people have little or no opportunity to influence policy, and their perspectives on the situation are systematically ignored by almost all theorists. For them the problem of development is one of the everyday life."

5. Local Communities are Treated as Passive Participants in Improvement and Bettering of their Lives

Most of the project personnel working in the villages return to the cities after their duty hours. The villagers cannot make their views known to them in cities. The result is lack of communication among them. When the project fails, it is intentionally ascribed to the obstinacy, fatalism, illiteracy or apparent irrationality of the poor people. The potential for community involvement has been seriously underestimated. We must encourage people's participation through all methods to promote development.

6. Absence of any Satisfactory Monitoring System to Measure the Regulated Performance during Implementation

Project control is the managerial function that helps the managers to keep the project functioning as scheduled. It is possible only if the realistic advance targets of output are fixed before implementation. This is not being done as is evident from the perusal of most of the projects studied. Monitoring if properly designed, projects can help the managers in keeping the process of implementation as scheduled. The project performance is compared at different intervals of time with the control indicators. Whenever deviations are located, causes of deviations are examined, solutions are found to correct the deviations. The following are the general causes of deviation:

(1) "Excessive optimism on the part of the project planners, resulting in unrealistic estimates in respect to:
- the time, funds, manpower or other resources required to do an activity, and
- the passability of achieving the expected results.

(2) Unfrozen resistance from or changes in the environment of the project (natural disaster, political changes, etc.).

(3) Decisions at higher, managerial levels to change the planned resources inputs of the project (change of a staff member).

(4) Inefficient administrative procedures.

If there is any unavoidable deviation beyond the control of the project authorities, we can think of alternative proposals immediately without wasting the future resources. If such timely action is taken, the developing countries can be sure of the success of the projects. More safely designing the control system means specifying who reports what to whom and when.

7. Unscientific Manpower Planning and Insufficient Utilisation of Project Personnel

The success of the project depends upon the quality and quantity of personnel associated with it. It was observed that in many projects, the projects personnel have their utilisation time as low as 20 per cent. This is highly serious as the resources are being consumed by the establishment rather than invested in the RCH programme. Because of the absence of manpower planning, personnel of the project utilize very little time. People in the area remarked about the workers appointed to motivate people to adopt family planning norm: "They are not available at all. They rarely devote any time for this work. They remain away from their work." It is essential to see through proper manpower planning that only needed persons are appointed and they are utilised to increase in the overall cost-productivity, efficiency and effectiveness. The projects should be so administered as to lead to overall improvement in its performance.

8. Lack of Clarification of Authority, Responsibility and Relationships

In the developing world, the persons responsible for implementation of the project do not work as a team as there is no clarification of authority, responsibility and relationships amongst them, i.e. the roles of the various participants are not often mutually understood. This result into friction among these persons. Most of the time of these persons are spent in their mutual disputes. It becomes very difficult for them to devote their whole attention to the project.

9. Private Sector Engaged in Merely Curative Services

Ninth Plan suggested the Private Sector participation in RCH. It is estimated that the private sector accounts for more than three quarters of all healthcare expenditure in India. Private sector provides MCH and family planning services also but to a lesser extent. It is increasingly recognised that the private sector represents an untapped potential for increasing the coverage and improving the quality of reproductive and child health services in the country. The challenge is to find ways and means to optimally utilise their potential. The major limitations in the private sector include the following:

(a) the focus has till now been mainly on curative services,
(b) the quality of services is often variable, and
(c) as the users have to pay for the services, the poorer sections of population cannot afford these services.

Some of the initiatives could be through collaboration between public and private sector in providing healthcare to the poorer segments of population who cannot afford to pay for health services. While organising the involvement of private medical practitioners in RCH care, it is essential to provide orientation training to all and ensure utilisation of their services is a cost-effective and sustainable basis.

Private/voluntary organisations providing healthcare to women are relatively small in number but they could play an effective role in the delivery of reproductive and child healthcare services at affordable cost, especially in certain specific locations such as urban slums. Giving the private sector and voluntary organisations appropriate incentives to broaden the range of activities and improve the quality of reproductive and child health-related services they offer are other avenues that require exploration. Continued collaboration, training and technical assistance by governmental agencies to private medical practitioners and private/ voluntary organisations may help in strengthening reproductive and child health services in remote or under-served areas.

10. Previous Implementation Experience of the Completed Project not Referred to

It was a great surprise to learn that there are no records of past experiences in relation to project implementation. One can always learn from the mistakes of others. Some of the project personnel remarks that "they do not know anything about the difficulties encountered by the project personnel and the causes of the failure of the project undertaken earlier." It is beneficial to examine how major projects have been managed in the past. It would also be better to identify those approaches which have been most successful. We can keep a record of good and bad points of the past project and this cumulative experience may be passed on to the present project managers. In this way, many of the difficulties likely to be encountered would vanish.

Frank A. Wilson in his article, "Planning for Project Management" in the *Journal of Administration Overseas* (July 1979) has rightly mentioned that, "Disappointing and inefficient project performance is a fact of life. . . . . Ex-post evaluation of existing projects can be the means by which we can systematically seek to analyse the potential for improving project management. Evaluation studies give the opportunity for developing a greater understanding of the way projects are managed and implemented."

11. Faulty and Cumbersome Administrative Procedures

Whenever a project is formulated, we do not pay much attention to the problems of communication, co-ordination, headquarters field relationship, supervision, etc. The purpose of these procedures is to help in the smooth functioning of the project. Without proper procedures developed most of the project personnel remain engrossed in preparing unnecessary reports. These procedures should be clarified in the initial stages of project management, so that no confusion arises later on. If there are already set procedures in a particular organization, these may be adopted otherwise new procedures may be adopted and made known to the project personnel. It must be clear that administrative procedures are an aid to help the efficient functioning of the project. The meticulous applications of these procedures may result into red-tapism and inefficiency.

The Five Year Plan (1978-83) has also indicated the technical, administrative and managerial problems which affect project efficiency. They are mentioned below:

(a) Inadequate investigation and data collection as a result of which the project appraisal, even when it is sought to be done in a systematic way, has to be carried out on the basis of wholly inadequate information, thus leading to wrong investment decisions.
(b) Inadequate detailed planning of projects in terms of their time schedule, input resource requirements and skills needed for project implementation.
(c) Lack of delegation of authority to subordinate organization levels.
(d) Delays in issuing sanction, approvals, fund authorisations and releases.
(e) Organizational weaknesses in planning and implementation at various levels.
(f) Lack of specific assignment of responsibility and accountability for results.
(g) Problems of industrial relations and inadequate motivation of personnel, lack of proper career planning and incentives and commitment to results.
(h) Inadequate share of representation of the weaker sections in elected bodies in the village, district and block levels and agencies.

We can improve upon the management of projects if we keep these difficulties or problems or obstacles in mind and try to reduce them to negligible proportions. Besides, there is a need of training project personnel in the art of project management.

CONCLUSION

The new RCH programme has been designed scientifically keeping in view the minor details meticulously. The programme is certainly better than the earlier Family Planning maternal and child health programmes aimed at specific activity. The RCH programme is operative in the whole of the country.

However, with the overall policy made by the Ministry of Health and Family Welfare, each district should design its own programme keeping in view the needs, resources, topography, quality of the peoples, facilities and infrastructure available as well as plan implementation and evaluation to inject flexibility as situations difference from district to district.

Radhakrishna Rao in his Article, "Towards Controlling the Numbers" in *The Daily Tribune* (31st January, 2000) rightly suggests that a target free approach has now become a part of the population control drive. To what extent this approach will contribute to the success of population control, no one is sure as yet. Sociologists, however, are clear in their perception that when literacy, health, hygiene and economic improvements get high priority, family planning stands a better chance of success.

The document prepared for the International Conference on Population and Development has recognised in its programme of action that "the main message for improving individual well-being comprises two elements: to provide contraceptive methods within the broader reproductive health services and to advance women's equal participation in education, health and economic opportunities."

Notes and References

1. Annual Report, Ministry of Health and Family Welfare, 1998-99, pp. 7-9.
2. State Family Welfare Bureau, DH and FWS, Reproductive and Child Health, Bangalore, July 1988, p. 1.
3. WHO, May-June 1994, p. 30.
4. State Family Welfare Bareau, Bangalore, *op. cit.*, pp. 19-20.
5. WHO, SEARO: Managing Essential Reproductive Healthcare, New Delhi, p. 5.
6. B.M. Ramesh, S.B. Ganiger and D.G. Satihal, "Family Welfare Programme under Target Free Approach: A Rapid Survey" in Belgaum District, Karnataka, 1998, Population Research Centre, J.S.S. Institute of Economic Research, Dharwad.
7. P.N. Mari Bhat, Target Free Approach to Family Planning Programme: A Rapid Survey in Dharwad District in Karnataka, 1997, Population Research Centre, J.S.S. Institute of Economic Research, Dharwad, pp. i-iii.

ANNEXURE 6.1

OF STATEMENT V

Guidelines to Prepare State Implementation Plan Under World Bank Supported Reproductive and Child Health Project

The categorisation of State have already been intimated to all the States. States are also aware that interventions under the proposed RCH project will be provided as per differential approach finalised with all States.

However, during the State Secretaries' meeting held in September 1996, some States requested that these interventions may be provided as per categorisation of Districts instead of States, as the districts in States can also be classified as Category A, B or C. Separately the problem of States under State Health Systems (SHS) project of World Bank also had to be resolved.

Some of the parameters earlier used for classification of States are not available district-wise from 1991 census data. Keeping in view differing needs and availability of reliable data at State and District levels as also available demographic parameters like CBR and female literacy rate district-wise (for major States only), the districts have been classified after computation of weightage and the same may be seen in enclosed *Statement A*. For some States/UTs where District-wise data is not available the State data has been used for classification.

Interventions have, generally, been provided for on District data except when it became necessary to restrict grouping under State Health Systems or under original classification of States. In some cases strengths available due to inputs under Social Safety Net Scheme for 90 demographically weak Districts have been taken into account.

2. Many interventions under the RCH Project will be made available to all States without any differentiation. These are:

- Orientation Workshops on RCH.
- Facilitation for operationalisation of Target Free Approach.
- Institutional Development.
- Preparation of Annual State and District Training (integrated training as per the plan and requirements of the RCH interventions), Logistics and implementation plans.
- Modified Management information system.
- Additional IEC activities under RCH on Team-Building and Community Sensitisation.
- Urban and Tribal Areas RCH as per the needs of the States based on the pilot studies. (Details to be intimated later).
- Local capacity enhancement, as per the projects submitted separately.
- Setting up of RTI/STI Clinics at left out District Hospitals at places where STD Clinic under AIDS/STD Programme has not,

yet been provided. The cost of drugs and equipment per unit will be Rs. 75,000.

3. There are some interventions which will be provided to the States on the basis of classification of the Districts and States mentioned at para 1 above. The facilities/interventions which are being considered for the different category of Districts are given below:

Facilities to be Provided in Category "A" Districts

- Provision of RTI/STI drugs at FRUs (*) (Not in the SHS Project States).
- Minor civil work/repairs/maintenance provisions of requisite inputs at FRU/PHC/SCs otherwise being covered under RCH Project @ upto Rs. 10.00 lakh per District for the project period.
- MTP equipments to all FRUs/CHCs not provided earlier will be given.
- MTP equipments in phased manner to all PHCs.
- Upto 2 Lab Teach. for FRUs on contract basis per District for operationalising RTI/STI screening and diagnostic interventions.
- Consultant doctor at PHC as per phasing on fixed day visit basis twice per month @ Rs. 500 per visit. (Government doctors can also be used for this purpose and paid an honorariam on the same term). The expected work of the Consultants during visit will be provided safe abortion services. This facility will be provided upto 75% of PHC only in the initial years with declining phasing as it is assumed that trained doctors are available at other facilities. By the end of 5 years, it is expected that with intensive training, the requirement of Consultant doctors will be reduced to 25% from 75%. Work load norms will be atleast 5 surgical interventions or assisted deliveries out of cases referred from periphery. Minimum of atleast 20 referred cases should be attended by the visiting doctor or each visit. Adequate advance IEC on expected date of visit of doctor should be announced.

Facilities to be Provided in Category "B" Districts

- Provision of RTI and EOC drugs at 1 FRU each (*) (Not in the SHS Project States).
- Minor civil work/repairs/maintenance provisions of requisite inputs at FRU/PHC/SCS otherwise being covered under RCH Project @ upto Rs. 10 lakh per District for the project period.
- Two Lab. Tech. at the FRU on contract basis for lab. diagnosis of STI/RTI apart from other work.

- All PHCs to get MTP equipments in phased manner.
- Consultant doctor preferably lady at PHC on fixed day visit basis twice per month @ Rs. 500 per visit. (Government doctors can also be used for this purpose and paid an honorariam on the same term) as per the phasing of MTP equipment and availability of appropriate facility. The expected work of the Consultants during visit is to provide safe abortion services MTP, ANC, PNC and other Family Planning and Family Welfare Services. This facility will be provided upto 75% of PHC only for the initial years with declining phasing as it is assumed that trained doctors are available at other facilities. By the end of 5 years, it is expected that with intensive training, the requirement of consultant doctors will be reduced to 25% from 75%. Work load norms will be atleast 5 surgical interventions or assisted deliveries out of cases referred from periphery. Minimum of atleast 20 referred cases should be attended by the visiting doctor of each visit. Adequate advance IEO on expected date of visit of doctor should be announced.
- SHS Project States viz. A.P., Karnataka, Punjab and West Bengal have already been strengthened upto Sub-District level. The average institutional deliveries in the districts in these states range around 50% as such, for the PHOs with low institutional deliveries (expected around 50%), the facility of the services of PHN/Staff Nurse will be provided in 50% PHOs to improve institutional delivery, ANC/PHC and screening and referral for RTI. This facility will be limited to the 30 identified Category B Districts in these States. They will be staying at the place of posting for round the clock services. Rental for residence @ upto Rs. 5000 per annum will be provided.
- PHC drug kit for management of essential obstetric care will also be provided to the PHOs where PNH/Staff Nurse have been appointed and are providing round the clock services.

Facilities to be Provided in Category "C" Districts

- Provision of EOC drugs at FRUs (*) (Not in the SHS Project States).
- Minor civil work/repairs/maintenance of FRU/PHC/SCs at Rs. 10 lakh per District for the project period.
- MTP equipments to all FRUs/CHOs not provided earlier.
- MTP equipments in phased manner to all PHOs.
- Two Lab. Tech. for selected FRUs on contract basis per District.
- Provision of PAN/Staff Nurse on contract basis in all the PHOs (for 30,000 population) in the 90 Social Safety Net Districts for providing institutional delivery, ANC/PHC, Family Planning and Family Welfare. They will be staying at the place of posting

for round the clock services and get rental for residence @ upto Rs. 5000 per annum. Under Social Safety Net Scheme provision was made for providing appropriate infrastructure for such PHCs where this was missing. While a perfect machine may not be feasible, it is expected that 35-40% PHCs in these districts would be having facilities which could not be used with provision of PHN/Staff Nurse for providing essential obstetric care.

- In other Districts, where delivery room and residential quarters have been built under various projects but remain unutilised, a PHN/Staff Nurse on contract basis will be provided at PHC (for 30,000 population). As per available information only about 25% PHCs in Category C Districts can avail this facility.
- Additional ANMs in a phased manner upto 30% of SOs @ Rs. 3600 p.m. will be provided to augment the ability to provide focused attention to safe motherhood in the less developed areas/blocks of these districts in 'C' category. This facility is being restricted to remote and for flung sub-centres in C category Districts of the 8 states originally identified as C category States, i.e. Assam, Bihar, Haryana, Madhya Pradesh, Nagaland, Orissa, Rajasthan and Uttar Pradesh.
- Nominal rental to facilitate the stay of these additional ANMs will be provided.
- A Pilot will be launched for assessing long-term feasibility of referral transport for pregnant women from below poverty line category for their obstetric emergencies to be carried out in 2-3 Cat. C Districts in the 8 States (originally identified as C States) with high infant and maternal mortality.
- All PHOs to get MTP equipments in phased manner.
- Consultant doctor (preferably lady) at PHC on fixed day visit basis twice per month @ Rs. 500 per visit. (Government doctors can also be used for this purpose and paid an honorariam on the same term) as per the phasing of MTP equipment and availability of appropriate facility. The expected work of the Consultants during visit will be provided safe abortion services MTP, ANC, PNC and other Family Planning and Family Welfare Services. This facility will be provided upto 75% of PHC only, as it is assumed that trained doctors are available at other facilities. By the end of 5 years, it is expected that with intensive training, the requirement of consultant doctors will be reduced to 25% from 75%. Work load norms will be atleast surgical interventions or assisted deliveries out of cases referred from periphery. Minimum of atleast 20 referred cases should be attended by the visiting doctor of each visit. Adequate advance IEC on expected date of visit of doctor should be announced.
- PHC drug kit for management of essential obstetric care will

also be provided to the PHCs where PHN/Staff Nurse have been appointed and are providing round the clock services.

(*) Identification of two FRUs per District is left to the States. However, it is advisable that these facilities (FRUs) be chosen (a) where availability of manpower is assured; (b) equipment kits were provided under CSSM or where these can be shifted from other facilities; (c) infrastructure is already available and Cesarian Section is being carried out; and (d) have good geographic advantage and have defined catchment area to provide referral services.

---

4. For proper implementation of some of the interventions, it is proposed to phase the interventions by selecting Districts under the Project, taking only those Districts for the interventions, which are prepared to receive the interventions. In the first year of the project, only those Districts should be selected which are able to start the proposed activity positively in the second half of the year of the project. All the pre-requisite activities like training, gaps in infrastructure, manpower, etc., should have been attended to under State MNP where relevant e.g., infrastructure. The phasing of the Districts for some of the major interventions are given at *Statement 'A-i'* and total number of Districts proposed under phasing is given at *Statement 'C'*.

5. While preparing the interventions for the States, assumptions used by this Ministry described in pre-paragraphs and below may also be kept in mind by States while preparing the State Implementation Plan and phasing of various interventions and districts over the five year project period.

Source: Department of Family Welfare, Government of India, Reproductive and Child Health, Vol. I, New Delhi, March 1997.

CHAPTER 6

INFORMATION, EDUCATION AND COMMUNICATION

"If genuine change is desired it will occur only through the social mechanisms for change which the community has established and to which it is accustomed. People are eager to change behaviour if they perceive the change as beneficial . . . . It is the fallacy of modernity that we believe, we communicate through bonds of mutual confidence. It is the prime task of the health communicator to facilitate a state of communal trust and also avoid Pseudo information."

—*World Health*

Information, Education and Communication

The creation of awareness is integral to the process of social development. The possibility for the power of communication to liberate the minds and potential of people to critical awareness is real in every field linked to human development, and the generation of public will hinges on effective communication of information and ideas that relate to people's needs, aspirations and capacities for progress in thought and action. In this sense, getting the development process started is largely the task of information, education and communication.

The communication aspect of a national family planning programme is generally termed as IEC-Information, Education Communication. The Year Book (1986-87) of Family Welfare Programme in India has rightly mentioned that the success of the Family Welfare Programme depends primarily upon the voluntary and widespread acceptance of the concept of small family and delayed marriages and well spaced and properly linked births are an effective way of achieving this objective. Mass education and Media activities, accordingly, were given multi-dimensional and integrated thrust through Information-Education-Communication activities in the form of a comprehensive package of social transformation . . . to bring behavioural and attitudinal changes in the people so as to enable them to adopt family planning as a way of life. In brief, we can simplify it, and can call it simply as communication function. Sometimes, the activities under IEG are also referred to as "Mass Communication", "Mass Education", "Mass Education and Media."

Donald J. Bogue has rightly said that IEG is a term widely used to identify the activities of family planning programme to inform the public and stimulate them to adopt contraception.[1] In every technical component of the Family Planning Programme provided by family planning workers, there exists a corresponding educational aspect, which has to be imparted more or less simultaneously, so as to enhance the continuing usefulness of the services provided at the time of need. This would have permanent value.

An added importance of communication in family planning resulted from the experience and studies which indicated that pure clinical approach did not bear fruit. A. Govindachari has mentioned some of the findings of the studies, which have brought to notice the limited impact of clinical approach. These are:

(i) The population reached by the clinics was very limited.

(ii) Education on family planning in the clinics was mostly through individual contacts. There was no organized community education.

(iii) The educational efforts were mostly directed towards women, since the clinics normally have female social workers. Husbands, who are important from the point of view of decision-making in family planning, especially in an Indian cultural context, were not given due attention.

(iv) Couples felt shy to visit clinics for fear of identification by their friends and neighbours.

(v) The working hours of the clinics were found to be inconvenient, especially for the low income groups.

(vi) There was a lack of social support for the programme due to inadequate involvement of the community.

(vii) People generally prefer to obtain contraceptives in an informal way which does not involve formal recording procedures and publicity. This was not possible in a clinic situation.

(viii) There was very little involvement of other supporting staff, like the village level workers, extension officers, etc., in the family planning programme.[2]

Today, Family planning programmes around the world are applying a broad range of service delivery and communication strategies. To make family planning services and supplies more accessible, conventional clinic-based programmes have been supplemented by innovative approaches to services delivery. These include community-based outreach, social marketing through commercial outlets at subsidized prices, and employment-based programmes organized or supported by employees or Unions. Extensive communication campaigns, combining a variety of modern and traditional mass-media are spreading family planning awareness and encouraging more people to seek out family planning services.[3]

INTRODUCTION

The Information, Education, Communication (IEC) component of National Family Welfare programme is mainly to create an effective communication strategy, to inform the masses about the means and measures of Family Welfare Programme, educate them about the perils of over-population and motivate and persuade them to adopt small family norm, using all possible channels of media.[4]

In a Family Planning organisation, external communication is very important in the implementation of its programme, as information about the utility and means of planned parenthood through appropriate choice and correct use of contraceptives by the eligible married couples is important. Moreover, communication being two-way process brings to the attention of the management the needs, reactions and complaints of the people concerned for necessary initiative or remedial actions. The external communication process needs to be guided by considerations of relevance of information, the choice of communication channels and the existing understanding capacity (education, etc.) of the people concerned outside the organisation. Moreover, it should not by any means be only one sided, i.e., from the organisation to the people. The reverse flow of information from the people to the organisation would make the latter to judge the impact of the programme as well as provide the basis for any changes in the strategies of the Programme. Here again, barriers and disruptions in the two-way communication process have to be dealt with appropriately.

Broadly speaking, communication is the means by which intentions of the programme are classified to ensure fruitful results. It may even be looked upon as the means by which special information inputs are fed into social systems. It is the means by which behaviour of the personnel engaged in the programme is modified; change is effected, information is made productive and goals are achieved.[5] Barnard has aptly viewed it as the means by which people can be linked together in an organisation to achieve the objectives of the programmes.[6] Communication is a universal phenomenon among living beings. Newman and Summer have viewed communication as an exchange of facts, ideas, opinion, or emotions by two or more persons.[7]

Family Planning Communication implies a number of actions starting with identifying the audience, assessing needs and channels for response, identifying specific messages especially in areas of resistance to change in attitude and behaviour, selecting complementary media for optimal combination, producing communication materials and refining messages and techniques after pre-testing, revision and re-testing, dissemination of communication, continuous support through stages of programmes implementation mainly to ensure community involvement and participatory monitoring and evaluation. Since, Family Planning is a challenging and arduous task, communication technology must be well planned. A successful communication effort blends the use of traditional communication media with the modern, brings together the channels of government communication with those of the community and of voluntary organisations and a variety of other groups, Family Planning ideology can be registered in the minds of the people not simply by providing the information on Family Planning, but because people can be told that they exist, shown that they work and encouraged (and empowered) to try them and make them work for themselves. This is the nature of the support which communication lends to a family planning programme.

ESSENTIALS AND ASPECTS OF MASS MOTIVATION CAMPAIGN

Essentials

Dr. John Hubley quoted by Gloria Gorden in his Article, "Let's Communicate" in *World Health* (January-Feb. 1989) has rightly described the essentials of Communication:

- Promote actions which are realistic and feasible within the constraints faced by the community.
- Build on ideas, concepts and practices that people already have.
- Repeat and reinforce information overtime, using different methods.
- Use existing channels of Communication such as songs, drama and story-telling, and be adaptable.
- Entertain and attract the attention of the Community.
- Use clear, simple language with local expressions and emphasize short-term benefits of action.
- Provide opportunities for dialogue and discussion to allow learner participation and feedback on understanding and implementation.
- Use demonstrations to show the benefits of adopting practices.[8]

E.M. Rogers mentions the following essentials:

(i) Family Planning Communication campaigns should be preceded by extensive planning of the strategies to be followed.

(ii) A Consumer Orientation in family planning communication activities will be more effective in achieving the objectives of the National Family Planning Programme.

(iii) A new family planning communication approach should be launched on a small scale pilot project basis.

(iv) Social research can perform an important function in more effective family planning communication, (a) by providing feedback for the design of communication messages through pre-testing; and (b) by yielding evaluative data about the efforts of communication activities.[9]

CHANNELS OF COMMUNICATION

(a) Radio

Radio has been in use since long. It has been effective as a means of communication. Since the start of the programme on a regular basis in May 1967 on All-India Radio, there have been many challenges as it was a new and sensitive issue. All types of methods have been tried on Radio and even today the importance of Radio as a means of popularising F.P. Programme is enormous. To quote G.K. Mathur, "It is through this common sense and realistic approach that All-India Radio is trying to create a massive awareness base which may serve as a take-off platform for ever widening acceptance of actual family planning methods. In all our programmes we have stressed that the family planning campaign is a people's programme for the total well-being of the family. It is from this angle that a distinction has been made between the programmes directed towards scarcely populated areas, like hill areas, desert areas, off-shore islands, etc. and programmes meant for over-crowded cities and densely populated areas. In order to avoid any possible resistance to the broadcast of family planning programmes on a fixed-time basis, they introduced the family planning themes in-between various programmes, thus taking the listener unawares."

All-India Radio produces and broadcasts in different formats such as group discussions, interviews, spot recordings, feature plays, etc. in different languages and areas. The Commercial Broadcasting Services (CBS) have been broadcasting the programme 'Haseen Lamhe' regularly, as well as one minute spots over various channels in Hindi and regional languages.

(b) Television

Television has become very popular. S.K. Sharma in an Article, "Role of Television in Promoting Family Planning" has rightly said that, "In fact, the potential impact of television, as a means of informing the people is greater than that of any other means of mass communication. With television, as with the motion picture film, we can hear what is to be done, can see it done and can see the results. Unlike the motion picture, television conveys the feeling of immediacy. In this sense, it combines radio's intimate quality with the motion pictures' ability to magnify the smallest detail which all can see.

(c) Films

Government of India, Publicity Division has been making documentary and other films on various themes of F.P. activities. Parmod Pati has mentioned that, Films Division has produced so far a number of films on subjects relating to family planning. A good number of films are now under production. A large number of news-reels have already exhibited slogans relating to family planning. Only a few of these are purely informational, for they are factual and principally of interest value without any attempt in conveying a specific educational message. They focus attention on food problem or housing *vis-a-vis* the rise in population. They talk of education facilities or employment and rise in population. But most of the remaining films are designed primarily to motivate, to encourage and inspire the audience to particular action in accepting new ideas and changing attitudes in accepting the norm of a small family or a means to space children or even to accept methods to completely limit further procreation. Some of the films help to put information about a particular means of contraception in the right perspective while the others keep on emphasising the massage, "if you have two that would do." Not all these films can be claimed to be outstanding. While an occasional film is made with a festival jury in mind, most of these films meet the needs of the communicator fully so far as family planning education is concerned.

An integrated IEG strategy, mixing inter-personal communication with multi-media contents was developed. Activities were given multi-dimensional and integrated thrust to increase the outreach and impact of Reproductive and Child Health and Family Welfare messages with the objective of bridging the gap between awareness and acceptance.

As part of the new strategy to utilise the services of eminent film-makers, the Ministry has assigned eminent directors, Shri Amol Palekar and Shyam Benegal's two feature films, i.e. 'Kairee' and 'Teri Godi Hari Bhari Rahe' respectively.

(d) Advertising and Visual Publicity

The Directorate of Advertising and Visual Publicity (DAVP) releases press advertisement and arranges exhibitions at various centres throughout the country. Special attention is given to the places of intensive multi-media campaigns.

(e) Song and Drama Division

To educate the masses about family welfare issues, Song and Drama Division organises live entertainment programmes like puppet shows, dance, dramas, folk recitals, mythological recitals, traditional plays, magic shows, etc. Special Programmes to sensitise people regarding the Pulse Polio Immunisation programmes are also being organised by the field units, so that greater number of people can bring their children up to the age of 5 years for the extra doses of Polio drops. More than 15,000 variety shows were organised during the year 1998-99 itself.

(f) Press Information

PIB conducts field visits of journalists for the coverage of family welfare activities. It organises special briefing and seminars for journalists. A Scheme to sensitise 'Opinion Leaders' by holding one day session on various aspects of family welfare issues, was instituted in 1993-94. Under this scheme, 10421 opinion leaders of various categories including members of Zilla Panchayats, panchs, private practitioners, teachers, etc. were exposed to family welfare issues. Now, it is proposed to be implemented through State/Regional Health and Family Welfare Training Centres.

(g) Personal Communication

Changes in knowledge, attitudes, behaviour, habits and customs can be brought about by personal as well as impersonal methods of FP education. These methods have certain advantages and disadvantages. While personal methods involve face-to-face interaction the impersonal methods do not require such a close personal contact. Personal methods are indeed more convincing and generally more successful. However, the success of personal methods greatly depends on the establishment of a good rapport between the FP educator and his recipients. The impersonal methods are relatively simpler and even less time-consuming. The radio, the newspapers, the posters, and the pamphlets, etc., can all play an important role in imparting FP education. Experience with personal and impersonal methods of FP education have revealed that if both the methods are used simultaneously one can obtain better results than simply using one or the other method. The most important aspect in the adoption of the programme is the use of inter-personal relationships.

Mr. Manu N. Kulkarni has rightly said that "the information transfer among the poor households takes place through indirect mechanisms like gossip among men in tea and bidi shops and gossip sessions of the women when they gather around a village well, pond, bathing ghats and temples. The health matters affecting poor women like pregnancy, maternity, child spacing, family planning, etc. are not talked out openly. When Public Health advertisement makes such information 'open', a sense of shyness and distrust is shown by these poor women and the "closeness" of information is lost. Unfortunately, glasnost does not work when it comes to information sharing on private health. Private health is not like DDT spraying for malaria eradication. The chances of Private health information sharing are better when it is shared through informal gossip sessions, inter-personal communication, folk media or street theatre. Commercial advertisements cannot penetrate the antenna of the poor and the deprived."[10]

Thus, we see that communication, i.e., dissemination of information is only one important element in FP education. The adoption or acceptance may not take place simply by communicating FP information. A study conducted by United States Public Health Services has revealed that, "unfortunately knowledge alone does not motivate a person to act in accordance with it. He may well know the correct answers to questions without really believing and accepting such information as the basis for his own action."

Dr. Gisela Gastrin, a Finnish physician mentions in his article, "How Education Helps." "People can be motivated to adjust their outlook towards health and disease, but before this can happen their negative attitudes have to be countered with factual information. Education needs to be a part of a comprehensive programme in which responsibilities involving the health authorities and others are clearly delineated and resources allocated."[11]

It was mentioned by Dr. E. Berthat in his article, "A new Role for Teachers" that besides information and motivation, action is indispensable. He said that "Information and motivation are not enough; it remains for governments to ensure that a good health infrastructure is available to all the people. Health education has to convince the men and women who are responsible for taking decisions that health is a basic raw material for their country's eventual social and economic development."[12]

A Family Planning educator as a persuasive communicator can make the best possible use of the personal methods of FP education. But he has to see that the messages which he is delivering get mentally registered with his recipients. Actually, he can present his message and then wait until he gets the requisite response from his recipients. D.F. Skinner has distinguished between two types of approaches to the learning situation, as 'operant behaviour' and 'respondent behaviour'. The two situations have also been described as involving instrumental learning and conditional learning. In 'instrumental learning situation', which involves 'operant behaviour', the FP educator will present his message and then wait for the receiver to make a correct response. When the receiver makes this response, the FP educator will attempt to fix the response by the appropriate award or reinforcement. On the other hand, in 'conditioned learning situation' which involves 'respondent behaviour', the FP education presents his message in such a way that he elicits the response that he wants from his recipients and thus the stimulus that originally served to elicit the response becomes the reinforcing or rewarding element in conditioning. Undoubtedly, conditioning is much more efficient than instrumental learning. It is, however, necessary for the FP educator to be aware of both kinds of situations since the condition for using 'respondent behaviour' may not be present in the persuasive situation. The FP educator has to be aware that the recipients of his messages differ in the ways in which they learn a given response. They may give different responses essentially in the same situation because of certain specific reasons.

Educational methods to promote family planning currently used by Health and Family Planning workers are often dialectic in character, prescribing "do's" and "don'ts" and are not a convenient medium for structured learning. Doubts have been raised about their effectiveness. They do not provide a learning environment within which people can examine whether the recommended procedures fit into their culture, are feasible in terms of cost and of lifestyles, and are not socially and psychologically counter-productive. In addition, family planning workers often use in appropriate and unrelated visual aids, which have been prepared without keeping in mind the local perceptual patterns of population groups or with insufficient regard to the relevance of these materials to the objectives they are intended to serve.

Everett M. Rogers[13] has maintained that most family programmes have taken too narrow a view of communication in the past They define the province of family planning communication in terms: (1) of only mass-media channels, and (2) of only the communication skills of producing family planning messages. Both functions, of course, are indeed the responsibility of the communication specialist. But, he should do much more, by engaging in activities that include: (1) inter-personnels, channels, and (2) the formation of communication strategies based upon social scientific understanding of behavioural change.

We know that the goals of family planning programmes cannot be reached by using mass-media channels alone. The audiences for such channels are too limited, the attention-getting powers are inadequate, and the motivating and persuading abilities of the mass-media are severely restricted. Research investigations consistently indicate that interpersonal channels are necessary to convince most individuals to adopt family planning methods. So, the province of family planning communication should include word-of-mouth interaction from peers who have previously adopted. By family planning communication, we do not just mean mass-media channels, they are often mediated and interpreted by opinion leaders to a large audience of receivers. So, mass media and interpersonal channels are impossible to separate in their functions and effects, even if we tried to do so.

(h) Local Community Groups

In this strategy, the doubts and misgivings hampering the promotion of family welfare measures are dispelled and popular support for the programme enlisted. Andreas Fuglessang, while admitting the role of information in motivating group action, has warned the need of guarding against Pseudo information. To quote him:

> "If genuine change is desired it will occur only through the social mechanisms for change which the community has established and to which it is accustomed. People are eager to change behaviour if they perceive the change as beneficial . . . . It is the fallacy of modernity that we believe, we communicate through bonds of mutual confidence. It is the prime task of the health communicator to facilitate a state of communal trust and also avoid Pseudo information."[14]

Mothers' Clubs in Korean villages play an important role, (1) in facilitating family planning communication, (2) in the general community development of these villages, and (3) in contributing toward women's equality. Local community groups could be important in reaching national family planning goals in other nations.

Mother's clubs for family planning communication are also being tried out on a pilot project basis in the Philippines and in Bangladesh, and are widely used in Colombia. Other types of local community groups can also be used for family planning communications, such as agricultural cooperatives, local units of political parties, farmers' associations, etc. Or, as in the "Extra Drive" approach used since 1971 in the province of East Java in Indonesia, strong local leadership in the village is used as a motivational force; here a local group with regular meetings is not used, but a temporary, once-only meeting of all target couples performs a similar function. The "group planning of births" in the People's Republic of China also depends for its success on encouraging the adoption of family planning methods and lowering fertility, on a once-a-year public meeting followed by continuous peer pressure to encourage parental implementation of the group birth plan.

All these examples illustrate a general proposition that local community groups can be an essential tool in family planning communication by providing motivation for the adoption of family planning methods and for their continued use to reduce fertility. In most Asian nations, there is presently no government development apparatus that reaches to the local level of social organisation in village. Local groups provide a mean for government to deliver services to the mass population and to change strongly-held beliefs and behaviour.

We must popularise such clubs in India and make trade unions, Mahila Mandals, Youth Organisations and students' associations active in this direction, as has been the experience in many other countries.

Donald J. Bogue rightly says that taking all factors into account, the group meeting in which some entertainment such as a film or film strip is shown, followed by group discussions, or comment by local leaders, combines many desirable features and is probably one of the best ways (if not the best) to bring information in family planning to a village or neighbourhood.

(i) Mahila Swasthya Sangh

Greater emphasis is being laid on inter-personal communication to encourage community participation, particularly for the women-folk through Mahila Swasthya Sangh (MSS) in villages with a population of over 1000 or 200 households in plain areas and for population of 500 or more in hilly terrain, including the North-Eastern States. The Auxiliary Nurse Midwife (ANM) is the member-Secretary of MSS. The MSS comprise five grass-root level functionaries and 10 prominent women from the village community. The field level functionaries of education are also the members of MSS. MSS are being constituted since 1990-91 at village level. A nominal amount of Rs. 1,200 per year is allocated for arranging its monthly meetings.

We can, thus safely say that in order to ensure the success of family planning programmes, the IEC activities must make use of all the communication skills and technology. P.T. Piotrow has rightly said that to enable couples to make informed choices, information about family planning methods must come through many media, leading ultimately to person to person contacts between clients and providers.[15]

CONCLUSIONS AND RECOMMENDATIONS

Without evaluating the impact of FP education programmes on the bulk of the people, one cannot possible identify positive as well as negative aspects of the programme. An objective evaluation of the FP education programme alone can help one improve guidelines for future action. Cost-benefit analysis should be an integral part of this evaluation, so that one may assess how available resources have been utilized. Through objective evaluation, one may also be able to curtail mass production of ritualistic FP education material as produced by various FP education bureaus. The amount thus saved can be effectively utilized for a more purposeful and meaningful health education programme.

FP education is the most difficult task as habits, usages and customs are deeply entrenched. But, FP administration would fail in its purpose, if it could not produce social change, as it is easier to destroy our villages than to change our customs. (Bosnian Proverb quoted in John I. Hanlon, Principles of Public Health Administration, St. Louis, 1960, p. 375). Professional training helps the FP experts to deal with the health changes effectively. Their pharmacopoeia in both fields must be strong in order to translate the findings of biological investigations into social application. So over and above each technical act, there is a corresponding education function which doubles the value of the act, increases its efficiency and endows it with real human and social value.[16]

We now give some concrete suggestions, which can enable effective communication and information

1. Strengthen Media to Cover Populous Areas Through Audience Segmentation

A recent study conducted by Monis Raza has indicated that the couple protection rate varies from 62 to 68 in different areas. Therefore, there is a need to segment the population areas so that more attention can be paid to low acceptability areas. To quote E.M. Rogers, "We conclude that audience segmentation strategies, which delineate sub-categories of the total audience and aim special messages at them, offer important potential for family planning communication effectiveness."

Joung Whang rightly stresses that sound communication strategies at the grass-roots level require segmentation of individual clients of the community into specific categories, according to geographical and social accessibility, kind of media available to identified clients, particular language and symbols familiar to them level of understanding, level of motivation already attained, level of aspiration, etc. There is a need of Audience research to get feedback, ready reference and analysis for programme planners on various aspects pertaining to audience composition, its habits, tastes, preference, exposure, extent of coverage, impact of the programme.

2. Adequate and Reliable Information based on Research in Bio-medical Aspects of Family Planning

The National Perspective Plan For Women (1988-2000 AD) has rightly stressed the need to educate and inform the people about Family Planning on the basis of genuine research and findings so that they can choose right methods. To quote the Perspective Plan:

> "It is unfortunate that the family planning policy is oriented towards fertility concerned with providing a means for women and men to have control on their own bodies. . . . Research studies have shed light on the fact that the knowledge regarding Family Planning/ Methods is low despite the huge amounts of money spent on propaganda. The only method known to all is sterilization. The high rates of abortion show the desire and need of the women for family planning and the failure of the family planning information and services to reach them in time. Laproscopic operations are being performed in several family planning camps without proper care and follow-up. Consequent problems tend to create apprehension among people. More intensive propagation of spacing methods together with innovative strategies for delivery of supplies has to be taken up and spread of information about temporary methods should be accorded high priority."

B.L. Raina has rightly mentioned that it is essential: (a) to understand human reproductive processes; (b) to find out means for modification, adaptation and control of these processes; (c) to know the complexity of human behaviours and its consequences; and (d) to mobilize our knowledge so gained for achievement of our social aims. The knowledge of reproductive processes is still limited. Species differences make the problem more difficult.

3. Research to make Mass Communication More Effective

There is a need of continuous research in the areas of FP Programme Communication activities. Reliance on mass media can reach only to those few who constitute the elite group. If the family planning programme was based only on elite participation, the public relations tools could have some utility because the rest of the population did not matter. But when the success of F.P. Programme is based on total participation, the public relations tools have got to be redevised. There has been no organized attempt to find out new tools and techniques of Public Relations based on a scientific study of the nature of the Public to be reached. The problem calls for intensive research programme to delineate channels of communication for reaching the public. To quote Dinesh Chandra Dubey and Kamla Gopal Rao, "With no pretence of giving a comprehensive review of needed research in mass communication for popularizing family planning, the foregoing review only seeks to highlight some of the important areas of research. While most of research findings in mass communication have been extracted from studies in highly urbanized, modern, western cultures, the authors feel strongly that the insights derived from these studies need to be tested out for their validity in the transitional societies and in developing societies."

4. Impart Training Programmes for Family Planning Education

S.S. Bharara has nicely said that 'The population programme essentially has multi-disciplinary and multi-dimensional characteristics. These disciplines fall within four categories, viz., (i) demography and statistics, (ii) biomedicine, (iii) social and behavioural sciences, and (iv) administration and programme planning. Accordingly, the personnel engaged in the family welfare programme are drawn from these disciplines and are demographers, statisticians, doctors, nurses and other paramedical workers; social scientists, social workers and extension educators; and planners, administrators, supervisors, evaluators, etc. Each discipline represented must be integrated into the whole of the programme in the most effective and efficient manner. Personnel from these disciplines have to be available in adequate number at the front line of action, as well as at other levels of administration, supervision and planning. It necessarily implies that the roles and responsibilities of these personnel will vary according to the level at which they function, even though the ultimate goal remains very much the same. All the personnel, therefore, become co-ordinated parts of a machinery, working as a team, in co-operation with each other, by fully synchronizing their activities. This is what a training programme has to cater to, and produce personnel who will be able to function accordingly.

The roles of each group of functionaries at different levels being so varied, training programmes have to develop correct role-perceptions among the workers and, accordingly correct role-expectations among their supervisors and those higher up in the echelons of administration. The higher the degree of role consensus, the lesser the chances of role conflicts, job dissatisfaction and frustrations.

5. Develop Effective Public Relations

One of the important functions of family welfare administrators is the development of cordial, equitable and harmonious relationships with the beneficiaries to ensure their welfare and participation. The public relations is the establishment of a climate of understanding. The purpose of public relations is not only to supply information, but also to encourage an understanding and co-operation between the social scientists, social workers and beneficiaries.

The management of any public agency should not only employ competent media specialists—those who handle press contacts, prepare news releases, write radio scripts, and carry on other information activities—but it should also create a favourable image of help both inside and outside the agency.[17] The family welfare programmes have not received desired publicity through the publicity media. Our inquiries have shown that the poor coverage was not due to apathy of the press or other media of publicity but due to lack of communication and inadequate release of information on the subject. Publicity is very useful or even essential not only to highlight the programmes and achievements of the organization but to enlist the cooperation of a large number of employees and the goodwill of public, in the implementation of family welfare programme. Many well intentioned and technically sound family welfare programmes, aimed at solving family welfare problems, have been frustrated by lack of popular acceptance and community participation. To quote a WHO Report, "It has been observed that such programmes are either not actively associated or passively ignored because they do not belong to the population they are designed to help; they are rather seen by the population as imposed external programme that belong to the government and consequently deserves and require little, if any, of the population's attention, action, or other response."[18]

Some of the measures which are suggested for improvement of public relations are:

- The help of local office of the press information bureau may be utilized to release photo-features from time to time.
- Local stations of All-India Radio be persuaded to include talks and discussions of family planning work specialists in the field of family welfare. Sometimes, discussions have much better effect than straight talks.

It is desirable to celebrate "Family Welfare Day" in the country every year during which, on a selected theme, publicity can be given through all available media of publicity. "Family Welfare Day" should be observed by all agencies in the field of family planning work from the village to union level on committed basis.

It may be worthwhile introducing printed "news letter" by every State, which can be sent to all State Boards, the Central Board and voluntary organizations concerned, highlighting the major events or developments in the field within their states during the month.

Another dimension of Public Relations in the area of Family Welfare is counselling the people and also those implementing Family Welfare Programmes. Primary Objective of all family services is to ensure that every individual becomes a well adjusted and productive member of a society. Effective delivery of these services depends, not merely on the material resources or well conceived programmes, but also on the quality of the personnel implementing them. So, there is a need of developing good rapport with the personnel responsible for implementation through counselling is defined in the "Encylopaedia of Social Work of India" as a professional activity associated with the process of helping individual or groups with their various problems and extending to developmental ends.

Successful Field Counselling depends on the following factors:

1. The counsellor should be a mature person, with broad outlook; wide interest and sensitiveness to the behavioural pattern and needs of the persons he/she deals with. These qualities are essential for development of a positive relationship, which is an indispensable tool, in addition to knowledge and counselling skill.
2. A field counsellor should have faith in voluntary and State action and their capacity to effectively render family welfare services.
3. A field counsellor is a dynamic and constructive leader with keen sensitivity to the community needs, feelings and attitudes and the capacity to stimulate the agency and the community to work towards goals, established through mutual and continued interaction between the two. He should be a catalytic agent of planned change, rather than a victim of the system.
4. Effective field counselling requires that the counsellor has knowledge of relevant family planning welfare activities of minimum standards for their family of other social services of National, State and Local levels and of Field Counselling Technique.[19]

Thus, public relations including counselling can help in promoting Family Welfare activities. Due care should be taken that the public relations should not degenerate into a propaganda machinery. "Public relations activities must be honest, truthful, open, authoritative and responsible, they must be fair and realistic; and they must be conducted in the public interest." Due safeguards are therefore necessary to make public relations effective for two-ways and authentic communication nerves of family welfare agencies. This traffic can be best organised by professional public relation men, but at the lowest levels of administration, the administrative personnel must do their own public relations. According to F.C. Gem, "It is not enough for mass media to be blaring forth statement in Government's policies and programmes. There must be deliberate and organised attempts also to assess the needs of people to listen to their grievances and to redress them. And the people, particularly the uneducated people must be treated with courtesy instead of being shouted at and compelled to shell out bribes."[20] All this requires dedicated, scientific and well-conceived public relations work.

6. Understand the Area of Operation

Before launching any F.P. programme, the family planning personnel must assess the local problems and must possess the knowledge about the beliefs, conceptions and misconceptions which the people have formed about F.P. activities. It needs to be stressed that the cultural context of F.P. education programme is of the greatest importance in the Indian situation. The social scientists can help the family planning workers through their studies and research.

7. Effective Administrative Machinery to Impart Family Planning Education

There is a lot of wastage and corruption in the conduct of Mass Education in F.P. Programme. Some activities like Drama, Folk Songs, Puppet shows remain only on the paper and thus the huge amount meant for the purpose is either wasted or embezzled. Vehicles supplied for this purpose are wrongly used.

After independence, the family welfare administrative machinery of India advanced considerably, both in magnitude and direction. Administrative efficiency is the most urgent demand of the day. Most of the grievances of the citizens are because of the apathy of the administration and lack of dynamic administration. An international group of public administration experts has also stressed upon this, "Dysfunctional and inapplicable administrative structures, systems and practices must be replaced. Nothing less than dynamic organizations, resourceful management and streamlined administrative processes will suffice . . . the torturous the consuming routines, special privileges, corruption, indolence and insolence often encumbering any governmental bureaucracies and civil services have no place in development administration. This calls for continuous action to foster honesty and integrity and to weed out corruption as well as to develop preventive measure."[21]

8. Develop Attractive Mass-Media Material

No doubt, a vast majority of our people is still unable to read and write. But, literacy is definitely spreading. More importantly, the printed word influences the literate opinion leader in the village like the teacher, panchayat chief, etc. who will be amongst the first to adopt family planning and who will be able to influence his untutored brethren.

9. Motivate Extension Personnel

The quality of the F.P. operations run by Government would be dependent to a great extent upon the quality of extension workers engaged in their operation. Personnel move the administrative machinery. To quote Mrs. Indira Gandhi: "If Government has to do more for the people, its employees must play a more dynamic and more creative role, as the instrument for implementing government policies and programmes."[22]

An extension group cannot work with their heart in it unless they are adequately motivated with reasonable remuneration and prospects of advancement. The emoluments paid to F.P. personnel have been less than those paid to professionals in comparable pursuits, while the task of successful extension is one of the most difficult. If the Extension workers are motivated, this would generate loyalty, co-operation and team work, essential for the achievement of the goals of F.P. Programmes.

Whenever there is a failure of the family planning programme, we generally attribute it to the illiteracy, ignorance and irrational attitudes of the people. On the other hand, we should make a fresh assessment of what the obstacles to family planning success actually are. In order to tackle these problems, IEC can help a great deal in promoting positive attitudes. The obstacles should not be considered as insurmountable barriers. Within each State and Union Territory, there is a need to set-up communication research project to provide information needed to replan the IEC activities to tide over the difficulties. Lyle Saunders has suggested the following change in IEC activities in future:[23]

(i) Family Planning communicators in the future are likely to be more focused on communities as audiences are more concerned with trying to change collective beliefs and values than with informing individuals;

(ii) They may find it necessary to spend more time providing information demanded by more strongly committed political leader, justifying and defending the spread of sterilization and abortion and developing public support for ideas and activities that may be initially unpopular;

(iii) They will be concerned with explaining new kinds of contraceptives and a variety of incentive and disincentive measures;

(iv) They will find themselves working more closely with other special interest communicators in efforts to integrate development programmes and trying to maximize the accuracy and reliance of family planning information provided by communicators with other major interests;

(v) They will have a role to play in changing the image of family planning as a health matter and may both contribute to and learn from the promotional activities of those on the commercial sector who are distributing contraceptives;

(vi) They will be helping to formulate and implement new communication strategies; and

(vii) They may have some new interesting tools to work with its current trends on communication technology.

10. Multi-disciplinary Integrated Approach to Promote Effective Communication

12th joint conference of central council of health and family planning suggested that the revised strategy predicates on multi-disciplinary integrated approach. Addressing the areas beyond family welfare and mobilizing all development agencies and sectors of society directly interfacing with the people to join in the task of family welfare promotion is a *sine-qua-non* for its success. The communication support for this work will now accordingly have to be through a multi-dimensional integrated thrust.

This requires a far broader vision for family welfare than has prevailed so far. On the one hand, family welfare communication will need to be embedded in primary healthcare messages and on the other, form an organic part of a core package of social development issues, particularly those relating to female literacy, employment status, age of marriage and child survival:

(i) Therefore, it is necessary that the State MEM organizations and State Education Health Bureau make more co-ordinated use of manpower and material to put out programmes and messages of health and family welfare in an integrated fashion, integration where possible and in any case functional co-ordination of these two units must be done immediately. Along side efforts must be initiated to ensure that health and family welfare IEC efforts link up and co-ordinate with the media efforts for women and child development, adult and non-formal education and youth activities. The budget for Health and Family Welfare IEC must be substantially enhanced.

(ii) The gap between widespread awareness and limited practice of family welfare also calls for different communication approaches which concentrate on effecting behavioural changes more rapidly. Therefore, at the present stage of the programme, greater use must be made of all inter-personnel channels and appropriate training and orientation of all developmental workers to bring about their involvement with family planning. Equally, the reorientation of Health and Family Welfare workers to enable an internalization of the broader perspective is important.

(iii) With the country presently going through a communication revolution, all media channels must be fully utilized to create an enabling ethos for the programme and as a means to vault the barriers of illiteracy and ignorance. Greater family welfare acceptance is noted where there is greater exposure to media. Towards this end, the Council recommends urgent steps to be taken to ensure greater access to television and radio for the most critical target groups, who presently form the media-deprived class. This is to be done through promotion of group listening and community viewing situations. A pooling of resources for all departments to create such an access must be considered. The greater use of television, film, radio and traditional media must be encouraged to create a synergy between mass media and inter-personal channels. In the case of television, which is a government medium, maximum support must be ensured to health and family welfare issues by earmarking minimum time for programmes on health and family welfare; weaving of appropriate messages in the regular serials and other-sponsored propagation of public service messages on health and family welfare at prime time.

(iv) Altogether, information must move to another plane from general to the specific, giving the how and why on what is required to be done so as to empower people to act on their own behalf. The spirit of family planning communication has to communicate information, not publicity and propaganda. The States may, therefore, like to ensure that the budget for media work are more effectively utilized on developing information, education and communication materials.

(v) As a part of the effort to bring about total mobilization of society and wider involvement of everyone in the programme, strenuous efforts must now be made to secure free publicity and promotion of the family planning programme and its objectives through every possible source. Free display at sports stadiums, bus panels and other commercial channels should be actively solicited and engineered.

(vi) All communication materials and messages must be pretested before application in the field. The pretesting should be done through quick and ready methods so that material can be corrected at appropriate stage.

(vii) Some immediate administrative measures are necessary to revitalize the IEC programme. There are large number of vacancies in the State media set-ups, particularly at the field level. These must be filled in the shortest possible time. The media staff working in the States should be utilized for intensifying IEC programmes, instead of deputing them for routine clerical jobs.

An efficient extension F.P. service, capable of winning people's confidence as their friend, philosopher and guide, takes decades to build up. Careful selection and training, morale-building, service conditions, rational organization—these are the bricks and mortars of the extension officers. Close co-ordination with research, input supply, marketing and guidance, and employment of an effective combination of communication techniques are prerequisites for the successful functioning of the F.P. service. Various management tasks involved in building up such extension service need strengthening.

Notes and References

1. Donald J. Bogue, "A Five Year Information—Education Communication Perspective to meet the Population, Health, Food Crises, 1975-80", in *Family Planning Resumed*, p. 117, Vol. 1, 1977, No. 1.
2. A. Govindachari, 'The Role of Extension Education in Family Planning', in *Aspects of Population Policy in India*, New Delhi, 1969, pp. 124-25, Population Reports Series, Number 35, November 1987, p. 2.
4. Annual Report of the Health Ministry of the Health and Family Welfare, 1998-99, p. 73.
5. H. Koontz and C. O'Donnell, "Principles of Management: An Analysis of Managerial Functions", London, McGraw Hill, Kogakusha Ltd., 1972, pp. 538-40.
6. Chester, I. Barnard, "Functions of the Executive", Cambridge; Harward University Press, 1968, pp. 226-27.
7. W.H. Newman and C.E. Summer, "The Process of Management Concepts Behaviour and Practice", Anglewood, Cliffs, N.J., Prentice Hall, 1961, p. 59.
8. *World Health,* Jan.-Feb. 1989.
9. F.M. Rogers in *Joung Whang*, ed., pp. 130-31.
10. *The Economic Times*, March 9, 1989.
11. WHO, *World Health*, Nov. 1975, p. 14.
12. *Ibid.*, May 1979, p. 25.
13. F.M. Rogers, Management of Family Planning IEC Activities, in *Joung Whang*, (ed.), pp. 116-17.
14. Andreas Fuglesang, "Fold Wisdom and Pseudo Information", in *World Health*, Jan.-Feb. 1989, pp. 6-7.
15. Population Reports, Series 1, Number 35, Nov. 1987, p. 16.
16. WHO Technical Report Series, 1954, No. 89, p. 4.
17. Felix, Nigro A., Modern Public Administration, *op. cit.*, p. 205.
18. *WHO Chronicle*, 30 (1976), pp. 177-78.
19. Central Social Welfare Board, Field Counselling Service, A Pilot Project, 1974, New Delhi, p. 13.
20. F.C. Gera, "Need for Public Relations in Administration", in *IJPA*, Vol. XXI, July-Sept. 1975, pp. 545-56.
21. United Nations Public Administration in the Second United Nations Development Decade, *Ibid*.
22. Presidential Address by Mrs. Indira Gandhi delivered on October 22, 1971, at the Annual Meeting of IIPA, New Delhi.
23. Lyle Saunders, Family Planning Resource, Vol. 1, No. 1, pp. 30-31.

CHAPTER 7

EDUCATION FOR GIRL: ESSENTIAL FOR HEALTH

Ensure equal access to education.
Eradicate illiteracy among women.
Improve women access to vocational training, science and technology, and continuing education.

Develop non-discriminatory education and training.

Allocate sufficient resources for and monitor the implementation of educational reforms.

Promote lifelong education and training for girls and women.

—*Strategic Objectives,* B.I. B.6 Platform for Action.

Education for Girl: Essential for Health

The Women of India have suffered neglect in the matter of education throughout the ages, seriously affecting their intellectual development and social status.

The constitution of India mandates universal and compulsory education for all. A number of programmes have been implemented and are still under implementation to improve the level of female literacy. Some States have made remarkable progress in this direction, but some have not. It is almost axiomatic to State that a literate mother is the greatest guarantor of education for the next generation with a great bearing on the socio-economic and cultural advancement of a nation.

Article 14 of the Constitution provides for equality before the law and equal protection of the law. Article 15 prohibits discrimination against any citizen on grounds of religion, race, caste, sex or place of birth. Article 16 guarantees equality of opportunity to all citizens in matters relating to employment or appointment to any office of the State and forbids discrimination on the basis of religion, caste, sex, etc., in matters of employment or appointment to any office under the State. However, Article 15(3) empowers the State to make any special provision for women and children even in violation of the fundamental obligation of non-discrimination on the basis of sex. This provision has enabled the State to draw up special policies and programmes to benefit women. [1]

First, let us understand the meaning and importance of Education in General for all whether male or female.

"Asato ma Sadgamya
Tamso ma Jyotirgamaya."

—Brihadaranyaka Upanishad

"Lead me from untruth to truth
Lead me from darkness to light."

Education has been of central significance to the development of human society. It can be the beginning, not only of individual knowledge, information and awareness, but also of a holistic strategy for development and change. Late Prime Minister Jawahar Lal Nehru rightly remarked, "Some people seem to think that education is not so important as putting up a factory. I may sacrifice any number of factories, but I will not sacrifice human beings and their education because it is the human beings who set-up factories and produce the things we want." UNESCO has described illiteracy as "the most monstrous of all the many instances of wasted human potential which still at the present time keeps more than one-third of the human race in a state of hopelessness, below the level of modern civilization." It is imperative to increase the literacy rate to bring about all round development. Education helps an individual to develop his potential to the full, to increase his productivity and to become a useful and productivity member of society. Education is holistic in concept and is multi-dimensional.

Education is a critical input in human resource development and is essential for the country's economic growth. Though the major indicators of socio-economic development viz., the growth rate of the economy, birth rate, death rate, infant mortality rate (IMR) and literacy rate, are all interconnected, the literacy rate has been the major determinant of the rise or fall in the other indicators. There is enough evidence even in India to show that a high literacy rate, especially in the case of women, correlates with low birth rate, low IMR and increase in the rate of life expectancy. The recognition of this fact has created awareness on the need to focus upon literacy and elementary education programme, not simply as a matter of social justice but more to foster economic growth, social well-being and social stability.[2]

"The general purpose and objective of women's education cannot, of course, be different from the purpose and objective of men's education. . . At the secondary and even at the university stage women's education should have a vocational or occupational bias."[3]

"In a democratic society where all citizens have to discharge their civic and social obligations, differences which may lead to variation in the standards of intellectual development achieved by boys and girls cannot be envisaged."[4]

"In the progressive society of tomorrow, life should be a joint venture for men and women. Men should share the responsibility of parenthood and home-making with women and women in their turn should share the social and economic responsibilities of men."[5]

"Women and mens' education should have many elements in common, but should not in general be identical in all respects, as is usually the case today. A women should learn something of problems that are certain to come up in all marriages, and in the relations of parents and children, and how they may be met. Her education should make her familiar with problems of home management and skilled in meeting them, so that she may take her place in a home with the same interest and the same sense of competence that a well trained man has in working at his calling."[6]

"The educational system must produce young men and women of character and ability committed to national service and development. Only then will education be able to play its vital role in promoting national progress, creating a sense of common citizenship and culture and strengthening national integration."[7]

Education was a state subject till 1976 and then was placed in the Concurrent list by the 42nd Constitutional Amendment. Placing education in the Concurrent List means a dominant role for the Central Government viz:

(i) to determine the policies, priorities and programmes relating to education,
(ii) to provide effective leadership to the states,
(iii) to provide funds for educational development in the States,
(iv) to take steps for minimizing regional imbalances in educational development and for equalization of educational opportunities in different States,
(v) to take steps for promoting national integration through education, and
(vi) to carry out uniform educational forms in the country.

Female Literacy Rate

The following Table 7.1 indicates the literacy rate in India and male and female literacy rates in the country from 1951:

TABLE 7.1

Census Year	*Persons*	*Males*	*Females*	*Male-female gap in literacy rate*
1951	18.33	27.16	8.86	18.30
1961	28.30	40.40	15.35	25.05
1971	24.35	45.96	21.97	23.98
1981	43.57	56.38	29.76	26.62
1991	52.21	64.13	39.29	24.84
2001	65.38	75.85	54.16	21.70

Source: Censes of India.

It is evident from the above table that the gap in male-female literacy rates of 18.30 percentage points in 1951, increased to 26.62 in 1981, but has improved since then. In 1991 this gap was reduced to 24.84 and in 2001

CHART 7.1

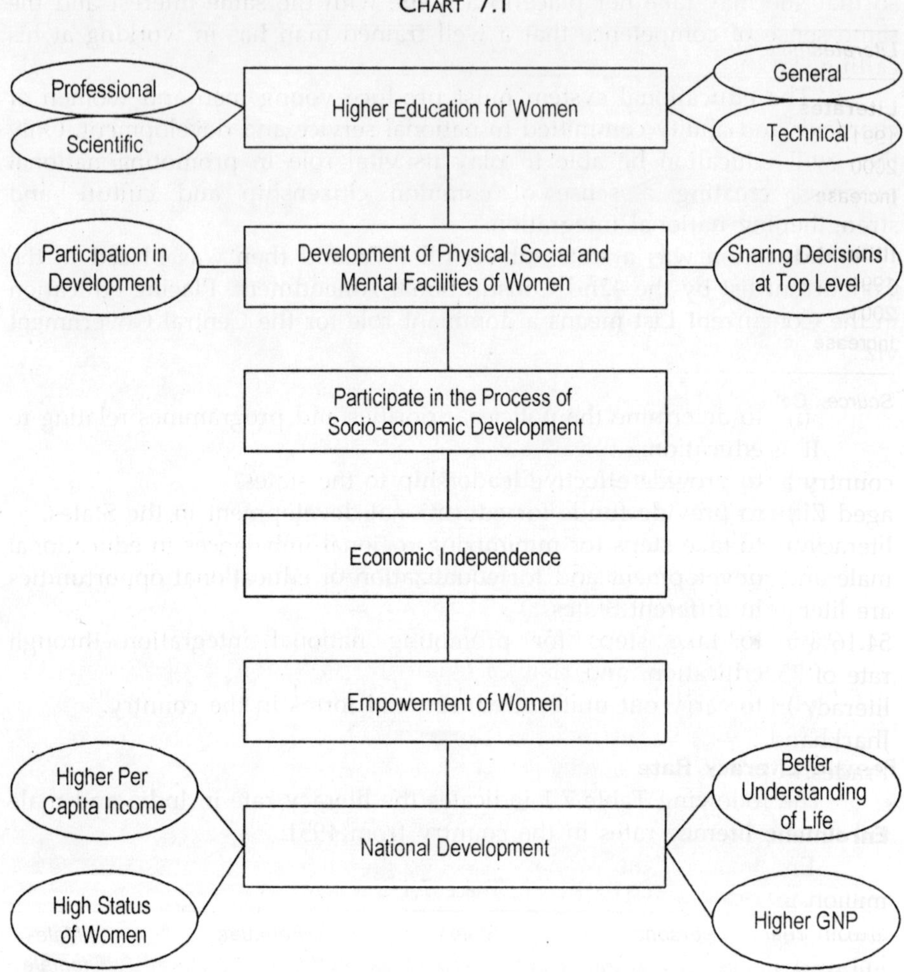

it has further gone down to 21.70 percentage points. These declines according to the Department of Elementary Education and Literacy are bound to be slow initially as a result of the continuing past legacy of a large number of adult illiterate women, but will show accelerated trends in the coming decade.

The following Table 7.2 indicates the number of literates and illiterates in the population aged 7 years and above, and their change from 1991 to 2001:

It is seen from Table 7.2 (see next page) that out of the 203 million added to the literate population during 1991-2001, 107 million were males and 95 million were females. On the other hand, during this period the contribution to the total decrease of 31 million among illiterates is dominated by males (21 million) as compared to the females (10 million).

TABLE 7.2

Literates/Illiterates	Persons	Males	Females
Literates			
1991	358,402,626	228,983,134	129,419,492
2000	562,010,743	336,969,695	225,041,048
Increase in 2001 over 1991	203,608,117	107,986,561	95,621,556
Illiterates			
1991	328,167,288	128,099,211	200,068,077
2001	296208,952	106,654,066	189,554,886
Increase in 2001 over 1991	-31,958,336	-21,445,145	-10,513,1991

Source: Census of India.

It is seen from the above Table 7.2 that the literacy rate for the country as a whole in 2001 works out to 65.38 per cent for the population aged 7 years and above. The corresponding figures for male and female literacy are 75.85 and 54.16 per cent respectively. Thus, three-fourths of the male and more than half of the female population aged 7 years and above are literate in the country today. Although female literacy has improved to 54.16% in 2001 from 39.29% in 1991, it is still far behind the male literacy rate of 75.85%. In fact, no State or Union Territory has an equal or greater literacy rate for women. Further, female literacy rate is very low in Jharkhand (39.38%), Arunachal Pradesh (44.24%), Bihar (33.57%), Uttar Pradesh (42.97%), Rajasthan (44.34%), and Jammu and Kashmir (41.82%).[8]

Enrolment Trends

Enrolment at the primary level (grades I to V) increased from 19.16 million in 1950-51 to 113.8 million in 2000-01. In comparison, the growth in enrolment at the upper primary level (grades VI to VIII) has been much more impressive, although it is still not adequate to attain the Constitutional goal of universal enrolment of children up to the age of 14. From 3.12 million in 1950-51, enrolment at the upper primary level increased to 42.06 million in 1999-2000, indicating a 13.5 times increase as against six times at the primary level. The percentage share of girls in total enrolment, both at the primary and upper primary levels, has increased consistently between 1950-51 (28.1 per cent) and 1999-2000 (43.6 percent). However, girls share in total enrolment at the upper primary level (40.4 percent) continues to be lower than their share at the primary level in 1999-2000.

The total enrolment at the primary and upper primary school levels in India witnessed a steady increase (Table 7.3) During 1999-2000 and 2000-01, the growth rate of enrolment for girls at the elementary levels was higher as compared to that for boys. Participation of girls at all levels of school education has improved appreciably over the years.

The Gross Enrolment Ratio (GER) at Primary and Upper Primary levels improved perceptibly in 2000-01 over the previous year (Table 7.4).

Out of the estimated population of 193 million in the age group of 6-14 years in 2000-01 nearly 81 percent attended school. In 1999-2000 nearly 79 percent in this age group attended school. The student retention rate at the primary and upper primary level have decreased over the years. At the primary level, the dropout rate increased from 40.3 percent in 1999-2000 to 40.7 percent 2000-01. At the upper primary level, the dropout rate decreased marginally from 54.5 percent in 1999-2000 to 53.7 percent in 2000-01. Though dropout rates at the elementary education stage have declined over the years, they are still relatively high especially in the case of girl students for whom the rates are 41.9 percent and 57.7 percent at the Primary and upper Primary Stages respectively in 2000-01.

In absolute terms, the number of teachers registered at the elementary level was 3.2 million in 2000-01. The percentage share of female teachers to total teachers was 36.7 percent in 2000-01. Despite the fact that the number of teachers has increased over the years. Pupil-Teacher Ratio (PTR) at the Primary education level worsened to 1:43 in 2000-01 although that at the Upper Primary level increased to 1:38 in 2000-01.

Within the education sector, elementary education has been given the highest priority in terms of sub-sectoral allocations and a number of schemes launched by the Central Government to meet the needs of the educationally disadvantaged viz. Operation Blackboard, District Primary Education Programme, Education Guarantee Scheme and Alternative and Innovative Education, Mahila Samakhya, Teacher Education, National Programme of Nutritional Support to Primary Education, Lok Jumbish, Shiksha Karmi Project, Janashala Programme and Pradhan Mantri Gramodaya Yojana.[9]

Elementary Education

Education has an intrinsic value for the development of the society and helps in the achievement of a better social order. Greater literacy and basic education help individuals to make better use of available economic opportunities. The Government has decided to make free and compulsory elementary education a fundamental right.

The need to impart value-based education to the children at the early stages of schooling can hardly be overemphasised. The essential elements of such education should be based on the development of concern towards the needs of society and the nation among the children. In this contemporary world, the value should also be based on the functional utility of education and should highlight the dignity of labour. The idea of creation of wealth should be incorporated into the education system.[10]

The Constitution of India has made it obligatory on the part of the Government to provide free and compulsory education to all children until they complete the age of 14 years. This was to be achieved by the year 1960, but could not be achieved and the target dates had to be repeatedly extended to 1990. The National Policy on Education, 1986 again extended the target date to 1995. The modified Education Policy, 1992 further revised

TABLE 7.3

Sex-wise Enrolment by Stages/Classes since 1950-51

Year	Primary (I-V)			Middle/Upper Primary (VI-VIII)			High/Hr. Sec./Inter/ Pre-Degree (IX-XII)		
	Boys	Girls	Total	Boys	Girls	Total	Boys	Girls	Total
1970-71	35.7	21.3	57.0	9.4	3.9	13.3	5.7	1.9	7.6
1980-81	45.3	28.5	73.98	13.9	6.8	20.37	7.6	3.4	11.0
1990-91	57.0	40.4	97.4	21.5	12.5	34.0	12.8	6.3	19.1
1991-92	5806	42.3	100.9	22.0	13.6	35.6	13.5	6.9	20.4
1992-93	57.9	41.7	99.6	21.02	12.9	34.1	13.6	6.9	20.5
1993-94	55.1	41.9	97.6	20.6	13.5	34.1	13.2	7.5	20.7
1994-95	60.1	45.1	105.1	22.1	14.5	36.4	14.2	7.9	22.1
1995-96	60.6	46.2	107.1	22.7	14.8	37.35	14.6	8.3	22.9
1996-97*	62.5	47.9	110.4	24.7	16.3	41.0	17.2	9.8	27.0
1997-98*	61.2	47.5	108.4	27.7	15.8	39.5	17.1	10.2	27.2
1998-99*	62.7	48.2	110.9	24.0	16.3	40.3	17.3	10.5	27.8
1999-2000*	64.1	49.5	113.6	25.1	17.0	42.1	17.2	11.0	28.2
2000-01*	64.0	49.8	113.8	25.3	17.5	42.8	16.9	10.7	27.6

* Provisional.

Source: Selected Educational Statistics, 2000-01, Ministry of Human Resources Development.

TABLE 7.4

Trends in Gross Enrolment Ratios in India

Year	Primary (I-V)			Middle/Upper Primary (VI-VIII)			High/Hr. Sec./Inter/ Pre-Degree (IX-XII)		
	Boys	Girls	Total	Boys	Girls	Total	Boys	Girls	Total
1970-71	95.5	60.5	78.6	46.5	20.8	33.4	75.5	44.4	61.9
1980-81	95.8	64.1	80.5	54.3	29.6	41.9	82.2	52.1	67.5
1990-91	114.0	85.5	100.1	76.6	47.0	62.1	100.0	70.8	86.0
1991-92	112.8	86.9	100.2	75.1	49.6	61.4	101.2	73.2	87.7
1992-93	95.0	73.5	84.6	72.5	48.9	67.5	87.7	65.7	77.2
1993-94	90.0	73.1	81.9	62.1	45.4	54.2	80.2	63.7	72.3
1994-95	96.6	78.2	87.7	68.9	50.0	60.0	87.2	68.8	78.4
1995-96	97.1	79.4	88.6	67.8	49.8	59.3	86.9	69.4	78.5
1996-97*	98.7	81.9	90.6	70.9	52.8	62.4	86.9	71.4	80.7
1997-98*	97.7	81.2	89.7	66.5	49.5	58.5	86.4	70.0	78.6
1998-99*	100.9	82.9	92.1	65.3	49.1	57.6	87.6	70.6	79.4
1999-2000*	104.1	85.2	94.9	67.2	49.7	58.8	90.1	72.0	81.3
2000-01*	104.9	85.9	95.7	66.7	49.9	58.6	90.3	72.4	81.6

* Provisional.

Source: Selected Educational Statistics, 2000-01, Ministry of Human Resources Development.

the target date so as to achieve compulsory education for all children upto 14 years of age by the end of 20th century. Inspite of the provisions having been made in the Constitution and the efforts made by successive Governments it has not yet been possible to universalise elementary education. Free and compulsory elementary education still remains a major challenge in most of the States.

Shockingly, of the 900 million illiterates in the world, almost one-third belong to India. In other words, Indians constitute the largest number of uneducated people in the world. It is a paradoxical situation in which the gains made in the realm of education since independence have been overshadowed by the presence of a huge population of illiterates, especially in rural India, and more so among girls. Admittedly, the massive increase in the population in the last 50 years has been one of the major reasons for the imbalance in the literacy-population ratio. But, this can hardly be a ground for absolving the nation of its responsibility for the failure in providing primary education to all children.

Inter-State disparities also exist in regard to the female literacy rate. The Committee feel that special measures should be taken in those States. Where female literacy rate is very low as compared to the all India average. These States are Jharkhand (39.98%), Arunachal Pradesh (44.24%), Bihar (33.57%), Uttar Pradesh (42.97), Rajasthan (44.34%) and Jammu and Kashmir (41.82%). The Government need to study the situation in these States with a view to identifying the precise reasons for the low female rates there, so that necessary steps could be taken in consultation and coordination with the respective State Governments, apart from vigorously implementing the Schemes/Programmes already in operation.

The Department of Elementary Education and Literacy have asserted that consistent efforts have been made to improve the participation of girls in the field of education in the last 50 years. According to them, the Gross Enrolment Ratio (GER) for girls has gone up from 24.8 per cent in 1950-51 at the primary level to 81.8 per cent in 1996-97. The Committee find that while the GER for girls at the primary stage in the country, as a whole and in most States, has improved, it is low as compared to GER for boys. A study of the progressive enrolment of girls and boys at primary and middle school levels points to a massive gender gap. Further there are a few States/ UTs where the (GER) is considerably low in respect of girl students. These are Bihar (54.6%), Jammu and Kashmir (53.1%), Uttar Pradesh (59.9%) and Chandigarh (62.1%). Similarly, the dropout rate in respect of girls is very high in some of the States such as Bihar (63.44%), West Bengal (55.59%), Tripura (56.65%), Sikkim (55.4%), Rajasthan (57.2%), Mizoram (56.95) and Meghalaya (62.46%).

The Committee are concerned over the lower Gross Enrolment Ratio and higher dropout rates among girls especially as compared to those in respect of boys. Low enrolment ratio and high dropout rates lead to children especially girls, lapsing into illiteracy, rendering futile, the efforts and investments made in improving literacy. The main reason for this situation in rural areas is that girls are engaged in household works such as fuel and fodder collection, fetching of water and care of siblings. The other reasons could be parent's lack of interest, poverty, absence of single sex schools, unsafe travel and lack of facilities in schools such as women teachers, separate toilets, etc.

The Committee strongly feel that there is urgent need to remove the constraints that lead parents to keep their daughters out of school. And once girls are in school, it must be ensured they are prepared for life, by developing curricula, textbooks and teaching attitudes that emphasise the life skills they will need. But the first step is for society to recognise that educating girls is not an option, but a necessity. This calls for a massive programme of awareness generation in the educationally backward areas of the country.

The Committee are of the firm opinion that the achievement of universalisation of elementary education is essential as it is an index of the general, social and economic development of the country. Primary education plays an important role in laying the proper foundation of the cultural, emotional, intellectual, moral, physical, social and spiritual developments of the children. The economic and social returns for education of women are, on the whole, greater than those of men. Education empowers girls by building up their confidence and enabling them to take firm decisions about their lives. By educating women we can reduce poverty, improve productivity, ease population pressure and offer the children a better future.

The Committee are informed that various schemes/programmes such as the National Literacy Mission, Mahila Samakhya, Operation Blackboard, Non-formal Education Lok Jumbish and District Primary Education Programme, have been initiated/undertaken for improvement of girls' education. These schemes are stated to have made enormous progress in terms of increase in number of schools, teachers and students in elementary education. The progress achieved in the female literacy rate during the last decade has been attributed to a great extent to the implementation of these schemes. The Sarva Shiksha Abhiyan (SSA) is stated to be another new holistic and integrated approach for universalising elementary education. Based on the experience of programmes for girls' education and women's empowerment, the proposed Sarva Shiksha Abhiyan, which is in mission mode, adopts many of the successful initiatives. The Sarva Shiksha Abhiyan has the objective of bringing every child in the 6-14 age group to school/back to school to an Education Guarantee Scheme Centre by 2003. It also aims at providing 5 years of primary schooling for all by 2007 and 8 years of elementary schooling by 2010. Mainstreaming of gender in all the proposed interventions through the District Elementary Education Plan (DEEP) is central to the proposed Sarva Shiksha Abhiyan. The Committee hope that vigorous efforts would be made under the aforesaid schemes/ programmes to ensure that the constitutional obligation of providing free and compulsory education for all children upto the age of 14 years becomes a reality.

The Committee on Empowerment of Women (2001-02), Sixth Report, Thirteen Lok Sabha desire that the following measures be taken on priority basis to achieve the objective of education for all and especially for girls:

(i) Universal enrolment of all children.

(ii) Provision of primary school, within one kilometer of walking distance.

(iii) Facility of non-formal education for school dropouts, working children and girls who cannot attend schools.

(iv) Reduction of dropout rates especially of girls.

(v) Achievement of minimum levels of learning by all children at the primary level, and introduction of this concept at the upper primary stage on a large scale.

(vi) Increased allocation of funds for various schemes/programmes initiated for girls' education and optimum utilization of allotted funds.

(vii) Taking up of intensive awareness generation activities for bringing about change in societal attitude towards girls' education.

(viii) Orientation of educational policies to take care of specific needs and requirements of girls and women, particularly in their socio-economic context.

(ix) Orientation of policies in other sectors for providing support and facilitating access to services like pure drinking water, fuel, fodder and crèches, thus freeing them from the drudgery of households chores, to help girls attend to their education.

(x) Gearing up of economic policies to improve employment of women and their earning capabilities so that they can relieve the girls' for educational activities.

(xi) Exploring the possibilities/potential of imparting distance education, through TV, to reach backward areas—SC/ST/Rural women/nomadic tribes/slum-dwellers of urban centers.

The Committee further recommend that to increase retention and reduce dropouts, the following measures may be taken by the Department in consultation with the State Governments:

(i) School should be made an attractive place, learning an enjoyable experience and teaching child centred and activity oriented, with text books made colourful and attractive from the child's point of view.

(ii) Early childhood education or pre-school education focuses on providing a learning environment for children under the age of six years. This fosters the natural process of initiating children into self-motivated education in which they learn as they play. Apart from enabling the all round development of children through child-centred play activities, this ensures that young girls are freed of their responsibility of sibling care enabling them to go to schools and thus contributing to universalisation of primary education. The Committee, therefore, emphasise the need for pre-school education as a significant input for providing a sound foundation for the growth and development of a child, especially from poor families. Government should pay special attention to this aspect.

(iii) The teachers should be motivated, dedicated and fully trained. NCERT should launch a pilot programme in close collaboration with State Councils of Education, Research and Training for the training of teachers. There should be provision for substitute full time teachers in all schools including Kendriya Vidyalayas when regular teachers go on long leave so that students do not suffer.

(iv) Instead of raw wheat/rice, cooked meals should be served to children.

(v) Free text books, uniforms and teaching/learning materials may be provided at the start of the academic session especially in rural areas for girls.

(vi) Proper toilets and drinking water facilities should be made available particularly in the girls' co-educational schools.

(vii) The children of the nomadic tribes, shifting cultivators, and construction workers are the most vulnerable group of school dropouts. Therefore, special attention must be paid to the target groups.

(viii) Vigorous steps are needed to associate the elected representatives of. the Panchayati Raj Institutions in the Literacy Programmes. The women elected to local bodies should be actively involved in such programmes and be provided sufficient protection while they act as supervisors of the educational institutions.

(ix) The Anganwadi Workers should also be involved to play an active role and should be the focal point for a number of activities and support services for the literacy programmes especially for girls.

(x) Basic education programmes such as Lok Jumbish and District Primary Education Programme have built in decentralisation as part of their management structures. The Committee desire that the local community, parents, women and local bodies should be associated in education through participation in the decentralised management structures like Village Education Committees, Parent-Teacher Associations, etc.[11]

ISSUES AND PROBLEMS OF ELEMENTARY EDUCATION

1. Less Coverage

In spite of the expansion of UEE, a large number of children especially female are outside the ambit of any educational programme. Besides, wide regional disparities exist in regard to the facilities of education at Primary and Middle School level. The policy-makers and Planners need to attend this seriously as it is a matter of great shame for the country.

2. Large Dropouts

A large number of students' dropout—the percentage reach to a great extent by Class V. This is more in case of female students. This results in wastage of resources. This need be checked.

3. Excessive and Uninteresting Curriculum

The curriculum is too much heavy that the child remains occupied with the school work both in school and at home. The curriculum is not linked with local needs and is uninteresting and devoid of skill formation. It is suggested that the curriculum need be less but interesting and related to needs.

4. Schools Lack Facilities

A school need be equipped with all the facilities like Play-grounds, lavatories, drinking water, etc. Fifth All-India Survey conducted by NCERT revealed that by 1996, drinking water was available in 46.6 per cent schools, urinals in 15 per cent schools, separate urinals for girls in 4.9 percent school, lavatory in 6.4 per cent schools and separate lavatory for girls in 2.9 per cent schools, usable conditions of playground in 34.54 per cent schools. The situation was poor in upper schools also but better than primary schools. How can a child learn without adequate facilities? It is suggested that the Government should not merely aim at expansion but should ensure full facilities to have good impact on the minds of children.

5. Lack of Supervision

It has been seen that many teachers do not attend regularly their duties. A good supervision need be made to ensure the regular functioning of schools.

Inspection of schools at all levels and at the primary level in particular is one of the weakest links in the chain. According to the findings of the Punjab Administrative Reforms Commission, the District Education Officer and other inspecting officers spend a larger part of their time in doing office work and meeting visitors than in travelling and inspecting schools. As a result, there is a constant problem of absenteeism among the teachers. There is also no monitoring of the utilization of funds provided to the schools.

Evidently, there is need to increase the number of inspection staff before monitoring can be undertaken in an effective manner and follow-up action taken where necessary. Another important issue is the lack of motivation among the teachers. Both these problems can be brought under control by involving local people in the running of the village schools. Once again, it should be emphasized that, by training teachers from rural areas and by drawing upon the communities' leadership for maintenance and management of primary schools, the state government would be able to build up a self-sufficient support and monitoring system for education at the micro-level.

6. Lack of Rapport between the School and the Community

It has been seen that School functions in isolation of the Community. The school and other educational infrastructure at District and State level need to encourage a good linkage between community especially women and school. This would help in generating extra resources from the Community. NPE, 1986 also felt this need for making the system work.

Besides, the Ministry of HRD may mobilise external resources for providing UEE. The World Conference on Education for all held in March 1990, in Jomtien, Thailand prompted the Ministry to formulate Education for all projects.

Eighth Five Year Plan suggests the following strategies:[10] (Eighth Five Year Plan (1992-97), p. 287.

The main strategy for achieving the targets would be:

(a) adoption of the decentralised approach to educational planning and management at all levels through Panchayat Raj (PR) institutions;
(b) combining this approach with a convergence model of rural development involving integrated utilisation of all possible resources available at Panchayat, Block and District level for activities relating to elementary education/literacy, child care/development, women's socio-economic empowerment and rural health programmes;
(c) large scale participation of voluntary agencies; and
(d) development of innovative and cost-effective complementary programmes including open learning system (OLS) supported by distance education techniques.

Suggestions

(i) Universal enrolment of all children, including girls and persons belonging to SC/ST;
(ii) Provision of primary school for all children within one kilometre of walking distance and of facility of non-formal education for school dropsouts working children and girls who cannot attend schools;

(iii) Improvement of ratio of primary school to upper primary school from the existing 1:4 to 1:2, this being a pre-condition for larger opportunity for widening girls participation at upper primary stage;

(iv) Reduction of dropout rates between Classes I to V and VI to VIII;

(v) Improvement of school facilities by revamped Operation Blackboard, to be extended to upper primary level also;

(vi) Achievement of minimum levels of learning by approximately all children at the primary level, and introduction of this concept at the upper primary stage on a large scale;

(vii) Local level committee, with due representation to women and teachers, to assist in the working of primary education and to oversee its functioning; and

(viii) Improvement of the monitoring system for universalisation of elementary education to see to the achievement of above mentioned goals.

SECONDARY EDUCATION

Secondary education serves as a bridge between elementary and higher education and prepares young persons between the age group of 14-18 for entry into higher education.

The impact of recent initiatives undertaken for the universalisation of elementary education is resulting in increased demand for expansion of secondary education. Unless steps are taken to expand the secondary education system, it would be difficult to accommodate the increasing number of upper primary pass-outs. While there has been an increase in the number of secondary schools, the spread has been uneven; there are regional disparities and variations in the socio-economic status of various states and Union Territories. The significant gender gap also has to be narrowed down.

The key theme in the Tenth Plan is imparting quality education at all stages of education and the pursuit of excellence. The on-going efforts in revision of curricula at the secondary education level, so as to make it more relevant, would continue in the Tenth Plan. The convergence of centrally sponsored schemes will help in imparting science, mathematics and computer education as well as environmental and value education in a more focused manner. There is a line of thinking which believes that subsidising students through a 'voucher system', as is the practice in some of the Latin American countries, is more effective than 'subsidising' institutions. The students will enrol themselves in reputed schools, letting the market forces weed out the inefficient and poor quality institutions.

Secondary Education prepares the students for future life career as the education at this level exposes the students to differentiated roles of science, the humanities and social sciences. Secondary Education Commission set-up in September 1952 under the Chairmanship of Dr. A.

Lakshmana Swami Mudaliar, suggested four aims of secondary education: (i) training of character and developing qualities essential for citizenship in a democratic social order, (ii) the improvement of vocational efficiency, (iii) personality development, and (iv) Leadership Training. There has been expansion in the field of Secondary Education.

Though a considerable degree of uniformity has been achieved in regard to common education structure of 10+2+3, there is a considerable diversity regarding the location of the +2 stage. In quite a few States it is not part of the School system.

Secondary Education is divided into two distinct sub-stages, i.e., secondary upto X Class which is the stage of general education and higher secondary (Class XI and XII) which is marked by differentiation and diversification.

Besides the Secondary Schools run by State Government, Government of India provides for different types of school systems. Let us mention briefly about them.

To provide good quality modern education to the talented children predominantly from the rural areas, Government of India have launched in 1985-86 a scheme to establish Navodaya Vidyalayas one in each district on an average.

The Central Tibetan Schools Administration was set-up as an autonomous organization in 1961 with the object to run, manage and assist institutions for the education of the children of Tibetan refugees.

Secondary and higher secondary education are important terminal stages in the system of general education because it is at these points that the youth decide on whether to pursue higher education, opt for technical training or joint the workforce. Educationists and experts have consistently recommended that education at these stages should be given a vocational bias to link it with the world of employment. The D.C. Kothari Commission, the recommendations of which form the basis of the 1968 National Policy on Education, felt that it should be possible to divert at least 50 per cent of the students completing Class X to the vocational stream, reducing the pressure on the universities and also preparing students for gainful employment. The vocational education scheme at the 10+2 stage came into existence in the late 1970s. However, only a handful of states and Union Territories took the lead in imparting vocational education.

The National Working Group on Vocationalisation Education (also known as the V.C. Kulandaiswamy Committee, 1985) reviewed the Vocational Education Programme (VEP) extensively and developed guidelines for the expansion of the programme. Its recommendations led to the initiating of the centrally sponsored scheme on vocationalisation of Secondary Education in February 1988.

The Programme of Action 12 (POA), 1992 suggests the following:

- The credibility of the programme should be established. This would depend on its quality, relevance and acceptability.

- Education-Employment linkage should be firmly established.
- Adequate infrastructure physical and academic should be provided.
- Assured supply of funds over an extended period of 5 to 10 years.
- Training programme for teachers—both pre-service and in-service.
- Training of teacher trainers.
- Effective management structures at all levels at the Centre and in the States/UTs and reasonable tenure for their functionaries.
- Equivalence among the vocational, technical and academic courses.
- Curriculum development in consultation with employers.
- Enlisting community involvement and participation of commercial establishments and industrial houses.
- Need for active co-operation of other Government Departments with the Department of Education at the Central and State level.

Vocationalisation, however, has not made much impact in practice. Krishna Jha in his article, "A Long way to Go" in *Hindustan Times* (6-2-1994) rightly mentions that "the growth of this programme was stunted from the very inception itself as there was no clear perspective about the availability of opportunities of employment or the type of expertise required for the same.

The scheme is being implemented through the state governments/ union Territory Administrations in the formal sector and non-government organisation (NGOs) in the non-formal sector. The main objectives of the scheme are to enhance individual employability, reduce the mismatch between demand and supply of skilled manpower and provide an alternative for those pursuing higher education without particular interest of purpose. During Ninth Plan, a Plan outlay of Rs. 1000 crore was provided under the scheme.

In the formal sector, the state governments implement the scheme at the +2 stage through approximately 6,700 schools. More than 150 courses are offered in six major disciplines: agriculture, business and commerce, engineering and technology, health and para medical services, home sciences and humanities. The ministry of human resource development (HRD) has taken up with the Department of Economic Affairs, in the Ministry of Finance the issue of nationalised banks and finance companies providing soft loans to help those who have completed vocational education to set-up their own enterprises.

In the non-formal sector, the scheme provides assistance to NGOs for taking up innovative programmes for promotion of vocationalisation of education on a project basis. A total of 168 NGOs have been financially assisted since the initiation of the scheme for taking up these projects which help rural unemployed youth and school dropouts.

As regards secondary education, the Committee consider it a bridge between elementary and higher education which prepares young persons between the age group of 14-18 years for entry into higher education. The Committee feel that the need for superior academic achievement is greater for girls as compared to boys, because of the prevailing socio-economic situation. The future of the girl child rests square on her educational achievements, and economic independence and are intimately linked to her educational advancement. It is no surprise that the National Policy on Education revised in 1992 *inter-alia* called for a planned expansion of secondary education facilities all over the country, higher participation of girls, SCs/STs, particularly in science vocational and commerce streams, etc. However, it is a matter of concern that there has been under-utilisation of funds allotted for Secondary Education in each of the years from 1995-96 to 1999-2000. The reasons attributed by the Department of Secondary Education and Higher Education for this, include slow utilisation of funds by State Government, delay in finalisation of Ninth Five Year Plan and delay in revision of some of the schemes. It is strange that while on the one hand experts recommend increased allocation for education, on the other hand funds earmarked for Secondary Education have remained unutilised. The Committee expect the Department of Secondary Education and Higher Education to ensure that timely action is taken to remedy the situation and ensure the proper utilisation of funds for education.

The Committee desire that adequate secondary schools be provided in the country particularly in rural, semi-urban and tribal areas. The Central School systems such as the Kendriya Vidyalaya Sangathan (KVS) and the Navodaya Vidyalaya (where one-third of the seats are reserved for girls) should be expanded. Further the National Open School (NOS) particularly for children who do not get the chance to go to the regular school system, such as, working children, children with disabilities and children from other marginalised groups such as rural youth, girls and women, SCs and STs, etc. should be strengthened.

Although education facilities have increased in recent years, yet they have not kept pace with the increasing demands of a growing population. Scarcity of resources is perhaps the main constraint in expansion of educational facilities. The people demand quantitative and qualitative improvement of education. The efforts of the Government need to be supplemented by private sector involvement and should be encouraged. The private sector can contribute not only in monetary terms but also in the form of expertise for quality improvement through effective management systems and investment in technical education. The Committee hope that the Department would explore the possibility of greater involvement of the private sector in the education system. Bureaucratic hurdles should be removed and the help of the private sector encouraged.

The Committee would like to point out that the Kothari Commission on Education (1964-66) stated that the investment on education should be gradually increased so as to reach a level of 6% of GDP. The National

Policy on education, 1986 also reiterated that the investment on education be increased to 6% of the national income against the then allocation of only 3.3%. However, it is a matter of deep concern that the current allocation for education is only 3.8% of GDP and falls far short of the target recommended by the Kothari Commission 34 years ago. The Department of Elementary Education and Literacy have admitted that in order to achieve the long cherished goal of universalisation of elementary education, there is an urgent need for increasing public expenditure on education to this level. Apparently no concrete steps have been taken by the Government all these years to step up the allocation. The Committee desire that the Planning Commission and Ministry of Finance should ensure increased allocation of funds for education in the immediate future. Further, since Education is a concurrent subject and is the joint responsibility of the Centre and the States, the States should also be associated in mobilisation of resources for achievement of the target of expenditure of 6% of GDP.[11]

India is home to the world's largest population of people aged below five years.

Approximately one quarter of the country's population comprises girls up to the age of 19 years. The developmental issues concerning women, therefore, are closely linked with the problems they face as children and adolescents. It is this crucial observation that has led India to increase its commitments towards the girl child through Constitutional provisions, policies, programmes and legislation.

India has also ratified the United Nations Convention, on the Rights of the Child (CRC), 1992. As a State party to the Convention, it submitted its first report to the UN Committee of Experts the Rights of the Child, in 1997. The policies of the Government also aim at preventing girl child labour and fulfiling the commitments made for her in the CRC.

Progress

- The enrolment of girls in elementary schools rose from 5.4 percent in 1950-51 to 5 percent in 1995-96:
  - o The National Plan of Action for the Girl Child for 1991-2000 was drawn up and Implemented as a response to the world summit on children in 1990, with 27 survival and developmental goals. The Government is implementing the National Plan of Action for meeting the objectives of the SMRC Decade of the Girl Child and so far 17 States have drawn up State Plans of Action. The plan recognises the right of the girl child to equal opportunities and to be free from hunger, illiteracy, ignorance and exploitation.
  - o Eradication of commercial and sexual exploitation of women and children.
  - o The Government participated in the drafting of the SMRC Regional Convention on Prevention and Combating

Trafficking in Women and Children Prostitution in 1998.

- o The Government has also finalised a Plan of Action for the same, and the State Governments and Union Territories Administrations have been requested to implement it.
- o The Central Advisory Committee on Child Prostitution will monitor that plan and it has also proposed that certain amendments be made to Immoral Traffic (Prevention) Act to make it more stringent and effective.
- o The Department of Women and Child Development has finalised the Government of India—UNICEF Master Plan of Operation (MPO) for that period from 1999-2002.
- o The National Policy on Education aims to include as many girl children as possible through the DPEP and through vocationalisation of education and through equal opportunities in institutions of higher and technical education. Non-Formal Education Programmes all over the country under the Balwadi programmes, address the girl child, in particular.
- o The Kasturba Gandhi Shiksha Yojana was announced in 1997 to provide State subsidies for the education of daughters.

- Innovative schemes like Lok Jumbish, Shiksha Karmi and Shiksha Samakhya especially aim the girl child.
- The DWCD has taken several initiatives for the girl child over the past decade.
- In 1992 the ICDS devised a special intervention for adolescent girls in the age-group of 11-18 years, to improve their nutritional and health status, literacy and other skills (in 507 blocks)
- Improved Healthcare for Adolescent Girls in Urban Slums Projects in Jabalpur, Madhya Pradesh, aiming to reduce morbidity and mortality Associated with reproductive health.
- The Girls' Primary Education Project (GPE) is underway in the States of Rajasthan and Uttar Pradesh. It aims to increase girls' access to education, in collaboration with local NGOs and community groups.
- The Balika Samriddhi Yojana, started in 1997, gives financial help to families below the poverty line to raise the status of the girl child.
- The DWCD and UNICEF jointly organised a National Consultative Meet on 23 September 1998, at New Delhi, as part of the run-up to the Girl Child Week from 22-26 September 1998.
- Efforts have been initiated to combat female foeticide and infanticide, for example through the Pre-Natal Diagnostics (Regulation and Prevention of Misuse) Act, 1995.
- The National Institute of Public Cooperation and Child Development (NIPCCD) is a well-known organisation concerned

with children's issues. It has undertaken several studies relevant to the Girl Child. One may mention here the studies on Girl Child in Adoption and on the Child Marriage Restraint Act.

- The National Council for Educational Research and Training (NCERT) has taken several steps to sensitise the educational system to the needs of the girl child.

Source: Progress Science, Beijing, Department of Women and Child Development, HRD, GOI, pp. 29-31.

CONCLUSION

Inspite of efforts, the number of girls per 100 boys is 77, 68, 62, 66 in Primary, Upper primary, secondary and Higher Education (Refer Table 7.5). The number of girls per 100 students in University Education is 80.1, 55.3, 46.1, 24.3 and 62% in Arts, Science, Commerce, Engineering, Medicine, respectively (Table 7.6). The number of dropouts in 1998-99 is 41.22, 60.09, 70.22 for girls in primary, upper primary and secondary education as compared to 38.62, 54.40 and 65.44 respectively for boys (Refer Table 7.7). The number of female teachers in primary, upper primary and secondary is 53.57, 50 respectively (Refer Table 7.8). Table 7.9 discuses the causes of children not attending schools.

Developing countries are committed to achieve education for all, and quality education through a decent Educational system from Pre-Primary to Higher Education, virtually within a short span of time. The base of the Pyramid of Educational system is the School education from Pre-Primary to Secondary Education. The School Education lack good administration entailing less output and low quality. Mr. Sher Singh, Former Union Minister of State for Education in his article "Education Sans Quality, Commitment" in the *Daily Tribune*, dated 18-1-1994 rightly senses that School Education in the Villages depicts a very disappointing and frustrating picture . . . there has been quantitative expansion, no doubt, but quantity without quality defeats the very purpose of education, the two have to be handled together. The need is to provide an efficient administration to manage School Education which can help in mobilisation of human and financial resources and generation of necessary changes. Educational administration reform and improvements need be carried out from time to time to keep the educational system efficient and effective.

The New Policy of Education and POA suggested the following strategy to improve education at Extending access to secondary education by setting up new schools in the unserved areas and by extending and consolidating the existing facilities, with particular emphasis on ensuring substantially increased enrolment of girls, the SCs and the STs.

- Progressively bringing in the higher secondary stage (and all its equivalents) as a part of the school system in all States.

TABLE 7.5

Number of Girls per 100 Boys Enrolled in Schools and Colleges

Year	*Primary (I-V)*	*Middle (VI-VIII)*	*Secondary (IX-X)*	*Colleges and universities for general education*
1950-51	39	18	16	11
1955-56	44	25	21	14
1960-61	48	32	23	21
1965-66	57	37	30	25
1970-71	60	41	35	27
1975-76	62	46	39	39
1979-80	62	48	41	42
1980-81	63	49	44	42
1981-82	63	49	43	46
1982-83	64	51	41	46
1983-84	64	51	43	46
1984-85	65	52	44	49
1985-86	67	54	44	51
1986-87	69	54	46	51
1987-88	69	55	47	46@
1988-89	70	55	50	46@
1989-90	70	56	50	48@
1990-91	71	58	50	50@
1991-92	72	62	52	48@
1992-93	72	61	51	50@
1993-94	76	66	57	50@
1994-95P	75	64	55	52@
1995-96P	76	64	57	56@
1996-97P	77	66	59	56@
1997-98P	77	67	60	60@
1998-99P	77	68	62	66@

P: Provisional.
@: Excludes professional, technical and special courses.
Source: Department of Education, Ministry of Human Resource Development, New Delhi.

- Formulating a National Curriculum Framework for the higher secondary stage as well as development of new curricula and instructional packages based on the semester pattern.
- Reviewing and revising the curricula of secondary education (Classes IX and X).
- Implementing a comprehensive scheme of examination reform.
- Improving considerably the physical and infrastructural facilities in secondary and higher secondary schools.
- Providing for diversity of courses in higher secondary schools.
- Reviewing afresh the existing system of pre-service teacher

TABLE 7.6

Number of Females per 100 Males in University Education in Major Disciplines

Year	Arts	Science	Commerce	Engineering	Medicine
1950-51	15.4	—	0.5	0.3	18.5
1955-56	14.9	—	0.7	0.2	18.9
1960-61	22.3	—	1.1	0.4	25.6
1965-66	36.9	—	4.9	2.2	29.4
1970-71	50.2	21.0	6.2	3.8	25.3
1975-76	44.7	27.1	9.9	5.2	22.0
1979-80	61.0	38.3	15.8	8.0	40.4
1980-81	59.7	38.9	18.5	6.8	40.4
1981-82	64.1	41.4	21.2	6.8	43.1
1982-83	63.0	41.6	22.9	6.8	46.1
1983-84	62.3	42.1	24.1	7.6	47.7
1984-85	66.8	45.8	25.9	8.6	51.4
1985-86	66.7	47.9	28.1	9.2	53.5
1986-87	65.6	47.5	29.2	8.4	43.4
1987-88P	64.5	44.3	27.9	8.6+	48.4+
1988-89P	63.9	47.t	28.5	8.6+	48.6+
1989-90P	63.3	56.8	30.0	11.9+	52.6+
1990-91P	65.5	58.3	31.6	12.2+	52.1+
1991-92P	65.3	45.7	33.8	9.5+	53.3+
1992-93P	64.7	48.0	35.9	11.9	52.4
1993-94P	64.7	49.1	36.5	12.5	57.5
1994-95P	65.5	50.1	38.9	15.1	51.2
1995-96P	70.3	56.8	40.8	16.6	52.7
1996-97P	70.7	54.2	41.4	17.4	54.8
1997-98P	70.6	55.4	44.0	20.3	56.5
1998-99P	80.1	55.3	46.1	24.3	62.1

— Not available.

\+ Only for degree level, not post-graduate..

P: Provisional.

Note: Arts and Science figures are combined for the years 1955-56, 1960-61 and 1965-66.

Source: Department of Education, Ministry of Human Resource Development, New Delhi.

education for the secondary stage and formulating and implementing an improved teacher education system.

- Institutionalising in-service teacher training.
- Transforming the role of the Boards of Secondary Education.
- Strengthening the academic institutions and bodies concerned with research and development in the areas of curriculum, instructional materials and equipment for secondary schools.[12]

TABLE 7.7

Dropout Rate (Percent) at Different Stages of School Education

Year	*Primary (I-V classes)*		*Elementary (I-VIII classes)*		*Secondary (I-X classes)*	
	Girls	*Boys*	*Girls*	*Boys*	*Girls*	*Boys*
1960-61	70.93	61.74	*	*	*	*
1965-66	70.49	63.17	*	*	*	*
1970-71	70.92	64.48	83.40	74.60	*	*
1975-76	66.18	60.21	82.80	74.30	*	*
1980-81	62.50	56.20	79.40	68.00	86.60	79.80
1981-82	57.30	51.10	77.70	68.50	86.81	79.44
1982-83	56.30	49.40	74.96	66.04	86.24	78.21
1983-84	53.96	47.83	75.27	66.10	84.79	76.41
1988-89	49.69	46.74	68.31	59.38	79.46	72.68
1989-90	50.35	46.50	68.75	61.00	77.72	70.99
1990-91	46.00	40.10	65.13	59.12	76.96	67.50
1991-92	44.30	40.30	62.40	56.10	75.87	68.55
1992-93	46.70	43.80	65.20	58.20	77.30	70.00
1993-94	38.60	36.10	63.40	58.40	75.40	69.70
1994-95P	37.79	35.18	56.53	50.02	73.78	67.15
1995-96P	41.31	37.92	61.70	54.99	74.07	66.36
1996-97P	39.37	38.35	51.89	52.77	66.82	73.04
1997-98P	41.34	38.23	58.61	50.72	72.67	67.65
1998-99P	41.22	38.62	60.09	54.40	70.22	65.44

P: Provisional.

*: Not Available.

Note: Total dropout during a course (stage) has been taken as percent of intake in the first year of the course (stage), Primary, Middle and Secondary stages consist of classes I-V, I-VIII, I-X.

Source: Department of Education, Ministry of Human Resource Development, Education in India, (Various Years).

TABLE 7.8

Number of Female Teachers per 100 Male Teachers at Different Levels of Education

Year	*Primary school*	*Middle school*	*High/higher secondary school*	*College and university*
1950-51	20	18	19	9
1955-56	20	19	23	12
1960-61	21	32	27	14
1965-66	24	30	30	16
1970-71	27	38	33	18
1975-76	29	40	36	20
1979-80	33	42	38	24

1980-81	33	42	38	24
1981-82	34	44	40	25
1982-83	34	44	40	25
1983-84	35	45	41	26
1984-85	35	46	42	29
1985-86	37	46	43	28
1986-87	38	47	44	28
1987-88	40	48	44	NA
1988-89	40	49	45	NA
1989-90	41	49	45	NA
1990-91	41	50	46	NA
1991-92	43	51	48	NA
1992-93	45	53	48	NA
1993-94	46	56	52	NA
1994-95P	45	53	51	NA
1995-96P	46	54	52	NA
1996-97P	49	56	54	NA
1997-98P	52	56	54	NA
1998-99P	53	57	50	NA

P: Provisional.
NA: Not available.
Source: Department of Education, Ministry of Human Resource Development, New Delhi.

TABLE 7.9

Reasons for Children not Attending School

Reason	*Rural*		*Urban*		*Total*	
	Male	*Female*	*Male*	*Female*	*Male*	*Female*
Main reason for never attending school						
School too far away	3.8	4.5	1.3	2.8	3.5	4.3
Transport not available	0.6	0.7	0.2	0.6	0.6	0.7
Education not considered necessary	7.8	13.1	6.1	12.9	7.6	13.1
Required for household work	6.7	15.5	4.6	9.6	6.4	14.9
Required for work on farm/family business	5.2	3.4	2.8	1.2	4.9	3.2
Required for outside work for payment in cash or kind	4.3	2.6	4.6	2.9	4.4	2.6
Costs too much	25.8	23.8	28.5	30.1	26.2	24.5
No proper school facilities for girls	0.0	2.6	0.0	1.1	0.0	2.5
Required for care of siblings	0.9	3.0	0.6	1.7	0.9	2.9
Not interested in studies	25.7	15.9	26.5	15.7	25.8	15.8
Other	17.0	12.8	21.9	18.6	17.6	13.4
Don't know	2.0	2.1	3.0	2.8	2.2	2.2
Total percent	100.0	100.0	100.0	100.0	100.0	100.0
Number of children	7081	12614	1107	1438	8188	14052
Main reason for not currently attending school						
School too far away	1.0	5.9	0.2	1.0	0.8	4.8
Transport not available	0.4	1.6	0.1	0.2	0.3	1.3

Futher education not considered necessary	2.3	4.3	2.4	5.4	2.4	4.5
Required for household work	8.7	17.3	5.7	14.7	8.0	16.7
Required for work on farm/family business	9.2	2.9	4.7	1.6	8.0	2.6
Required for outside work for payment in cash or kind	9.9	3.7	11.3	3.0	10.3	3.5
Costs too much	13.3	11.4	15.2	17.0	13.8	12.6
No proper school facilities for girls	0.0	3.5	0.0	1.2	0.0	3:0
Required for care of siblings	0.6	2.3	0.2	1.5	0.5	2.2
Not interested in studies	40.0	24.8	42.5	30.2	40.6	26.0
Repeated failures	5.3	3.7	6.0	6.1	5.5	4.2
Got married	0.2	8.5	0.1	4.9	0.2	7.7
Other	5.3	6.2	5.8	8.2	5.5	6.6
Don't know	3.8	4.0	5.7	5.1	4.2	4.2
Total percent	100.0	100.0	100.0	100.0	100.0	100.0
Number of children	5475	6121	1852	1747	7327	7868

Note: Percent distribution of children age 6-17 years who never attended school by the main reason for never attending school and percent distribution of children age 6-17 years who have dropped out of school by the main reason for not currently attending school, according to residence and sex, India, 1998-99.

1. For chidren who have never attended school.
2. For chidren who have dropped out of school.

Source: National Family Health Survey-II, 1998-99.

Notes and References

1. Lok Sabha Secretariat, Committee on Empowerment of Women (2001-02), Sixth Report, Thirteenth Lok Sabha, Education Programmes for Women, Ministry of HRD, Dec. 2001, p. 1.
2. GOI, Planning Commission, Xth Plan (Draft), 2002-07.
3. First Five Year Plan, Government of India, 1951, Chapter XXXIII.
4. Report of the Secondary Education Commissio, Government of India, 1953, Chapter IV.
5. Report of the COmmittee on Differentiation of Curricula for boys and girls, Government of India, 1954, Chapter IV.
6. Report of the University Education Commission, 1949, Government of India, Chapter 12.
7. National Policy on Education, Government of India, 1965.
8. Committee on Empowerment of Women, 2001-02, Sixth Report, 13th Lok Sabha, *op. cit.*, pp. 107.
9. Economic Survey, 2002-03, GOI, New Delhi, pp. 233-35.
10. Xth Five Year Plan Draft, *op. cit.*, p. 40.
11. Committee on Empowerment, Sixth Report, 13th Lok Sabha, *op. cit.*, pp. 26-30.
12. GOI, Planning Commission, XIth Plan (Draft), 2002-07, New Delhi, p. 23.

CHAPTER 8

HIGHER EDUCATION AND WOMEN'S DEVELOPMENT AND EMPOWERMENT

> Ensure equal access to education.
> Eradication illiteracy among women.
> Improve women's access to vocational.
> Training, science and technology, and continuing education.
>
> Develop non-discriminatory education and training.
>
> Allocate sufficient resources for and monitor the implementation of educational reforms.
>
> Promote lifelong education and training for girls and women.
>
> —*Strategic Objectives*, B.I-B.6
> Platform for Action suggests for 21st Century

Higher Education and Women's Development and Empowerment

Provision of educational opportunities for girls and women has been a part of the national endeavour since Independence. The Constitutional of India is clearly committed to the cause of education and unequivocally endorses State intervention to redress an adverse educational scenario. The Supreme Court has given the right to education, the status of a fundamental rights.

The Constitution directs the State to provide free and compulsory education to all children upto the age of 14. The Supreme Court has held that the right to education of children upto the age of 14 years is a fundamental right.

The National Policy on Education (NPE) reformulated in 1992, is committed to a "well conceived edge in favour of women." The NPE recognizes that the empowerment of women is possibly the most critical precondition for the participation of girls and women in the educational process. The consequent Programme of Action which includes Education for Women's Equality, looks at the role of education as an instrument to bring about change in the status of women. Departing from the First National Education Policy of 1968 which was committed to the provision of equal education opportunity, the NPE brought the fundamental issue of women's equality center-stage.[1]

Seventh Five Year Plan has rightly pinpointed the linkage between Education and development. To quote the Plan, "Human resources development has necessarily to be assigned a key role in any development strategy, particularly in a country with a large population. Trained and educated on sound lines, a large population can itself become an asset in accelerating economic growth and in ensuring social change in desired directions. Education develops basic skills and abilities and fosters a value

CHART 8.1

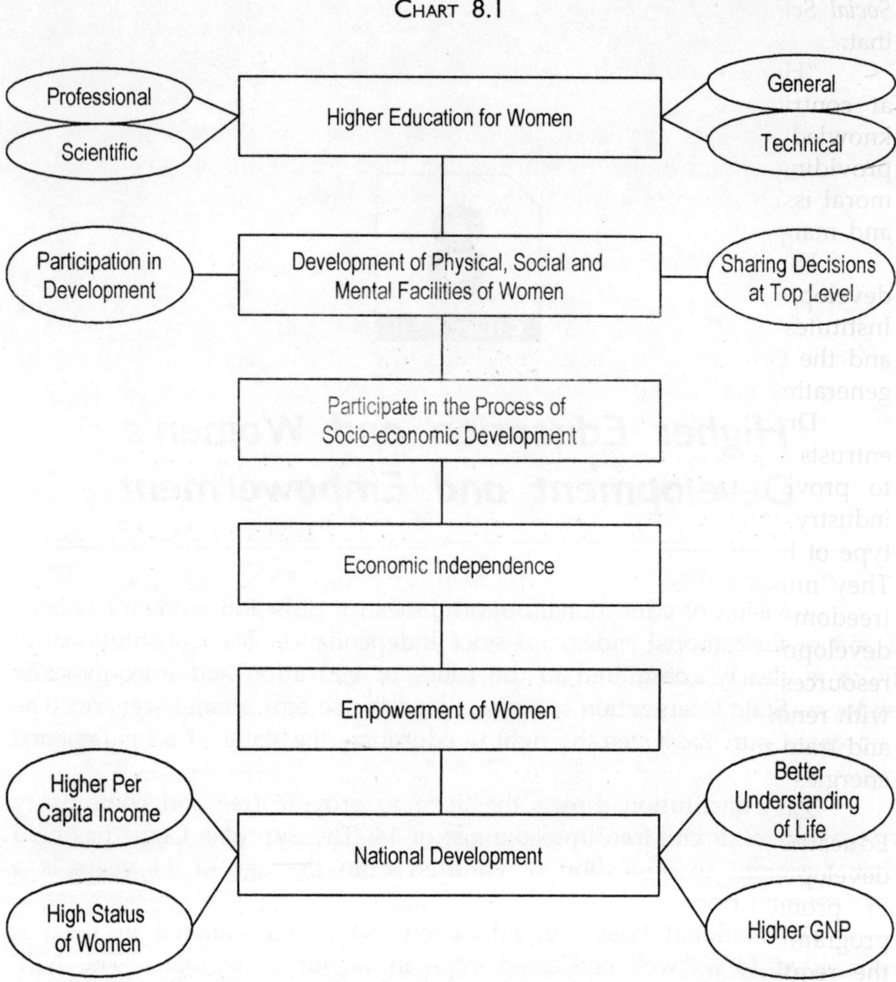

system conducive to, and is support of national development goals, both long-term and immediate. In a world where knowledge is increasing at an exponential rate, the task of education in the diffusion of new knowledge and at the same time in the preservation and promotion of what is basic to India's culture and ethos, is both complex and challenging."

"In a world based on Science and Technology, it is education that determines the level of prosperity, welfare and security of the people."

Dr. K.L. Shrimali, the then Minister of Education while addressing the First Conference of Vice-Chancellors held from 30th July to 1st August, 1957 at New Delhi, remarked, "A state, which does not finance higher education liberally undermines the very basis of civilization. Whether we look from the point of view of the cultural growth of the individual or practical necessities of social life, higher education is vital for the society."

S. Gakhar in her article "Higher Education: Some Reflections" in

Social Sciences Research Journal, Vol. 2, Nos. 1-2, July-Dec. 1993, mentions that:

"Higher Education, a sub-system of the larger societal system, aims at contributing to national development by way of dissemination of knowledge, skills and attitudes; excellence of standards of achievement; providing opportunities to reflect upon the social, political, economic and moral issues facing the country; and its key role in generating leadership and manpower resources."

Higher Education is of great significance for the all round development of a country especially a developing country like India. The Institutes of Higher Education can act as bridge between the Community and the Government. These can serve as the brain of the Government in generating creative ideas and creative people.

Dr. S. Radha Krishnan in his report to the Education Commission entrusts Universities with major responsibilities. To quote him; "They have to provide leadership in politics and administration, the professions, industry and commerce. They have to meet the increasing demand for every type of higher education Iiterary and scientific, technical and professional. They must enable the country to attain, in as short a time as possible, freedom from want, disease and ignorance, by the application and development of scientific and technical knowledge. India is rich in natural resources and her people have intelligence and energy and are throbbing with renewed life and vigour. It is for the universities to create knowledge and train minds who bring together the two-material resources and human energies."[2]

Zakir Hussain has stressed the positive relationship between Higher Education and Development, "Education is an important input for development, and towards this end the universities are the key institutions in promoting the process of national development through their programmes, of teaching, research, and extension. The universities provide the required trained and educated manpower to implement activities/ programmes relating to national development."[3]

A report on Standards of University Education published by UGC in 1965 mentions that the pursuit of liberal values should be a perennial activity. The universities have to preserve and communicate the existing knowledge and to advance the frontiers of knowledge. They should try to develop in students a modern Indian outlook which requires a reinterpretation and adaptation of our traditional values in the context of the contemporary situation. A national outlook and purpose has also to be cultivated by a deliberate pursuit of national ends in preference to local interests.

The National Policy on Education, 1986, had emphasised "Education for Women's Equality", envisaging that the National Education System would play a positive interventionist role in the empowerment of women. The National Policy on Education saw education as an agent for change in the status of women, and their empowerment as a critical pre-condition for their participation in the development process. Education must function as an equaliser in providing equality of opportunities in education so that no individual is denied access to quality education, solely on account of personal attributes or primordial identities. However, inequality of educational opportunities exists throughout the world and more so in India. The Committee therefore, desire that equal opportunities be ensured to all citizens and nothing be allowed to obstruct their path to development, particularly of the underprivileged, the disadvantaged, the disabled and women.[4]

NPE, 1986 laid special emphasis on "Education for Women's Equality." In fact, women's education was presented by the policy in the perspective of an overall strategy for securing equity and social justice. Paras 4.2 and 4.3 of the Policy in particular strongly brought out the "intervening and empowering" role of education. The parameters and strategies specifically envisaged in the Policy were:

- Gearing the entire education system to play a positive interventionist role in the empowerment of women.
- Encouraging educational institutions to take up active programmes to enhance women's status and further women's development in all sectors.
- Widening women's access to vocational, technical and professional education levels, breaking gender stereotypes.
- Creation of dynamic management structure that would respond to the challenges posed by the mandate on enhancing women's status.[5]

The POA viewed the empowering role of education in terms of several value/skill parameters—enhancing the self-esteem and self-confidence of women, building up positive image about them by due recognition of their contribution to society, polity and economy, capability to think critically, making informed choices in areas like education, employment and health including reproductive health, equal participation in developmental processes, acquisition of information, knowledge and skill for economic independence, legal literacy, etc.

ROLE OF UGC IN PROMOTING WOMEN DEVELOPMENT AND EMPOWERMENT

History

Before the University Grants Commission (UGC) was set-up, the Inter-University Board set-up by Indian Universities in 1924 served as an advisory agency. This was taken over by the University Grants Commission set-up in 1945 in response to the recommendations of the Sargent Report. Its main function was recommendatory, i.e. recommended grants of Central Universities to the Ministry of Education. The University Education

Commission (1948-49) recommended the creation of University Grants Committee with funds of its own. The Commission suggested "the first and most essential change is that the Committee shall have power to allocate grants within total limits set by the government, instead of merely recommending their allocation to the Finance Ministry which may or may not agree. In a democratic country, the decision of how much public money can be made, and ought to be made, only by the Government, it is political decision and a part of their yearly budgetary proposals. But once that decision is made, the detailed allocation of the money must be left to an expert body, not merely non-political, but as rigidly protected from politic or personal lobbying and pressure as the Constitution of the country can make them."

From a Committee, it became a Commission in 1953 through an executive order of the Government of India based upon the recommendation of the University Education Commission for the purpose of allocation and disbursement of grants to the Universities as well as for the purpose of coordination and maintenance of standards of higher education in India. With the passage of University Grants Commission Bill, 1956 of Parliament, it became a Statutory Body. C.D. Deshmukh was appointed its first Chairman.

Education must aim at breaking gender stereotypes and refashion curriculum to build a positive image of women by recognizing their contribution to society, polity and economy. It would thus facilitates the enhancement of self-esteem and self-confidence among women.

The Commission consists of the Chairman, Vice-Chairman and ten other members appointed/nominated by the Central Government. The UGC has been implementing various schemes/programmes devised for college sector through its seven Regional Offices located at Hyderabad, Pune, Bhopal, Ghaziabad, Kolkata, Guwahati and Bangalore. The UGC Regional Office at Ghaziabad, has been shifted to New Delhi and converted into Northern Region College Bureau (NRCB) of the UGC (Head Office).

The main objective in the Tenth Plan is to raise the enrolment of women in higher education of the 18-23 year age group from the present 6 percent to 10 percent by the end of the Plan period. The strategies would focus on increasing access, quality, adoption of state-specific strategies and the liberalization of the higher education system. Emphasis would also be laid on the relevance of the curriculum, vocationalization, and networking on the use of information technology. The Plan would focus on distance education, convergence of formal, non-formal, distance and IT education institutions, increased private participation in the management of colleges and deemed to be universities; research in frontier areas of knowledge and meeting challenges in the area of Internationalization of Indian education.[7]

The UGC, the apex body responsible for the development of higher education in the country, has been providing financial assistance to all eligible central, state and deemed universities, both under Plan and non-Plan heads, for improving infrastructure and basic facilities. The grants-in-aid would be used for setting up central universities especially in states that do not have one, more autonomous colleges and providing support to private colleges. Attempt would be made to ensure that the socially, economically and geographically disadvantaged sections are able to access higher education. To encourage more women to pursue higher studies, the number of counselling/study centers, day care centers for children and hostels will be increased during the Tenth Plan. Similar steps will be taken for scheduled castes/scheduled tribes (SCs/STs) students and minorities. Besides, the activities of distance/open universities will be supported to increase access for the north-eastern and backward areas.

FACILITIES BY UGC FOR WOMEN IN HIGHER EDUCATION

1. Introduction of Technological Courses for Women in Universities[6]

During Ninth Plan period, the Commission has introduced a new scheme, "Technological Courses for Women in Women Universities" with an objective to provide an opportunity for women in areas perceived to be prestigious and lucrative and also to reduce gender imbalance in the sphere of Engineering and/Technology. Under the scheme, the UGC has been providing financial assistance for introduction of Under Graduate (UG) Courses in emerging areas under Engineering and Technology under recurring and non-recurring items for a period of years from the date of implementation of the course.

During the Ninth Plan period, the Commission considered the proposals of three Universities under the above scheme viz. (i) S.P. Mahila Visvavidyalayam, Tirupati, (ii) Avinashilingam Institute for Home Science, Coimbatore, and (iii) SNDT Women's University, Mumbai, out of which the Commission approved the proposal of SNDT Women's University for establishment of Department of Technology with the following three courses:

(i) B.E. (Electronics and Communication)
(ii) B.E. (Computer Science)
(iii) B.E. (Information Technology)

The grant released so far to the SNDT Women's University for the Department of Technology is as under Table 8.1

In the Tenth Plan proposals formulated by the Commission, it has been decided that the technological courses for women universities may be extended to all the Universities and has formulated a new scheme 'Promotion of Professional Education for Women'. Even Xth Plan is devoting more attention to vocationalisation.

The UGC propose to promote quality and relevance in higher education in the Tenth Plan by initiating complementary skill-oriented courses. The career development of students will be promoted through courses with a professional focus. A major programme of vocationalisation

TABLE 8.1

Grants Released

(Rs. in lakh)

Year	*Allocation*	*Grants released*
1997-98	100.00	Nil
1998-99	100.00	94.00
1999-2000	100.00	200.00*
Total	300.00	294.00

* The excess amount released was adjusted within the overall allocation.
No grant was provided under the scheme during the year 2000-01 and 2001-02.
Source: Annual Report UGC, 2001-02, p. 294.

of education has already been initiated in 35 subjects at the under-graduate level. In the Tenth Plan, new courses including vocational courses, relating emerging areas such as information technology, biotechnology, biomedicine, genetic engineering, applied psychology, tourism and travel, physical education and sports would be introduced in more and more universities. The UGC has been continuously updating curriculum and the process has been completed in 30 subjects in different disciplines. The Administrative Staff Colleges (ASCs) have proved to be good instruments for teacher training and orientation. Many courses in these ASC's is run in the area of Women Studies. Efforts will be made to widen and enhance the range and scope of ASCs and set-up more ASCs to achieve a uniform regional spread. Steps have been taken from time to time for making accreditation of institutions mandatory.

2. Special Scheme for Construction of Women's Hostels

With a view to increase enrolment by providing a safe environment and to encourage the mobility of women students to pursue higher education in the universities and colleges of their choice, the Commission introduced a special scheme during the latter half of the Eighth Plan period for the construction of women's hostels. It has been decided to continue this scheme during the Ninth Plan period also. Although the scheme is very much in demand, it was not possible to increase the amount to provide more accommodation in each hostel due to shortage of funds. Therefore, the colleges/universities and deemed universities provided assistance limited to 60 per cent of the total cost of the hostel and subject to ceilings give below: (Table 8.2)

The Commission has made slight modification in its norms concerning this scheme giving relaxation of Women's enrolment by 10% to all of those Universities and Colleges located in tribal, hilly and border areas (State Government notified for the purpose) all over the country.

TABLE 8.2

Hostels

(Rs. in Lakhs)

Women's Enrolment	*Amount*
(a) Up to 250	7.00
(b) 251 to 500	10.00
(c) More than 500	15.00

Source: Annual Report of UGC, 2001-02, p. 295.

During the year 2001-02, two eligible State Universities were provided part grants under the scheme amounting to Rs. 17.25 lakhs, the UGC released grants amounting to Rs. 29.95 lakhs to Universities, Rs. 320.37 lakhs to Colleges (by Head Office) and Rs. 803.04 lakhs to affiliated colleges (by Regional Offices).

3. Promotion of Studies on Women in Universities and Colleges

The UGC programme for promotion of Women's Studies envisages financial assistance to universities and colleges for setting up centres and cells for Women's Studies. The Centres/Cells are required to undertake research, develop curricula and organize training and extension work in the areas of gender equity, economic self-reliance of women, girls' education, population issues, issues of human rights, social exploitation, etc. These activities are expected to contribute not only to social awareness and change but also to academic development. However, the Women's Studies Centres are not expected to be like other conventional departments of university, in that they are not required to run courses that lead to an undergraduate or postgraduate degrees, although they could do so.

Under the Programme, the UGC set-up Women's Studies Centres in 34 universities (21 old Women Studies Centres continuing from Seventh Plan and 13 new Centres approved during Ninth Plan). These Studies Centres are only established in such universities which come under the purview of the UGC Act, 1956 and these are only beneficiary institutions. No college was considered for setting up Studies Centres during Ninth Plan.

The UGC allocated an amount of Rs. 1.00 crore for the promotion of women's Studies for the year 2001-02. A total grant of Rs. 97.62 lakhs was released to the existing study centres from 1.4.2001 to 31.3.2002 for carrying out their activities/programmes and salary of project staff appointed on contractual basis.

A. Kalpana in her article, "Women's Studies Programmes and Higher Education" in *University News* (Dec. 21, 1998) states that the general query from most people would be what would a department devoted to women's studies in an university do. It is an extension of home science or does it have a distinct role and obligation? What is the benefit of having such a department when most women-related issues and dealt with, by various government and non-government agencies? The role of the women's studies department is to conduct research and teaching in all areas pertaining to women, society and their inter-relationship. The department is also expected to attempt to understand the nature of oppression and subjugation undergone by women in the contemporary society. Women's studies programmes should help women to learn to feel for themselves and understand their role in society. It should explicate women's contribution to the social processes; evaluate women's perception of their own lives in the broader social perspective; and explain the role and status of women in various social, economic, political, legal, educational and historical processes. A good women's studies programme should help raise questions from faculty as well as students pertaining to the role and status of women.

The University Grants Commission in their Policy frame on higher education recognized extension as the third dimension of the institutions of Higher Education, in addition to the earlier two-fold dimensions of Teaching and Research in the following words. "If the University system has to discharge adequately its responsibility to the entire education systems and to the society as a whole, it must assume extension as the third important responsibility and give it the same status as research and teaching. This is a new extremely significant area which should be developed on the basis of high priority.

Women's studies programmes has 4 dimensions—teaching, research, training and extension. In teaching, the following activities can be taken up:

(i) Incorporation of issues relating to women's status and role in the foundation course proposed to be introduced by University Grants Commission for all undergraduate students;
(ii) Incorporation of the women's dimension into courses in different disciplines;
(iii) Elimination of sexist bias and sex stereo-types from text books.
(iv) To expand the concept, theoretical perspectives and practical application of gender issues through women study centers based on interdisciplinary approach.
(v) Identify social, political, educational and economic resources that enhance the self-respect and confidence among women and remove obstacles like violence, etc.
(vi) Identify social and historical reasons biases and prejudices that interfere with growth and development of a gender just society and make efforts to remove them.
(vii) To develop a resource center through documentation of new researches and other references materials on women to disseminate information on these issues.
(viii) Highlighting women's contribution in the developmental process and convince policy-making authorities to provide more resources to women development.

(ix) To establish and strengthen networking among governmental and non-governmental agencies with the center for women studies concerned with women's issues and development.

(x) Strengthening UGC study centres.

(xi) Women Study centres can promote the following:
- Creating mass awareness about women's rights,
- Motivational campaign about women's health and education,
- Involvement of women in their own welfare,
- Preparation of material for girls for personality development, developing self-confidence and vocational training, etc., and
- The university can undertake monitoring programme for various activities relating to women's studies and women's movement run by Government Agencies, PRI system and voluntary organization and find out the strengths and weakness of the programme and can suggest to concerned agency for better implementation of women's movements.

Under research, the following steps can be taken:

(i) Encouraging research on identified areas and subjects which are crucial in advancing knowledge in this area and to expand the information base.

(ii) Critical appraisal of existing tools and techniques which have been responsible for the disadvantages suffered by them and where necessary reformation of research methodology.

(iii) To create awareness, knowledge, problems, and sensitivity in the society about the problems and issues affecting women, especially women from underprivileged sections of society.

(iv) To publish pamphlets for women attending these programmes.

(v) Suggesting the UGC policy actions to restore women's status.

(vi) UGC Researches conducted by different study centres may be consolidated.

The following measures can be taken under training:

(i) Dissemination of information and interaction through seminars/workshops on the need for Women's Studies and its role in University education.

(ii) Orientation of teachers and researches to handle women-related topics and to incorporate women's dimension into general topics.

(iii) Workshops for restructuring the curriculum.

(iv) Involving women of the Area.

(v) UGC should engage itself in training women of PRIS through colleges and universities.

Under extension, we need to encourage educational institutions to take up programmes which directly benefit the community and bring about the empowerment of women.

These would include actual implementation of development programmes directly aimed at women's empowerment such as adult education, awareness building, legal literacy, informational and training support for socio-economic programmes of women's development, media, etc. For this UGC may make a scheme to involve colleges and universities in a well-planned manner to provide extension services. UGC is also funding Adult Education Department in universities, Women Studies Centre can take the help of Adult Education Programmes.

4. Growth in Enrolment of Women in Higher Education

There has been a phenomenal growth in the number of women students enrolled in higher education, since independence. Women enrolment was less than 10 per cent of the total enrolment on the eve of Independence and it rose to 39.84 per cent in 2001-02.

The pace of growth has been particularly faster in the last two decades. As the data in Table 8.3 show that the number of women enrolled per hundred men registered a five-fold increase during the period 1950-51 to 2001-02.

TABLE 8.3

Women Students Per Hundred Men Students

Year	*Total Women Enrolment (000's)*	*Enrolment Per Hundred Men*
1950-51	40	14
2001-02	3514	66

5. Distribution of Women Enrolment by State, Stage and Faculty

(a) State-wise Distribution of Women Enrolment

Distribution of women enrolment by state shows that there has been a marginal increase of 2.19% in the enrolment of women as a percentage of total enrolment in all the states during 2001-02 over the preceding year. Among the states, Kerala with 60% topped in terms of women enrolment as a percentage of total enrolment in 2001-02, followed by Goa (58.6%), Punjab (52.9%), etc. There were 18 states which had higher enrolment of women than the national percentage of 39.84 per cent. In the rest of the states, the percentage of women enrolled was less than the national level, with Bihar recording the lowest women enrolment of 23.0 per cent only.

(b) Distribution of Women Enrolment by Stage of Education

During the decennial period 1992-93 to 2001-02, the enrolment of women as a percentage of total enrolment has been consistently going up at all stages of education—Graduate, Post-graduate, etc. (Table 8.4)

A noteworthy of women enrolment is that their incidence is the highest at the Post-graduate level as compared to other levels.

TABLE 8.4

Stage-wise Percentage of Women Enrolment to Total Enrolment

Year/Stage	*Graduate*	*Post-Graduate*	*Research*	*Diploma/ Certificate*
1992-93	33.0	34.9	37.4	26.0
2001-02*	40.9	42.2	38.9	35.8

* Provisional.

Source: Annual Report of UGC, 2001-02, p. 298.

(c) Distribution of Women Enrolment by Faculty

The faculty-wise distribution of women enrolment during 2001-02 is as given in Table 8.5.

Table 8.5 shows that women enrolment in the Faculty of Arts has been 51.79 per cent of total women enrolment, followed by the faculty of Science (19.90%), the faculty of Commerce (16.56%), etc. There was no much change in the percentage of women enrolled in any faculty in 2001-02 as compared to 2000-01.

TABLE 8.5

Women Enrolment by Faculty: 2001-02

Sl. No.	*Faculty*	*Enrolment**	*Percentage*
1.	Art	18,20,134	51.79
2.	Science	6,99,376	19.90
3.	Commerce/Management	5,81,993	16.56
4.	Education	59,394	1.69
5.	Engineering/Technology	1,31,792	3.75
6.	Medicine	1,23,006	3.50
7.	Agriculture	9,137	0.26
8.	Veterinary Science	3,163	0.09
9.	Law	56,934	1.62
10.	Others	29,521	0.84
	Total	35,14,450	100.00

Source: *Ibid.*

CHART 8.2

Distribution of Men and Women Enrolment in Universities and Colleges: 2000-01

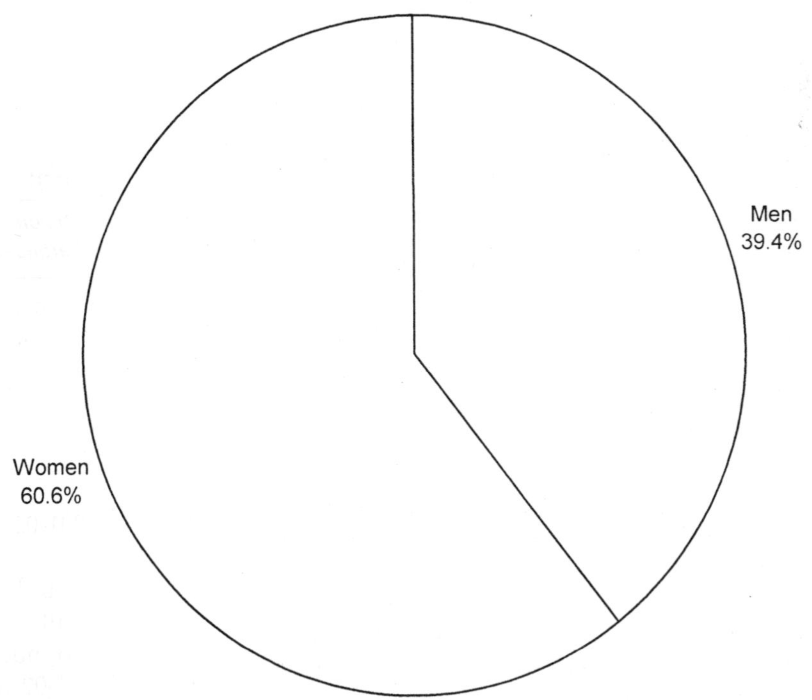

Source: UGC.

6. Women Colleges

The number of women colleges, as shown in Table 8.6 shows that there has been a substantial increase during the last decade, i.e. 1992-93 to 2001-02 and thus resulting in increase of women enrolment as a whole.

7. Cells to Combat Sexual Harassment

In addition to the above, the UGC has issued two circulars dated 30.5.2001 and 2.5.2002 to all the Indian Universities to set-up a permanent cell in each university for combating sexual harassment to women in the university campus as per the directives of the Supreme Court of India. Only 20 universities have so far informed the UGC that they have constituted a permanent cell in the university and rest of the universities have been reminded to set-up such a cell to combat on the issues of violence and sexual harassment against women in the university campuses.

8. Part-time Research Associateships for Women

The scheme of Part-time Research Associateship for Women is

TABLE 8.6

Number of Women Colleges during 1992-1993 to 2001-02

Year	*Number of Women Colleges*
1992-93	994
1993-94	1033
1994-95	1107
1995-96	1146
1996-97	1195
1997-98	1260
1998-99	1359
1999-2000	1503
2000-01	1578
2001-02	*1600

Source: *Ibid*., p. 299.

intended to provide opportunities to the women, who are employed or unemployed, to take up research work in Humanities including Languages, Social Sciences, Sciences, and Engineering and Technology independently and on project basis. The duration of the associateship is five years with no further extension.

The Part-time Research Associateship for Women existed in Eighth Plan. The scheme was revised in the Ninth Plan with certain modifications. Earlier, the scheme was meant only for unemployed women. The revised scheme is opened to unemployed as well as employed women. Under the revised scheme, selections were made in the year 1999. The scheme is suspended for the time being.

No physical target was set for this scheme as well. During the first selection in the year 1999, 165 candidates were selected and 162 are working at present. During 2001-02, an amount of Rs. 135.32 lakhs was released from the allocated budget of Rs. 150.00 lakhs. The year-wise position of release of grants to Part-time Women Research Associates during the Ninth Plan period is as shown in the Table 8.7.

9. Day Care Centres in Universities

Under the scheme, day care facilities are provided at the campuses for children of three months to six years age group, whose parents (university employees/students/researchers) are away from home for the day. During the year 2001-02, grants amounting to Rs. 12.00 lakhs were released to six State Universities and Rs. 6.00 lakhs to three Deemed to be Universities.

TABLE 8.7

(Rs. in Lakhs)

Year Grants	*Released*
1997-98	160.39
1998-99	190.62
1999-2000	129.26
2000-01	137.50
2001-02	135.32
Total	753.09

ISSUES AND PROBLEMS

1. Women Study Centers are Located in most of the Universities in Metropolitan and Semi-metropolition Cities

Need of setting up women study centers in universities in rural areas. The women in urban areas are mostly educated and understand about women's issues and how to pursue them. The study centres in Chandigarh, Bombay, Delhi serve limited purpose. There is a need of setting up study centres by UGC in rural universities like Bhagalpur, Chitterkut, Dharbhanga, where women do not know a fringe of their rights. These centres would be very near the women who need them. UGC, in Xth Plan should set-up new centres in rural areas, tribal areas, backward areas to make the maximum impact.

2. Lack of Clear-cut Objective

Need of defining in details the objectives. Women study centers must have clearly spelt out objectives, functions, and targets and not leave the matter to the discretion of study centres. These centres are a basic necessity for rural areas. We must set-up new centres or even transfer some of the centres from urban to rural areas. Women faculty members appointed to head these centres. Different centres work differently to suit their purposes. There is a need to spell out guidelines so that comparative studies can be made. A little bit flexibility may be allowed to suit the area. UGC at headquarter must draw a blue print for these women study centres in detail with the help of experts from Department of Women and Child Development, National Council for Women, etc. After this, training may be imparted to all the heads of these study centres so that they understand the rationale, Philosophy and purpose of these centres. The UGC headquarter may design a performa through which monitoring can be done and through this exercise, centres not performing well may be advised accordingly.

CHART 8.3

Number of Total Colleges and Women Colleges in the Country since 1980-51

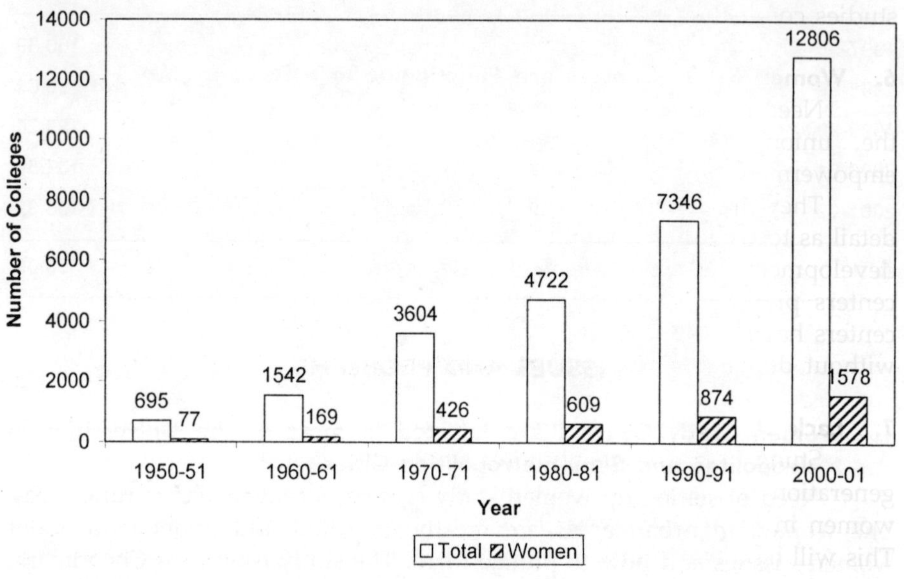

Source: *Ibid.*

3. **The Heads of Study Centers are mostly Engaged in Building a Self-image by Inviting Influential Ladies to Preside over the Functions in Selected Gathering of well-off Women, i.e. who are already Empowered: Need of Fresh Thinking**

Prominent ladies invited add to the grace of the occasion but are a great burden on UGC as they travel by Air and need excellent arrangements. In addition, they are nothing to give through their example. They cannot motivate the women. There is a need to invite such women who are self-made and really respect and honour the problems faced by other women. A discussion with the Vice-Chancellors and Registrars revealed that the heads do of these centers have made an exchange programme to enjoy holidaying. If one head of a women study center visits another, the clearance of UGC must be mandatory.

4. **Courses conducted through Academic Staff Colleges or by the Center directly do not result in Multiplier Effect as the Topics are Repeatedly the same and Teachers as Students are Non-receptive**

Need of making the course attractive. The course should be made interesting. The topic is changed to suit the speaker and not *vice-versa* causing disinterestedness among participants. A field visit can create enthusiasm and make the participants understand the trend issues.

5. Lack of Co-ordination: Need of Linkages

There is no coordination between UGC, National Council for Women, Department of Women and Child Development resulting in duplication and over-lapping. UGC can get the money from NCW for getting the research studies conducted through their women study centers.

6. Women Study Centers are Functioning in a Routine Way

Need to develop innovative methods which may be path breaking for the union and state governments in women development and empowerment.

They are repeating what all others are doing. UGC may enquire in detail as to what has been the contribution of these centers towards women development and empowerment. As a member of UGC, my visit to these centers presented a pathetic outlook as some women incharge of these centers have made it their monopoly. They are arranging the programme without doing any cost benefit analysis.

7. Lack of Interest of Women Study Centers

Study centers in training, capacity building and awareness generation to women elected in PRI system. Need of building through women in villages training. This will strengthen rural local environment. This will be a real contribution of women study centers of UGC. Ten years have elapsed when seats were reserved for women in PRIS but still they lack competence and confidence.

8. Lack of Monitoring

UGC should exercise effective monitoring of the Women Study Centers after giving them a clear cut policy and plan with some local flexibility.

Monitoring should not be done in a hurry by UGC officials. It should be got done by chairperson of center of UGC of these centers with some other eminent scholars in depth. If they find irregularities, women managing these centres must be changed. At present, university authorities are appointing them resulting into the patronage to the Vice-Chancellor. UGC should use this prerogative and appoint the women teaching staff in universities. There is a need of some change as at present as many of them are working for the last 10-15 years.

9. Need for Multi-disciplinary Approach

As has been recommended in Beijing Conference in 1995, women issues should be integrated in all discipline (areas relevant to that discipline). It would be better if we take up 12 areas identified by Beijing conference.

10. Need for Centres of Excellence

UGC may give more grants to girls colleges and declare some of them doing excellent work as colleges of excellence. They may be given extra financial resources.

11. Need for Affirmative Action

Universities may be encouraged to give preference to women candidates whether it may be the case of admission or appointment or scholarship.

12. Women as Decision-makers

UGC should appoint women on search panels to select Vice-Chancellor so that they can recommend the names of women Vice-Chancellors whose number is negligible.

UGC should associate more and more women as experts in all the areas of activities under the purview of UGC.

Central universities had not women Vice-Chancellors which is within the purview of Union Government. It is a strange matter. UGC should send letters to Chancellors describing them the real facts about Vice-Chancellors and request them to encourage women Vice-Chancellors.

In UGC, if the Chairman is a man, then Vice-Chairman must be a woman or *vice-versa*.

Sneha Joshi and Pushpandham K. in their Article,[8] "Empowering Women for Educational Management" in *University News*, January 22,2001 rightly discuss that we need to deliberate on how to ensure adequate representation of women in positions of leadership in education? What changes in policies and professional training may be required to attract and retain women in educational leadership positions.

The following are the suggestions to altar the prevailing situation and as responses to the questions raised above:

- Promoting the advocacy concerning the access of women to higher education and their participation in management.
- Establishing and promoting gender management systems at national levels to main stream gender into national sectorial policies by increasing capacity in gender training and gender policy appraisal.
- Considering women's rights as human rights, elimination of violence against women, protection of the girl child and outlawing of all forms of trafficking in women and girls.
- There is a need to make special provisions for women with young children at the work place especially regarding time. This would require that we openly acknowledge and help women combine having a baby with their career.
- Recent advancement of information technology, be it the cordless telephone, computer, fax machine, e-mail or paging, has freed the executive from having to be confined to the office for operational purposes. Women manages with children could operate from the home. Real productivity has to be measured. And not the time spent in the office. Flexible office hours may become the order of the future.

- There is a need for scientific and systematic career planning and career advancement policy that will enable aspiring, committed and qualified women to rise to top positions in their career without any discrimination against them on the basis of gender. The prevailing perception is that women's commitment to careers is not taken seriously by many. A reversal of this mindset will be brought about only when the numerical strength of career women in the country goes up in the years to come.
- There is a need to encourage young career women to be more mobile rather than remain in the first job that they land in. In order to quickly rise in the hierarchical ladder one needs to move quite a bit, at least initially.

13. Poor Linkage between Education and Modernization: Need of Developing Linkages

Modernization aims at creating an environment of socio-economic development wherein all people can enjoy a decent standard of living. This is in addition to spiritual values and self-discipline. Education Commission (1964-66) has rightly said that, "The most important and urgent reform needed in education is to transform it, to endeavour to relate it to the life, needs and aspirations of the people and thereby make it a powerful instrument of social, economic and cultural transformation necessary for the realization of the national goals. For the purpose, education should be developed so as to increase productivity, achieve social and national integration, accelerate the process of modernization and cultivate social, moral and spiritual values."

The self-reliant and indigenous character of an economy can only be maintained when competent people are available to foresee, plan and execute research and development activity, necessary to keep India abreast of developments elsewhere in the world. (Challenge of Education, p. 34)

It is a paradoxical situation that on the one hand there are large number of educated people without any job while on the other hand, there are many jobs without suitable manpower. The report of the Education Commission (1964-66) laid stress on this aspect in the following words:

"Quantitatively, education can be organized to promote social justice or to retard it. History shows numerous instances where small social groups and elites have used education as a prerogative of their rule and as a tool for maintaining their hegemony and perpetuating the values upon which it has rested. On the other hand, there are cases in which a social and cultural revolution has been brought about in a system where equality of educational opportunities is provided and education is deliberately used to develop more and more potential talent and to harness it to the solution of national problems. The same is even more true of the quality of education. A system of university education which produces a high proportion of competent professional manpower is of great assistance in increasing productivity and promoting economic growth. Another system of higher education with the same total output but producing a large proportion of indifferently educated graduates of arts, many of whom remains unemployed or even reemployable, could create, social tension and read economic growth. It is only the right type of education, provided on an adequate scale that can lead to national development; when these conditions are not satisfied the opposite effect may result."

An Enlightened Woman is a source of infinite strength: "Sanskrita Sri Prashakti" Shikha Misra and Subhash C. Agarwal in their article, "Gender Sensitivity and Barriers in Education—An Overview" in *University News*, January 19, 1998 observes that although much has been achieved, much still remains to be done. Significant inroads have been made in field as diverse as aviation and academics, politics and entrepreneurship, yet all around the world and especially in developing countries, the statistics are truly horrifying. Girls are aborted or killed as infants and the surviving few grow up in an atmosphere of neglect and abuse. Of the 100 millions children worldwide between the ages of 6 and 11 who do not attend school, 70% are girls. Of the one billion illiterate adults an estimated two-third are women. Under these circumstances the importance of education for women cannot be over-emphasized. It is the first but an essential step towards rehabilitating, restoring and equalizing step towards rehabilitating, restoring and equalizing the power balances for women who for centuries have been forced to be submissive and docile to whimsical and irrational laws of patriarchal authority. Traditional behavioural patterns today are in a state of flux all over the world. We, in India, have to emerge from the old system of rigid social stratification and become part of a new order in which social status is based on personal achievement. The stringent criteria of age, sex, family membership must of necessity lose their weight in determining a person's place and her treatment in society. The need of the times is greater freedom for the women and her assessment on personal merit—or in the words immortalized in the constitution of India, "prohibition of discrimination on grounds of religion, race, caste, sex or place of birth."

H. Kalpana in her Article, "Women's Studies Programmes and Higher Education in University", Dec. 21, 1998—The general query from most people would be what would a department devoted to women's studies in an university do. Is it an extension of home science or does it have a distinct role and obligation? What is the benefit of having such a department when most women-related issues are dealt with, by various government and non-government agencies? The role of the women's studies department is to conduct research and teaching in all areas pertaining to women, society and their inter-relationship. The department is also expected to attempt to understand the nature of oppression and subjugation undergone by women in the contemporary society. Women's studies programmes should help women to learn to feel for themselves and understand their role in society. It should explicate women's contribution to the social processes; evaluate women's perception of their own lives in the broader social perspective; and explain the role and status of women in various social, economic, political, legal, educational and historical processes. A good women's studies programme should help raise questions from faculty as well as students pertaining to the role and status of women.

Though there have been achievements but the success of the WSCs have been very limited. Some of the hindering factors are:

- Status and position of the Director.
- Selection of Directors left to Vice-Chancellor.
- Lack of dedication and Enthusiasm.
- Too small faculty to be viable and ensure full justice
- Provision of very meager resources to provide extension services.
- Lack of monitoring by the UGC as no guidelines have been issued under which these function.
- Lack of autonomy and accountability for the centers.
- Lack of understanding and support from the university authorities about these centres.
- No interest among other departments in the university as they consider it superflous.
- Vested interest created in arranging its activities.
- No original research has been done.
- Stationery wasted through publishing useless material.
- No expect involved during teaching. Only favourite are considered a special privilege prompted and not a duty.

What is needed is that UGC should take a serious note of these centres as these are consuming money and time. It is high time to ensure that these centres run efficiently and the UGC should provide leadership to strengthen women services along with Union and State Government agencies. UGC can show the way to Government improve the status of women through its many schemes and women study centres.

IMPLICATIONS AND SUGGESTIONS

NPE claims that "Education will be used as an agent of basic change in the status of women in order to neutralize the accumulated distortions of the past." While the objective is laudable, mere rhetoric will not yield the desired results. Mere quantitative expansion by setting up new colleges without concern for the quality and type of courses offered will not lead to the achievement of the goal of empowerment or raising the status of women. Some of the emerging policy implications and suggestion are:

- Priority and funding to be made available for starting science courses, courses in emerging areas, vocational courses in women's colleges;
- Adequate funding to be allocated for providing and expanding

hostel facilities for women students, especially in rural and backward areas;

- Principals of both co-educational and women's colleges need to be sensitized and trained for creating a gender positive climate in colleges and initiate activities for capacity building and empowerment of women students;
- Teachers, both men and women, to be oriented towards the special needs of women students and trained to incorporate measures for empowering women students;
- Foundation course incorporating women's issues to be made mandatory for all undergraduate students;
- Curriculum in all subject to be revised to include women's issues;
- Women's studies centers to be strengthened for undertaking relevant research, training, extension, curriculum development, developing teaching materials, documentation and publications. In brief, to act as resource centres for women's development;
- Colleges to be networked with women's study centres who should provide consultancy and guidance in setting up women's cells of counselling programmes in colleges;
- Organize legal education and other life skill and capacity building programmes for women students in colleges; and
- Provide special funding for promoting these gender positive initiatives in colleges.

Distance Education

Keeping in mind the declaration of SAARC Decade of Girls Child, greater thrust was given to the introduction of open school, distance education system and other innovative educational programmes, especially for girls in rural/remote areas and urban slums. It has been observed that a large number of girls are beneficiaries of correspondence courses and also appear as private students.

Technical Education

During the past five decades, there has been a phenomenal expansion of technical education facilities in the country since technical education is considered one of the significant components of human resource development.

Polytechnic Education

Participation of women students in polytechnics was one of the thrust areas under the World Bank assisted Technical Education Project, which was implemented in two phases, Tech. Ed. I and Tech Ed. II in 19 states and UTs Women's participation has grown considerably in polytechnics from 11 per cent in 1990 to 29 per cent in 1999. During the year 1998-99, 60,104 girls were enrolled in polytechnic institutes of different states and UTs, as against 2,97,070 boys. All the boys' polytechnics have been converted into co-educational polytechnics. Besides, in existing and new Women Polytechnics, 9,535 additional seats have been created for girls and additional hostels to accommodate 7085 girls have been provided.

Community Polytechnics

The scheme of Community Polytechnics is aimed at bringing community rural development through science and technology applications and through skill-oriented non-formal training focused on women, minorities, SC/ST/OBCs and other disadvantaged sections of the society. Since the inception of the scheme, i.e. from 1978-79, about 9 lakh persons have been trained in various job-oriented skills. As per the study conducted by Technical Teachers' Training Institutes in 1996-97, it was estimated that 43 per cent of the total beneficiaries were women. As in April 2000, there were seven degree-level institutions and 116 diploma-level technical institutions in the country exclusively for women.

Initiatives of All India Council for Technical Education

All India Council for Technical Education (AICTE) has constituted a Board on Women Participation in Technical Education for developing strategies to induct more women in technical education. Special incentives like scholarships, stipends, etc. are to be provided to attract women in professional education.

Mahila Samakhya

Provision of educational opportunities for women has been an important part of the national endeavour in the field of education since independence. Though there have been some significant results, however, gender disparities continue to persist with uncompromising tenacity, more so in rural areas and among disadvantaged communities. The National Policy on Education, 1986 (as revised in 1992) is landmark in the field of policy on women's education in that it recognises the need to redress traditional gender imbalances in educational access and achievement. It was decided that education would be used as an agent of basic change in the status of women. the Mahila Samakhya (MS) programme was started in 1989 with Dutch assistance to translate the goals mentioned in the NPE into action. The MS programme recognises the centrality of education in empowering women to achieve equality. Mahila Samakhya has adopted an innovative approach which emphasises the process rather than mere fulfilment of targets. It seeks to bring about a change in women's perception about themselves and the perception of society with regard to women's traditional roles. Under this programme, education is understood as a process of learning to question, critically analysing issues and problems and seeking solutions. The Mahila Sanghas endeavour to create an environment for women to learn at their own pace, set their own priorities and seek knowledge and information to make informed choices. This involves enabling women (especially from socially and economically disadvantaged and marginalised groups) to address and deal with problems of isolation and lack of self-confidence, oppressive social customs and struggle for survival, all of which inhibit their learning. It is in this process that women become empowered. The Mahila Sanghas in all the states have taken initiatives to address issues/problems ranging from—

- Meeting daily minimum needs;
- Improving civic amenities;
- Gaining control over their health;
- Actively accessing and controlling resources;
- Ensuring Educational opportunities for their children, especially girls;
- Entering the political sphere through participation in Panchayats, etc.;
- Articulating their concerns and tackling social issues like violence against women, child marriage; and
- Seeking and obtaining literacy and numeracy skills.

The Mahila Samakhya Programme helps to provide a greater access to education; forge links between teachers and the Mahila Sanghas; provide specialised inputs for vocational and skill development; for strengthening women's abilities to effectively participate in village-level educational processes.

Several evaluation studies have shown that the MS programmes has:

- Helped generate a demand for literacy;
- Increased women's recognition and visibility, both within the family and the community;
- Given women the strength and ability to demand accountability from Government delivery systems;
- Increased women's participation in Panchayati Raj bodies; and
- Created an awareness of the need to struggle for a gender-just society.

The Committee would like to highlight the main deficiency in the education system due to which a large number of degree and diploma holders in our country remain unemployed. Students come out of universities with high expectations, which are often belied. It is indeed tragic that planners have confined their duties to only providing degrees to thousands of students every year, without linking them to employment generation which in turn leads to frustration. It is, therefore, essential that curriculum at the secondary school level should be such that it also technically equips students so that they are able to get jobs easily and quickly. The need for vocational education and computer literacy cannot be ignored. the Committee desire that the requisite changes/Modifications should be effected in the existing curricula to make the courses more professional and job-oriented. Certification should be provided to students who pass the eighth class to enable them to take up academic or vocational courses according to their aptitude.

Another shortcoming of the existing educational system is that it has distanced our younger generation from moral, social and ethical values. Although, it is claimed that character-building should become an inherent part of any education system, hardly anything is being done in this regard. The Committee are of the firm view that instead of loading the students with unnecessary, too detailed and extraneous curricula, the need of the hour is to inculcate in them social and moral values which would make them honest, law abiding citizens and social and civilised human beings.

In additions, special provision through Distance Education and Adult Education may be made for women to provide functional literacy.

CONCLUSIONS

The bold decision to declare 'Education as the Fundamental Right' reflects the Government's concern and commitment to ensure that everyone born in this country is literate/educated and thus fulfil the Constitutional commitment of 'Education for All' by 2007. Through the specially targeted programme of Sarva Shiksha Abhiyan (SSA), launched in 2000, efforts will be made to reach the un-reached women and the girl child. Thus, all out efforts will be made during the Tenth Plan to ensure that the SSA achieves its commitment within the time targets set.

The Tenth Plan will further endeavour to consolidate the progress made under female education and carry it forward for achieving the set goal of 'Education for Women's Equality' as advocated by the National Policy on Education, 1986 (revised in 1992) by reducing the gender gaps at the secondary and higher education levels. Also, special attention will be paid to the already identified low female literacy pockets and to the women and girl children socially disadvantaged groups viz. Scheduled Castes (SCs), Scheduled Tribes (STs), Other Backward Classes (OBCs), Minorities, Disabled, etc. as they still lag behind the rest of the population with female literacy rates as low as 5 to 10 per cent, while the national average of female literacy stands at 54.16 per cent in 2001.

Recognizing the fact that the application of science and technology is vital for the advancement of women and technology is vital for the advancement of women, the Tenth Plan will encourage women to participate in science and technology activities, especially in rural areas as it reduces the drudgery of household chores and provides a better quality of life. These will include measures to motive girls to take up subjects of science and technology in higher education and ensure that development projects with scientific and technical inputs involve women fully. Efforts to develop a scientific temper and awareness will also be stepped up. Special measures will be taken to train women in areas where they have special skills like communication and information technology. Efforts to develop appropriate technologies suited to women's needs as well as to reduce their drudgery will be made through the on-going programme of 'Science and Technology Project for Women'. Also, special efforts/provisions will be made to cover the existing gap in disseminating and reaching the technologies to rural women for whose benefit these were designed.

Further, to encourage more and more girls to enter into the mainstream of higher education, the Tenth Plan endeavours to put into action the governmental commitment of providing free education for girls upto the college level, including professional courses, so as to quicken the process of empowerment of women. All these efforts will continue during the Tenth Plan with the strength and support of the National Policy on Education, as it extends the most positive interventionist role in empowering women.

We may not be pessimistic. We should hope that the present momentum of women study centers built-up since by UGC would continue. The Central and State Governments, the mass media and educational institutions, teachers, students, youth, voluntary agencies, social activist groups, and employers, who must reinforce their commitment to literacy campaigns, awareness among about the socio-economic reality and the possibility to change. We should not hesitate to bring about innovative changes to make the programme realistic. We cannot afford to allow the programme to go slow as the programme is a source of strength to all other schemes of socio-economic development, whatever may be their immediate goal.

Notes and References

1. Department of Women and Child Development, Plato from for Action, *op. cit.*, p. 16.
2. The Report of the University Education Commission, Ministry of Education, GOI, New Delhi, 1962, p. 33.
3. Zabir Hussain, The Dynamic University, Asia, Bombay, 1965, p. 103.
4. National Policy of Education, 1986.
5. Education Policy, 1986.
6. *Ibid.*
7. GOI, Planning Commission, Tenth Five Year Plan (Draft) 2002-07.
8. *University News*, January 22, 2001.

CHAPTER 9

HEALTH EDUCATION AND HEALTH DEVELOPMENT FOR WOMEN

> ". . . the principle which regulates the existing social relations between the two sexes—the legal subordination of one sex to the other—is wrong in itself, and now one of the chief hindrances to human improvement; . . . it ought to be replaced by a principle of perfect equality, admitting no power or privilege on the one side, nor disability on the other."
>
> —*J.S. Mill and Hariet Taylor Mill*

Health Education and Health Development for Women

Health Education is the sum of experiences which favourably influence habits, attitudes and knowledge relating to individual, community and racial health.

Health Education has been an integral part of the functions of health personnel since time immemorial to educate the people pertaining to factors which influence their health. We have been engaged in the 20th century in finding out new technology and medicines to tackle the problems of health. That is why super speciality hospitals have come up in a big way. However, we have ignored the role of health education in preventing killer diseases resulting from faulty lifestyle, use of alcohol, smoking, drugs, etc. Let us analyse these health hazards which are causing great misery to individual, families and society.

(I) (i) Defective Lifestyles

Muhammad Al-Khrateeb[1] in his Article, "New Lifestyles' New Diseases" rightly remarks that Recent Social Development—such as bigger incomes and greater availability of a wide variety of commodities—have led to changes in lifestyles that threaten health. Coronary diseases are on the increase because of changes in diets; people are eating more fats, carbohydrates and animal proteins; fast-food restaurants offer hamburgers, hot dogs and fried chicken; the intake of salt from canned food is rapidly increasing; access to transport facilities reduce physical exercise; and stress is common in their daily life.

(ii) Non-availability of Balanced Diet

On the other hand, there is a large population in the developing countries especially India which is suffering from a number of diseases caused by malnutrition and under-nutrition. Some of the diseases are protein-energy malnutrition-related diseases e.g., low birth weights, Iodine deficiency disorders, Vitamin A deficiency disorders, iron deficiency, Anaemia, etc. These diseases do not require super specialists' interventions but timely Primary healthcare and education of mother and simple medicinal interventions.

The International Conference on Nutrition (ICN) in 1992 enunciated the following goals: (1) reduce severe and moderate malnutrition among children under five years of age by half of the 1990 levels, (2) increase the percentage of newborns having an adequate birth weight (2500 grams or more) to 90%, (3) reduce to less than 10% and possibly eliminate iodine deficiency disorders, (4) eliminate Vitamin A deficiency and its consequences including blindness, and (5) reduce iron deficiency anaemia.

Drawing up an integrated national strategy for the prevention of non-communicable diseases is both advisable and economically justifiable. But prevention of such diseases cannot be achieved through the efforts of health officials alone. Health education has to be made accessible to the entire population and non-health institutions and various mass media should be mobilized to this end. Research data yielded by national as well as international studies show that early intervention can make the prevention of diseases possible.[2]

(2) Use of Excessive Alcohol, Smoking and Drugs

World Health, July-August 1995 has published figures about prevalence of alcohol, tobacco and drugs which are quite alarmings.[3] In developed countries, typically 70-90% of adults consume alcohol. Studies in a number of industrialized countries suggest that 5-10% of drinkers are dependent on alcohol.

For several diseases, including cancers of the mouth, Oesophagus and pharynx, as well as for many forms of injury including motor vehicle accidents, industrial accidents, drowning, falls, suicide and homicide, the contribution of alcohol is well known, the risk increasing steadily with the amount consumed.

World-wide, there are about 1100 million smokers with 800 million in developing countries and 300 million in developed countries. About 6000 million cigarettes are smoked every year. In developed countries, about 41% of men and 21% of women regularly smoke cigarettes. In developing countries, about 50% of men but only about 8% of women smoke.

Tobacco causes about 3 million deaths a year now, with about one-third of them in developing countries. If current smoking trends persist, tobacco is likely to kill approximately 10 million people a year in 30-40 years time, with about 70% of them in developing countries.

If current smoking trends persist, about 500 million people currently alive (about 9% of the world's population) will eventually be killed by tobacco, and half of them will be in middle age when they die, losing about 20-25 years of life.

In many developing countries heroin and cocaine use is becoming more common and increasingly problematic. In several countries heroin use is increasingly replacing traditional patterns of substance use including opium smoking.

In many developing countries drug injecting is becoming increasingly common, and in these countries injecting often means the sharing of injecting equipment, with the risk of HIV, hepatitis and other infections.

One crude estimate suggests that, world-wide, between 160,000 and 210,000 deaths every year are associated with drug injecting.

Norman Sartorius in his Article, "Putting a Higher Value on Health" in *World Health,* June 1986 has cautioned about the negative effects of the use of these horrible drinks in excess. To quote:[4]

> "The abuse of psychoactive substances including alcohol, tobacco and narcotic and psychotropic drugs causes enormous damage to the health and productivity of nations. It undermines the quality of life of individuals and their families, and threatens the welfare of communities. The health consequences of abuse are also grave, and range from violence and delinquency to liver cirrhosis, brain damage and lung cancer."

Dr. H. Mahler, Former Director-General of World Health Organisation in his Article, "Smoking or Health: The Choice is Yours" rightly stated,[5] "Smoking increases the risk of lung cancer, heart disease and respiratory infections of all kinds. In fact, many of the diseases associated with smoking have become current only in the last few generations, when the habit of smoking factory made cigarettes became widespread."

The latest report of South-East Asia Region on Health situation in 1994-97 has clearly brought out the consequences of the use of these substances. A major problem with the use of alcohol is its impact on the health and well-being of the family. A study carried out in India in 1996 reported that drinking families from lower income groups spend from 15% to 45% of their income on alcohol. A high proportion of hospital beds are occupied by the physically and mentally damaged victims of alcohol dependence. Many beds occupied by accidents affected patients are because of alcohol.

The causal relationship between tobacco use and diseases such as cancers, cardiovascular diseases, and chronic respiratory disorders is increasingly being studied in most countries of the Region. In India, the number of avoidable cases of chronic heart and obstructive lung diseases has been estimated at 12 million per year. Cancer incidence data reveal that almost 50% and 25% of cancers in men and women respectively are related to tobacco use. The incidence of oral cancer caused by chewing tobacco is estimated to be one of the world's highest, at about one-third of all cancer cases. Annually, tobacco-related conditions are reported to cause 635,000 deaths in India.[6]

The basic question is how to tackle these non-communicable

diseases? How to motivate the people using these substances not to do so? What can be done by health experts? The only answer to these questions is the need of strengthening Health Education intensively. Muhammad Al-Khateeb[7] suggests that drawing upon integrated national strategy for the prevention of non-communicable diseases is both advisable and economically justifiable. But prevention of such diseases cannot be achieved through the efforts of health officials alone. Health education has to be made accessible to the entire population, and non-health institutions and various mass media should be mobilised to this end. Research data yielded by national as well as international studies show that early intervention can make the prevention of disease possible.

Achieving 'Health for All' requires much more than just setting up a health centre in every district and providing a high standard of medical care within easy reach of everyone.

A key element in the primary healthcare approach to Health for All is health education, which seeks to bring about a change in behaviour patterns by making essential health information available to all people in a simple, direct and effective manner. It is hoped that people will thus be motivated to evaluate their habits and practices, and will modify them according to the requirements of health protection and promotion.

Behavioural change, however, is too complex a process to be initiated simply by providing a set of facts. The motivation to break a habit must be much stronger than the force of habits or the pleasure derived from a certain practice. The spiritual dimension can be highly influential in this process of behavioural change.[8]

In spite of overwhelming evidence linking tobacco consumption and various diseases, including cancer, the consumption of cigarettes in nearly all countries of the world is increasing. The rise in tobacco consumption is especially seen among women and the youth. Non-smoking campaigns over the past years have been less than successful. This is mainly because of the aggressive advertisements and counter-attacks by the tobacco industry and the fact that nicotine is addictive. Moreover, most governments are reluctant to take a strong stand on this issue considering that tobacco is a source of revenue and of foreign exchange.

The need for heightened global advocacy for tobacco control has been stressed by Dr. Gro Harlem Brundtland, WHO Director-General, in her statement to the Fifty-first World Health Assembly in May 1998. To quote her:

> "I am a doctor, I believe in science and evidence . . . Tobacco is a killer, Tobacco should not be advertised, subsidized or glamorized."

Of late there is a move to ban Tobacco companies from sponsoring Sports events in India leading to a major debate as to whether it would be at the cost of the Sports activity and so on.

MEANING, NATURE AND SCOPE OF HEALTH EDUCATION

The most important aim of Health Education is to alter behaviour which may have directly or indirectly influenced occurrence of spread of diseases in a given cultural setting. A culturally relevant health education programme can be planned only after understanding the behaviour in all its manifestations. One of the best definitions of Health Education was offered by Wood in 1926: "Health Education is the sum of experiences which favourably influences habits, attitudes and knowledge relating to individual, community, and racial health."[9]

Different authorities have differently viewed the aims of health education. According to one source:[10]

> "The aim of health education is to help people achieve health by their own actions and efforts. Health education begins therefore with the interest of people in improving their condition of living, and aims at developing a sense of responsibility for their own health betterment as individuals and as members of families, communities or government."

Another source[11] highlights that, "Health education aims at promoting the greater possible fulfilment of inherited powers of the body and the mind and the happy adjustment of individual to society. It is the educational approach to health problem and as such is concerned with practical measures for the promotion of health and the control and treatment of disease."

Unfortunately, the experts and development planners have failed to improve the lives of the people as they do not understand properly the science to communicate effectively with each other or with the people are trying to help. Most of the people in authority today, who are guiding the people in this field, have not realised the urgency of such education and the benefit it can generate; consequently governments have not taken any substantial steps in this direction.

Health education does not mean merely removal of ignorance. On the contrary, it involves four important things:

(i) It provides a person with appropriate knowledge to enjoy decent health and also the knowledge about the occurrence and spread of disease thus enabling him to adopt relevant preventive measures;

(ii) It creates in him an interest in his own health and well-being;

(iii) It even creates in him an interest for the health of other members of his family as well as of those living in his surrounding; and

(iv) It creates in him a desire to support health education programmes in his area.

Besides, Health Education should make the people understand the benefits that they can derive from modern medicine. K.S. Sanjive, Professor of Medicine has said:

> "It will not be an exaggeration to say that the paramount step in the effort to take modern medicine to every corner of the country and every citizen is health education. Health education in its widest sense of getting every one to understand what modern medicine can do to diminish disease and death and to be properly motivated to utilise this knowledge in their daily lives, requires the simple quality of sincerity more than highly specialised techniques."[12]

Neglect of health education is one of the main reasons why scientific medicine is not taking root in the country and people are steeped in ignorance and superstition.

ESSENTIALS OF HEALTH EDUCATION

Health education would be possible only if the health educator and the receiver are in constant dialogue with each other. It is not wholly correct that the purpose of health education is to manipulate the receiver. What might be more appropriate is a circular diagram in which the parties to the "Communication Contract" as it is sometimes called, function dually as senders and receivers.

This model would avoid the possibilities of misinterpretation. We know that even well-planned campaigns can end in failures if there is no proper monitoring or feed-back to make sure that the wrong effect is not being created by the communicator, however innocently.

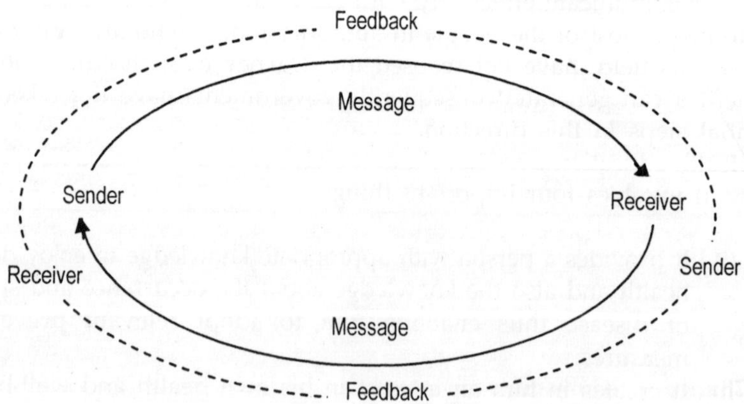

In a democratic society, the dynamic power which impels governments to action is the voice and enlightenment of the people. People can only pressurise their executive or legislative machinery to undertake suitable health measures when they themselves are aware of the means of warding off disease and promotion of positive health. This knowledge (Health Education) is therefore a pre-condition and prerequisite to creating the demand for health and setting the pace of implementation of environmental sanitation and the total health policy.

FUNCTIONS OF HEALTH EDUCATION PROGRAMME (See Chart 9.1)

No health education programme can function in isolation. A health education programme has to be an integral part of various other development programmes. Functionally, a health education programme should aim at bringing about the following changes:

CHART 9.1

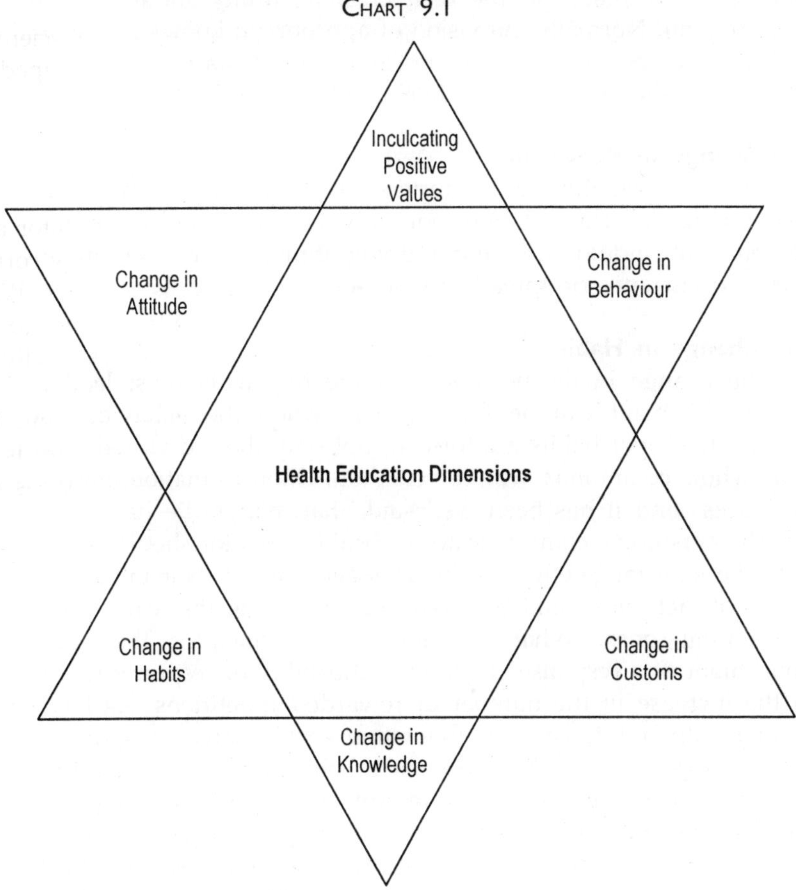

(1) A Change in Knowledge

The most important need which health education programme can serve is to provide appropriate knowledge about health and diseases to the people. This knowledge should be provided in such a way that the recipients do not find it hard to accept it. How to provide this knowledge in an acceptable way? This is the first challenge faced by a health educator.

Meaningful responses are relatively easier to learn than the meaningless ones. The health educator can do a lot better by making his demands on the response of receivers which are meaningful. For instance, the health educator who gives a big lecture to the mother on the value of practising family planning without indicating its benefits to her as an individual would be showing inadequate understanding of this principle, for she has to look into her own benefits first. Vigorous efforts would be required to proliferate suggestions that are realistic and meaningful.

(2) A Change in Attitude

A change in attitude is possible only when the new knowledge that is offered is acceptable to the recipients. Its utility should also be well known to them. Normally, provision of appropriate knowledge should lead to formation of positive attitudes not only towards a person's own health but also towards the health of other members of the community.

(3) A Change in Behaviour

Once positive attitudes are formed, these must reflect in the behaviour of the recipients. They should not only become mindful of their past behaviour but should also avoid doing things which can in any way influence occurrence or spread of diseases.

(4) A Change in Habit

The change in the behaviour of the recipients must lead to habit formation. A habit can be formed only when the behaviour becomes repetitive. If proper habits are formed, not only the individuals concerned but the whole community will be benefited. Habit formation, however, is a slow process and it has been well said, that 'habits die hard'.

The persuasive communicator or health educator should be interested both in the long range effects of his messages and in their initial effects. As a matter of fact, he should be interested in turning the learned responses into habitual ones. What are the other principles that guide the establishment of a response? First, the probability of response will increase with the increase in the number of rewarded repetitions. As long as the stimulus with reinforcement following each correct response is not adequately repeated, it will not become a habitual response. Many messages are short-lived because of lack of reinforcement and are likely to become extinct. Second, in order to establish habit patterns, it would be necessary to have a shorter interval between response and reward. Third, habit formation is easier when stimuli are presented in isolation. A nutrition message when unaccompanied by another message such as sanitation message facilitates habit formation. Fourthly, timely increase in reinforcement will further strengthen habit formation. Fifth, receiver's original level of motivation will also influence her habit formation. The mother having a better level of motivation from the beginning will find habit formation much easier. Sixth, providing timely information about receiver performance would lead to further improvement in performance. Providing selective information to a mother on the positive aspects of her performance will also improve her performance. Thus, communication of health ideas can yield the desired result if the above principles are followed religiously.

(5) A Change in Customs

Acquisition of positive attitudes leading to appropriate habit formation must sooner or later, evolve into customs. Only when a substantial number of people in a given cultural setting start behaving in a customary manner, one can say that behaviour has become a part of their customs.

Don Palmer in his article, "Social Health: A True Story, Culture and Tradition as Medicine" in the *Daily Tribune* dated 26th January 2000, rightly stresses "the need of health education. Modern urban life, devoid of the goodness of social health, can be particularly tough for young indigenous inhabitants of developed countries. Some kill themselves, while many more drift into drugs, alcohol and crime. Now a prison programme is helping in rehabilitation of aboriginal offenders by reintroducing them to their cultural traditions."

It needs to be re-emphasised that health education is a slow process and that it proceeds gradually—a part of the process may get established without any problem but additional efforts may be required to complete the whole process. This process may be directed towards the following important programmes: (See Chart 9.2)

(a) Personal hygiene.
(b) Knowledge of modern medicine, i.e., use of health services.
(c) Nutrition.
(d) Mental health.
(e) Prevention of communicable diseases.
(f) Care of children.
(g) Environmental sanitation.
(h) Human physiology.
(i) Lifestyle diseases.
(j) Education about Alcohol and drugs.

Health education must be imparted keeping in mind latest developments in the field of health. Life is changing fast and the individuals must be educated in the new technology—its role and limitations. Mr. V. Tatochenko, a member of the WHO Expert Panel on Maternal and Child Health in his Article on "Education for Health" said, "Rapid changes in lifestyles and the evolution of views on health and disease call for new departures in health education. A quick glance of health education material of even one generation ago will show how fast it tends to get out of date. Medical facts, it has been estimated, get outdated

CHART 9.2

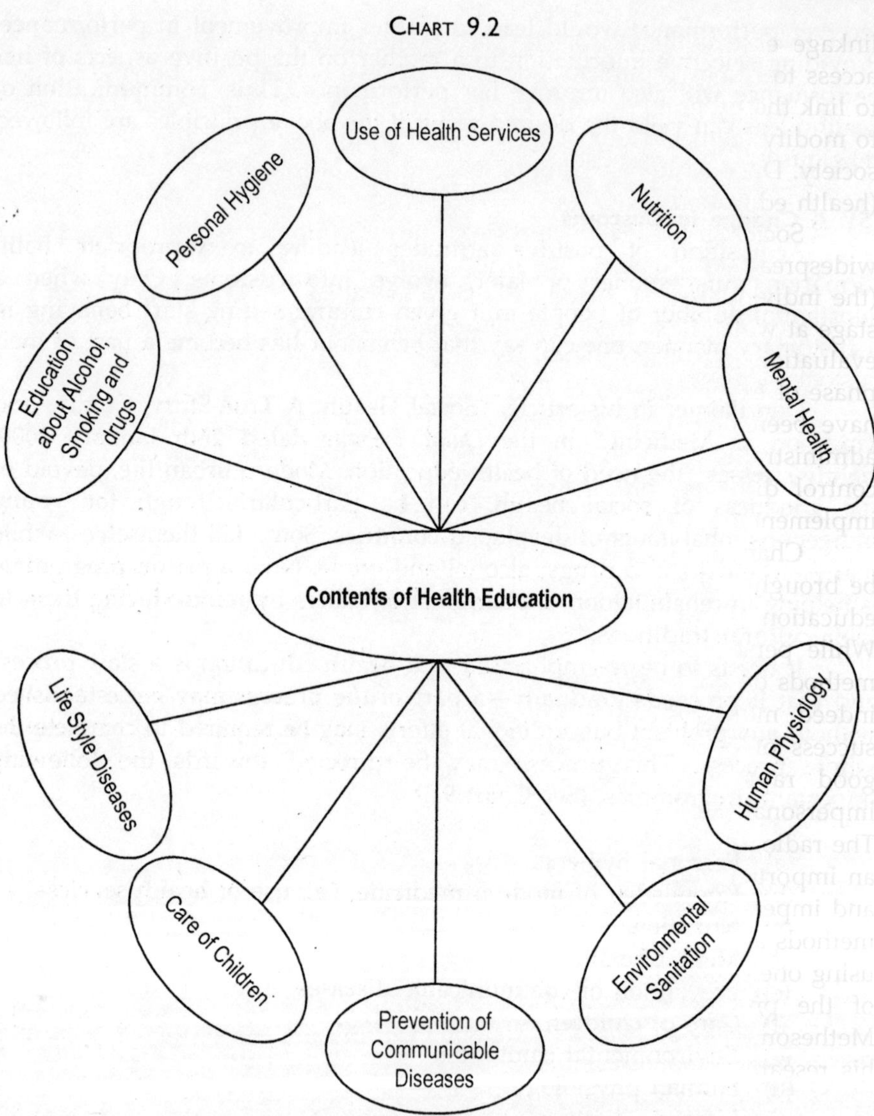

within a decade or so. Effective health education, therefore, requires a continuous stream of knowledge, development of the people's ability to absorb it, and decisions taken on the basis of a constantly changing body of information.[13]

METHODS OF HEALTH EDUCATION

Health organisations are set-up to promote positive health. A good health organisation must establish environmental linkages—points of interactions with the environment. These can be classified into four categories: enabling, functional, normative and diffused. The enabling linkage ensures and protects the organisational authority to operate its access to resources and its power to achieve results. Functional linkage is to link the programme with the task environment. Normative linkages try to modify the behaviour of the people into the existing value system of the society. Diffused linkages imply reaching the clients through public relation (health education).

Sociologists have categorised diffusion process which leads to a widespread acceptance of the programme into five critical stages awareness (the individuals first introduction to a new idea or practice), interest (the stage at which he actively seeks further information and background data), evaluation (the stage of assessment on critical grounds), trial (a limited phase of experiment), and finally acceptance or adoption. These processes have been occurring for centuries. The need of the present day health administration is to accelerate adoption of the health programmes and to control diffusion process in a short span of time to achieve effective implementation of health programmes.

Changes in knowledge, attitudes, behaviour, habits and customs can be brought about by 'personal' as well as 'impersonal' methods of health education. These methods have certain advantages and disadvantages. While personal methods involve face-to-face interaction, the impersonal methods do not require such a close personal contact. Personal methods are indeed more convincing and generally more successful. However, the success of personal methods greatly depends on the establishment of a good rapport between the health educator and his recipients. The impersonal methods are relatively simpler and even less time-consuming. The radio, the newspapers, the posters, and the pamphlets, etc. can all play an important role in imparting health education. Experience with personal and impersonal methods of health education have revealed that if both the methods are used simultaneously one can obtain better results than simply using one or the other method. The most important aspect in the adoption of the programme is the use of inter-personal relationships. Alastair Metheson, Deputy Director of UNICEF's division remarks on the basis of his research that:

> "To get people to act in ways that conform to new values almost always requires that mass communications to be reinforced by personal influence."[14]

Thus, we see that communication, i.e., dissemination of information is only an important element in health education. The adoption or acceptance may not take place simply by communicating health information. A study conducted by United States Public Health Services has revealed that, "Unfortunately knowledge alone does not motivate a person to act in accordance with it. He may well know the correct answers to questions without really believing and accepting such information as the basis for his own action."

Dr. Gisela Gastrin, a Finnish physician mentions in his article, "How Education Helps"; "People can be motivated to adjust their outlook towards health and disease, but before this can happen their negative attitudes have to be countered with factual information."

Education needs to be a part of a comprehensive programme in which responsibilities involving the health authorities and others are clearly delineated and resources allocated."[15]

For effective health education, people's involvement is essential. Eric R. Ram[16] in his article, "Information is Power" in *World Health,* rightly says that making people aware of their rights and responsibilities helps them to determine their own health priorities and take part in solving their own health problems, a step so essential in the process of empowerment of the people. We have to employ all credible channels of communication, including the traditional methods of story-telling and drama, in order to reach all people. Films, radio and television whenever available can be useful, but we have to recognize their limitations; they are useful in creating awareness among people in their communities, but to bring about a real change in health practices, people have to decide for themselves and take responsibility for their own health.

It was mentioned by Dr. E. Berthat in his article, "A New Role for Teachers" that besides information and motivation, action is indispensable. He said that "Information and motivation are not enough; it remains for governments to ensure that a good health infrastructure is available to all the people. Health education has to convince the men and women who are responsible for taking decisions that health is a basic raw-material for their country's eventual social and economic development.[17]

A health educator, as a persuasive communicator can make the best possible use of the personal methods of health education. But he has to see that the messages which he is delivering get mentally registered with his recipients. Actually, he can present his message and then wait until he gets the requisite response from his recipients. D.F. Skinner has distinguished between two types of approaches to the learning situation, as 'operant behaviour' and 'respondent behaviour'. The two situations have also been described as involving instrumental learning and conditional learning. In 'instrumental learning situations', which involves 'operant behaviour', the health educator will present his message and then wait for the receiver to make a correct response. When the receiver makes this response, the health educator will attempt to fix the response by the appropriate award or reinforcement. On the other hand in 'conditional learning situation' which involves 'respondent behaviour', the health educator presents his message in such a way that he elicits the response that he wants from his recipients and thus the stimulus that originally served to elicit the response becomes the reinforcing or rewarding element in conditioning. Undoubtedly, conditioning is much more efficient than instrumental learning. It is, however, necessary for the health educator to be aware of both kinds of situations since the condition for using 'respondent behaviour' may not be present in the persuasive situation. The health educator has to be aware that the recipients of his messages differ in the ways in which they learn a given response. They may give different responses essentially in the same situation because of certain specific reasons.

TRAINING OF PERSONNEL FOR HEALTH EDUCATION

We can divide the personnel for health education in two categories, i.e., Health Workers like teachers, social workers, physicians, nurses, etc., and Specialists, i.e., the persons specially trained for this function.

Objectives of training for Health Workers are:

(1) To create an awareness and understanding of the health education aspects of health work and of the principles and procedures to be considered in achieving these purposes;
(2) To foster an interest in health education in all health personnel;
(3) To teach the right way to communicate with individual families, community groups, and the general public;
(4) To stress the importance of team work for the realisation of effective health education; and
(5) To strengthen the aspects of health education in the curriculum of medical education.

The main objectives of training health education Specialists are:

(a) To establish professional standards to secure public confidence. It is essential that such specialists possess an ethical code and technical competence which govern their behaviour and standards of performance.
(b) To prepare specialists to encompass health education planning, organisation, coordination, dissemination, training, studies and research.

The health education Specialist should acquire through his basic education and post-graduate training the following qualities:

(a) A high degree of competence involving a thorough understanding of the importance and implication of cultural, economic and social influences in relation to health.
(b) Special competence in planning, organisation, administration, evaluation, etc., of health education aspects of health programmes.
(c) The ability to give technical leadership in planning and conduct of health education, training for health workers and workers in closely related fields (content, methods, planning, etc.).
(d) Skill in giving technical guidance and consultation on planning, preparation, pre-testing, production, and use of visual materials.

(e) The ability to assume technical leadership in cooperation with others in planning and execution of studies and research on major health education problems.
(f) Thorough knowledge of educational principles and methods involved in planning and arranging of seminars, conferences, meetings, courses, teaching units, etc.
(g) They should acquire latest information from research in teaching and learning relevant to health education.

THE ROLE OF UNION AND STATE GOVERNMENTS IN THE PROMOTION OF HEALTH EDUCATION IN INDIA

Imparting of health education is the responsibility of all professions, i.e. teachers, community leaders and parents. Central and the State Health Departments have instituted a separate bureau or division or section to provide expertise to health education programmes and assist in the training of health workers at various levels of health administration. There is also one premier institute—All India Institute of Hygiene and Public Health, Calcutta to provide training in the field of Health Education. Health Education forms part of all types of training courses in public health subjects.

CENTRAL HEALTH EDUCATION BUREAU (CHEB)

On the recommendation of the Planning Commission, the Government of India set-up a Central Health Education Bureau in the Directorate-General of Health Services under the Ministry of Health and Family Welfare, New Delhi, in 1956. It was entrusted with the following functions:

(1) To interpret the plans, programmes, and achievements of Health Ministry.
(2) To train key health and community welfare workers in health education and research methods and to evolve effective methodology and tools of training.
(3) To design, guide, coordinate and conduct researches in health behaviour, health education and aids.
(4) To prepare and distribute 'typed' health education materials to states and other agencies.
(5) To render technical and other assistance to official and non-official agencies engaged in health education work and to coordinate their programmes.
(6) To cooperate and collaborate with international agencies in promoting health education activities.

The Central Health Education Bureau—an apex Institute in Health

Education—imparts in-service training to all categories of personnel in health and related sectors at the state and district levels. They in turn disseminate the message of health education in the community at large. The Bureau, also continues to provide up-to-date information on current issues and development in health education, besides communication and training. The Bureau achieves its objectives through eight technical divisions, namely, Training, Media, Editorial, Health Education Services, Research and Evaluation, Field Study and Demonstration, Centre and Health-Related Vocational Courses. The Training Division runs a post-graduate Diploma Course in Health Education of two years' duration at the University of Delhi; Media personnel training course of eight weeks' duration; Certificate courses in Health Education for para-medical professionals, medical officers, teachers and key trainers; district-level medical officers' course, etc. Besides, about 25 orientation courses of one-day duration are held for Nursing, para-medical professionals and international visitors.

The Media Division is the Information, Education and Communication unit of the Bureau. The Editorial Division brings out three periodicals, namely, *Swasth Hind* (English monthly), *Arogya Sandesh* (Hindi monthly) and *Swasth Siksha Samachar* devoted to important public health problems, plans and policies of the Ministry of Health and Family Welfare. It also prepares and produces printed materials like folders, pamphlets, etc., on important public health subjects. The School Health Division promotes health education in the school system. The Health Education Services Division renders technical guidance to State Health Education Bureau and assists government and non-government agencies in promoting health education in the country. It also co-ordinates with international and national agencies.

The CHEB is a nodal agency for promoting Health-Related Vocational Courses (HRVCs) at the stage of education in the country in collaboration with the Department of Education. The HRVC Division develops curricula and textbooks for various HRVCs and persuades the States/UTs to start these courses. The Research Division conducts Behavioural Studies on various aspects of health problems that serve as a basis for launching health education campaigns. It also conducts Social Science Research Methods Courses. The Field Study and Demonstration Centres of the Bureau are field laboratories to test and evaluate methods and the media of health education which can be adopted elsewhere.

It may not be an exaggeration to say that all these contributions of CHEB have failed to produce the desired impact on the health status of the people. It is unfortunate that some of the 'good' workers who were earlier associated with the CHEB left it in favour of highly remunerative assignments with the World Health Organisation. If the CHEB has to prove its utility in a meaningful manner then it has to have suitably trained persons on its staff. Otherwise, the CHEB, without technically qualified people, is likely to become a rehabilitation centre for the relatives and friends of highups in the Government.

The state of Health Education Bureaus in different States of India is no better. Most of the literature produced by them lacks the necessary appeal for the rural masses. It has little or no relevance to the realities of the health situation. Many a time the authorities of these bureaus derive a sense of satisfaction by merely distributing pamphlets to the people. No effort is made to evaluate its impact on the health behaviour of the people. It is common knowledge that a substantial part of this literature goes to the junk shop where its value is judged only in terms of its weight. Unless, those responsible for producing the health education material also become seriously involved in knowing how it is used, very little is likely to be known about utility to the people for whom it is meant. A visit to a District Hospital in North India will show how irrelevant is the health education material which gets displayed on the walls of the ward or in the OPD in the hospital. While one may find an excess of posters on a disease like smallpox, which is no longer a problem, one may not see any poster on common problems as measles and diarrhoea.

Thus, a lot depends on how the Central and State Ministries of Health plan and implement their health education programmes. Actually, planning and implementation of health education programme at the Centre, State and District levels also depends on the available financial resources. Health education programmes for the hospital and for the health centers do not have any separate funding. In practice, the money allocated for health education either lapses at the Head Office or is not made available at these places. It is necessary for a developing country like India to attach the highest importance to health education. Without planning appropriate health education programmes, one can hardly hope to bring about a positive change in the existing health condition. "Planning of health education should be an integral part of the overall national health planning."[18]

HEALTH EDUCATION IN HOSPITALS

Gone are those days when people used to feel frightened at the thought of going to a hospital. Hospitals were considered as sordid places where people waited for death. Today, the image of hospitals has vastly changed. People expect hospitals to be well organised so that all the services offered by them are well received by the clients. Somehow, the modern hospitals, both teaching and non-teaching, continue to attach the highest importance to providing curative services. The teaching hospitals, in particular, assign a great prestige and value to medical education and research activities. Thus, the medical scientists remain 'wedded to curative medicine rather than to preventive medicine.' A developed country, like the United States of America, had a couple of decades back, recognised the need of combining curative aspects of diseases with preventive aspects. Such a recognition had led to the opening of some of the best schools of hygiene and public health in the world in some of the prestigious American

Universities like the Harvard, John Hopkins, North Carolina and California. Thus, for a developing country like India, there is not only a need for combining curative services with preventive services but there is also the need for introducing effective health education programmes in the teaching as well as non-teaching hospitals.

In February 1977, India organised a national workshop with WHO's collaboration on health education in hospitals which was attended by sixty hospital and health administrators and health educators. This is going to be extended to cover other hospitals in the country. The efforts of Sri Lanka are noteworthy in this direction. Most of the country's larger hospitals have accepted health education as one of their functions. Each of these hospitals has been equipped and the staff have been trained in health education. Educational work is undertaken in wards, clinics and out-patient departments. These activities are coordinated with those in the communities.

The functions, which the teaching and non-teaching hospitals can perform in the modern times need to be defined properly. At present, no effort has been made to study the functions of these hospitals in relation to the needs of the people. Even among the staff members of these hospitals there is a great deal of confusion about individual's role, perception, role expectation and role performance. The health administrators have differently perceived the roles of the different members of the teaching hospitals. These hospitals, no doubt, can play a significant role in imparting health education to the patients because they have certain basic facilities available to them in the form of staff members like physicians, nurses, social workers, photographers and artists and they also have various audio-visual aids.

The object of health education, as defined by WHO is to help people attain not just freedom from disease or infirmity but a state of complete mental, physical and social well-being. If this object is followed seriously then the hospitals cannot escape the responsibility of organising relevant health education programmes with the help of experts in the field of health education. The hospitals provide an extraordinary opportunity to the medical staff to communicate modern concepts and ideas about health not only to the patients but also to their relatives who accompany them to the clinic for moral support. In fact, health education can be provided at the out-patient departments in the special clinics, in the wards and even at the registration counter. The Departments of Obstetrics and Gynaecology and Pediatrics can play a special role in organising suitable health education programmes for their clients when they come to them for ante-natal and post-natal care. Actually, the immunization activities can also be combined with certain well-planned health education activities. At the Primary Health Centre level too, there is a great scope for imparting health education to the patients and their attendants, but unfortunately, the medical staff there rarely uses this opportunity to educate them by providing certain basic knowledge about prevention of diseases. Similarly, the in-patients provide a tremendous opportunity to the medical staff to talk to them about various health protective, preventive and promotive measures. If these situations were utilized properly to educate people who come to the hospitals for seeking medical care, the general health of the Indian people would have been much better than what it is today. As long as the specialists and the super-specialists working in the teaching hospitals will not realize that they themselves have to become health educators rather than leave this task to the paramedical only, one can hardly hope for a positive change in the health status of the Indian people in the near future. The specialists like the general surgeons, orthopedic surgeons, obstetricians, pediatric surgeons, eye surgeons, dental surgeons, plastic surgeons and the like can all, in their own distinct ways, play an exceedingly important role of providing specific disease-related health education to the patients when they come to them for treatment. No one can deny that a person involved in an automobile accident can understand the value of wearing a helmet much more quickly if he is told about it by an orthopedic or plastic surgeon to whom he has approached for the treatment of his head injury. Similarly, a pediatrician, treating a case of neo-natorum tetanus can use this opportunity of educating the mother about the devastating effect of the traditional practice of applying cowdung on the umbilical cord.

The kind of value and respect which the patients attach to the word of a medical specialist is virtually beyond the domain of a para-medical like the present day community health workers who just have a three-month training at a health centre. Unfortunately, not many teaching hospitals provide good examples of working in teams. The specialists succumb to a certain tendency of working in their own closed compartments. Thus, the higher the specialisation, the greater the possibility of compartmentalisation. Health education can have its impact only when it becomes the responsibility of the entire team of specialists. If all of them equally realise the importance of health education, they can create a desirable preventive atmosphere in the hospitals. The most frequent complaint against the hospital administration are lack of sympathy and courtesy on the part of medical and administrative staff. This is particularly the case in the OPD's and Emergency Ward as the patients and their attendants are already in a state of agony and tension. It is suggested that the medical and administrative staff must spare some time to console the patients and their relatives. This would provide a great psychological and moral satisfaction to patients. The hospital authorities must foster goodwill, trust and understanding among the patients and their relatives. This would operate genuine climate and real situation where health education can be imparted to the people. In this way the functioning of the hospital would not be limited to its four walls but would infiltrate in the whole community served by the hospital. This would create a good relationship between the hospital and the community it serves.

CONCLUSIONS AND RECOMMENDATIONS

Without evaluating the impact of health education programmes on the bulk of the people, one cannot possibly identify positive as well as negative aspects of the programme. An objective evaluation of the health education programme alone can help one improve the guidelines for future action. 'Cost-benefit' analysis should be an integral part of this evaluation, so that one may assess how available resources have been utilized. Through objective evaluation; one may also be able to curtail mass production of ritualistic health education material as produced by various health education bureaus. The amount thus saved can be effectively utilised for a more purposeful and meaningful health education programme.

Health education is the most difficult task as habits, usages and customs are deeply entrenched. But health administration would fail in its purpose if it could not produce social change through health education. That is why it has been said that "it is easier to destroy mountains than to change our customs."[19] Professional training helps the health experts to deal with the health changes effectively. Their pharmacopoeia in both fields must be strong in order to translate the findings of biological investigations into social application. So over and above each technical act; there is a corresponding education function which doubles the value of the act, increases its efficiency and endows it with real human and social value.[20] G. Borkar in his book, "Health in Independent India" writes that all progress in public health depends ultimately on the willing assent and cooperation of the people and their active participation in measures intended for individual and community health protection, considering how much of illness is the result of ignorance of simple hygienic laws or indifference to their application. In practice, no single measure is productive of greater returns to outlay than health education.[21] Thus, health education can influence the lives of people for many generations. WHO conducted an interview of a Mongolian Feldsher. He stated that "conducting continuous health education is my first duty, prevention is our basic principle. Every effort is made to raise the health knowledge of the people. Child care, correct feeding and vaccinations are among the most important topics for health education."[22]

In order to improve the functioning of the administration of health education at the Union and State levels in India, the following facts and suggestions may be taken into consideration:[23]

1. Effective Role for Hospitals in Health Education as Patients are Amenable to their Advice

Hospitals within the country are not serving as agencies of health education. Health education can be imparted to mothers when they come to hospitals with their babies. During their stay in the hospital, mothers can be taught how to care for their children during sickness and how to feed them correctly. The mental field is also full of promise. Hospital physicians can do much in this direction by their own attitude to patients, give them simple instructions and, above all, treat them as persons rather than cases.

2. Modernise Health Education Institutes

Those very institutions responsible for imparting health education courses are lacking in standards for sanitary facilities. It is difficult to see how the concepts of sanitation can be effectively imparted among trainees, under such conditions. The curricula and contents of health education need careful planning. The educational methods for health education used in a country or community should be regularly evaluated and revised in line with socio-economic development. Health education should be oriented to health consciousness and not disease consciousness.

3. Constant Research and Evaluation

There is the necessity of research in behavioural sciences for the improvement of health education. Dr. B.S. Sehgal, Director, CHEB, New Delhi, said, "It was essential to conduct research on the behavioural sciences, in order to build-up a body of knowledge for meeting the challenges posed by the health programmes."[24]

4. Special Attention to Training of Trainers

Training for trainers needs re-orientation and re-examination. We should supplement classroom-based academically oriented training strategy in health education with the actual practice based on models of social change. The emphasis should be on learning by doing and nor by listening alone. To quote a UNICEF/WHO study:

> "Efforts in health education have often been limited to giving information dogmatically, as if this alone would bring about a transformation. Inevitably, the outcome has been disappointing. The pattern of existing resources—economic, human and cultural—has been forgotten and this too has contributed to health education's failure."[25]

5. Creation of Womens' Club as in Democratic Republic of Korea (DRK)

Women can be effectively approached only by women workers. The experiment of mother's club has been sufficiently rewarding and useful in the People's Democratic Republic of Korea as agencies of socio-economic development. The process of social and economic development is a process of human development for people is the target as well as essential variable in development. Communication being a two-way process, provides for participation at whatever stage of enlightenment the individuals composing a society find themselves. Mother clubs if established in India in right earnest can be the key factors in both the communication and development process since they can be the instruments for getting facts to the people upon which decisions can be based.[26]

6. Understand Local Social-cultural Issues

Before launching any programme of health education, the health educator must assess the local problems and possess the knowledge about the beliefs, conceptions and misconceptions which the people have formed about diseases, their causation and cure. This is possible provided the multi-disciplinary studies of rural communities are encouraged. Such studies would throw light about the cultural background of the people. He can arrange his programmes accordingly and this will save him from antagonism and hostility.

7. Create Good Relations with Mass Media

There is less coordination between health education and the means of mass media communication which needs strengthening on positive lines.

It needs to be recognised that most of our health education programmes and activities are so ritualistic in nature that they rarely correspond to the realities of the situation. In most situations the health educator's knowledge of the cultural content of health education programme is often so deficient that they find it hard to deliver the health education messages in a culturally acceptable manner. It needs to be stressed that the cultural aspect of health education programme is of the greatest importance in the Indian situation. Anthropological and sociological studies in the area of health education are so few in our country that health educators find it extremely hard to understand the many changing aspects of the communities they deal with. There is, thus, an urgent need to study the social and cultural context of health and disease, and to design health services in such a way as will gain the acceptance and support of the people involved. The social scientists can help the health educator in the following ways:

(1) to understand the role of socio-cultural factors in health, including people's beliefs about etiology, diagnosis and therapy of prevalent diseases;
(2) to understand the food culture including people's belief regarding consumption or rejection of various foods on socio-cultural considerations;
(3) to understand people's attitudes towards acceptance or rejection of health education programmes; and
(4) to help them plan and develop culturally relevant health education programmes.

South-East Regional Office of WHO has also expressed its dissatisfaction over the lack of importance to health education in its report, "Health Situation in the South-East Asian Region, 1994-97", (p. 72).

Despite these achievements, health education and promotion practices are faced with major constraints—the low priority accorded to health education at the policy level, high illiteracy levels, inadequate resources, poor social status of women, and limited capacity for health promotion research are but only a few examples. To overcome such constraints, new thinking and innovative approaches are required. As we move into the 21st century, the challenges for health promotion go beyond the wider articulation of the concept of health promotion, to building infrastructure and achieving adequate levels of resources both technical and financial, in order to respond effectively to the increasing demands for health promotion in the Region. "Settings for health" represent the organizational base of the infrastructure required for health promotion.

Partnerships which effectively respond to the health needs of specific population groups, such as workers, women and school children, need to be more vigorously pursued. Healthy public policies need to be developed to ensure supportive environments for individual and community health action, and to protect people from lifestyle-related problems such as those due to tobacco and alcohol. Documentation and dissemination of health promotion outcomes are also critical to the legitimization of the cause of health promotion in the Region.

New health challenges mean that new and diverse networks need to be created to achieve intersectoral collaboration. Such network should provide mutual assistance within and among countries, and facilitate the exchange of information about which strategies have proved effective. All countries need to develop the appropriate political, legal, educational, social and economic environments required to support health promotion. In this venture of health education, mass-media if properly used can help solve the problems.

Health promoters and educators need to be convinced that the mass-media can operate in the public interest and should play a critical role in social affairs, including health issues. The health concerns of readers, listeners and viewers are very much the concerns of the print and broadcast journalists. The basis of the relationship between the health and media sectors should therefore be one of partnership, not one of user-helper.

Health and media are not naturally inclined to work in unison. Historically, medical scientists trained in the methodical and meticulous search for knowledge have been somewhat skeptical of any effort at popularizing their work. Some doctors even view the media with suspicion and ambivalence. Media people, on the other hand, need to have their source material in language understandable to the layman; they have motive to dwell on technical details and often lose patience with lengthy scientific nappers.

Yet media and health in a close partnership have much to contribute to the public's welfare. Without the involvement of the media, the health sector cannot hope to inform the public on health issues or to help stimulate a community's involvement, which is critical to the success of any health effort. Without the technical input of the health sector the media cannot fulfil their obligations to serve the interest of the public and these public interests certainly include health.

The complexity of the media, with their obsession for meeting dead lines and their own technical constraints, is little appreciated or understood by health professionals. Those in health who work in partnership with the media need to acquire a rudimentary knowledge of how media works—not in order to become media specialists but to be more empathetic in their dealings with the journalists and broadcasters. This in turn will call for a good hard look at the core curriculum of the training of health promoters and educators.

Whether the health professionals can play their rightful role in battling successfully against lifestyle-related illness—including AIDS and whether health education and promotion practitioners will enter the 21st century adequately prepared for the communication challenges, will depend on the actions that health authorities take now.[27]

In the new millennium, we need to harness all the resources especially the mass-media in a planned manner. This would require active collaboration between media and health specialists. Jack Ling[28] in his article, "Health and the Media" has rightly stressed that the health sector should focus on making technical subjects digestible and understandable to the layman. In particular, the health professionals should identify existing, credible channels of communication, including traditional ones, in order to reach the public. The media offers the public health community more than just access to air-time and newspaper space; they are also a source of communications expertise that is needed to ensure the success of large-scale health promotion campaigns and transmit technical information about health to a mass audience.

What is more useful is the follow-up of media-transmitted message that can be effected by village health workers. For instance, primary healthcare workers can be an effective channel of communication by delivering in person the same messages that have been delivered to a target audience in print or over the radio, thus increasing the overall impact of the educational drive.

A dialogue has to be initiated between decision-makers in media and in public health. The object of that dialogue should be to heighten awareness among the media personnel about the important responsibility they hold for the health and well-being of their people, and equally to alert health professionals to their own responsibility for ensuring that their health initiatives reach all people. Without this whole-hearted backing from the media in conveying health messages to the greatest number of people, we risk having only Health for Some and not Health for All.

However, the success of health education would depend in the long-run upon the shoulders of the providers of healthcare to the people. They should be motivated to do this job as a part of their medical duties. S.S. Sooch in his Article, "Revamping Healthcare" in the *Daily Tribune* (26 January, 2000) rightly remarks that there is a general feeling that most of the healthcare providers in the government-run hospitals are indifferent, apathetic and insensitive and a few even outrightly arrogant in their behaviour. A sense of compassion and human touch is simply missing. A series of crash courses should be arranged to expose the entire staff to the art of public relations.

Health Education is vital to provide health to all in 21st century.

This is the cheapest and most effective tool of healthcare. The success of Primary Healthcare in 21st Century depends upon the identification of community needs through community needs assessment surveys and later on providing health education to the community so that they can solve their health problems themselves.

Notes and References

1. Muhammad Al-Khateeb, 'New Lifestyles, New Disease" in *World Health,* July 1989, p. 23.
2. *Ibid.*
3. WHO, *World Health,* July-August 1995, p. 16.
4. *World Health,* June 1986, p. 2.
5. *World Health,* Feb.-March 1980, p. 1.
6. WHO, SEARO: Health Situation in the South-East Asia Region, 1994-97, New Delhi, 1999, pp. 149-51.
7. *World Health,* July 1989, p. 23.
8. Abdulmoneim Aly: Health Education Through Religion, in *World Health,* July 1989, p. 27.
9. John J. Hanlon, Principles of Public Health Administration, St. Louis, 1960, p. 402.
10. WHO, *Technical Report Series,* No. 89, p. 4.
11. WHO, *Ibid.,* No. 156, p. 3.
12. K.S. Sanjiva, Planning India's Health, Orient Longman, New Delhi, 1971, p. 64.
13. WHO, *World Health,* Feb.-March 1979, p. 24.
14. UNICEF, *UNICEF News,* "Communication: A Tool for Development", Issue 84/ 1975/12, p. 18.
15. WHO, *World Health,* Nov. 1975, p. 14.
16. *World Health,* Jan.-Feb. 1989, p. 9.
17. *World Health,* May 1979, p. 25.
18. WHO: *Technical Report Series,* No. 89, 1954.
19. Bosnian proverb.
20. WHO: *Technical Report Series,* 1954.
21. Borkar, Health in Independent India, p. 217.
22. WHO, *World Health,* April 1977, p. 20.
23. Based on personal discussion and interview.
24. WHO, SEARO: SEA/RC 23, p. 88.
25. UNICEF, Health and Basic Services, Keys to Development, *op. cit.,* p. 46.
26. For further details refer to author's article, "Role of Communication in Family Planning Setting up of Mother's Club in PEN, Family Planning Association of India, Haryana Branch, May 1977.
27. Jack C.S. Ling, "The Media its Role," in *World Health,* January-Feb. 1989, p. 25.
28. Jack Ling, "Health and Media" in *World Health,* March 1986, p. 15.

APPENDIX 9.1

WOMEN AND HEALTH

The approach to women's health has evolved over the 90s from a target-oriented approach into a more holistic, integrated lifecycle and need-based approach. The challenge is to ensure that women's health throughout the life cycle, from birth to old age, is a public health priority; and that it is viewed in a holistic manner that encompasses decline in the incidence of diseases; improvement in access to, and the quality of services; and empowers women to make informed choices. Improvement in the health status of women is sought to be achieved through access and utilisation of health, family welfare and nutrition services with special focus on the underprivileged segment. The Government of India is engaged in considering ways and means of fostering active community involvement in the population and reproductive health programme. Bringing down the incidence of maternal mortality is a priority. The progress is evident from the data, which shows fall in maternal mortality rate (MMR) from 437 in 1993 to 407 in 1998. The total fertility rate (TFR) stood at 3.2 in 1998 and the objective is to bring this down to 2.1 by 2001 Infant Mortality Rate (IMR) for girls was 70.8 in 1999 and 69.8 for boys. Latest data suggests that the IMR in 2002 stood at 65 for girls and 62 for boys. The crude birth rate fell from 29.5 to 25.0 and the crude death rate from 9.8 to 8.1 between 1991 and 2002 respectively.

Maternal mortality, despite the fall in the MMR remains high. In Uttar Pradesh and Rajasthan, it is 707 and 670 respectively. Other states in which MMR is above the national average of 407 are Madhya Pradesh, Bihar and Assam. Causes of maternal death include haemorrhage, sepsis, obstructed/prolonged labour, unsafe abortion, anaemia, etc. Factors responsible include poor healthcare facilities, lack of access to healthcare units, poor nutrition, early marriage, frequent and closely spaced pregnancies.

Access of the poor to integrated health services is limited, especially in rural areas, despite the fact that the poor face a disproportionate disease burden. The resurgence of communicable diseases is a challenge. The Common Minimum Programme of the present government commits to increase public health expenditure to 2-3% of GDP. The government proposes to launch a National Rural Healthcare Mission throughout the country to improve healthcare delivery over the next five years. Key measures include a national scheme for health insurance for poor families, special attention to poorer sections, food and nutrition security, focused population stabilization programme in high fertility districts, replication of success of the southern states, and availability of life saving drugs at reasonable prices.

Policy framework

The National Health Policy 2001 promises increased access to women for basic healthcare and commits highest priority to funding programmes relating to women's health. The National Population Policy 2000 addresses issues of ensuring universal access to healthcare options and stabilising population. It recognises links between socio-economic development and health. The policy provides a framework for advancing goals and prioritising strategies during the next decade, to meet the reproductive and child health needs of the people of India and to achieve net replacement levels of total fertility rate by 2010. The immediate objective of the policy is to address the unmet needs of contraception, health infrastructure, health personnel and to provide integrated service delivery for basic reproductive and child healthcare. The hallmark of India's National Population Policy is its emphasis on improving the quality of reproductive healthcare by working more closely with community-based organisations and women's groups.

A national level resource committee has been constituted to guide the states in formulated their population policies. Some state governments have already formulated their state policies with specific strategies, goals and programmes. These states are Andhra Pradesh (1997), Rajasthan (1999), Madhya Pradesh (2000), Uttar Pradesh (2000), and Gujarat (2002). At a Colloquium on Population Policy-Development and Human Rights, organised by UNFPA with the NHRC and the Department of Family Welfare in January 2003, it was agreed that a rights-based approach would inform the formulation of population policy.

On December 5, 2002, the Parliament approved the bill to amend the Medical Termination of Pregnancy Act (MTP), 1971. This law is meant to strengthen the right to terminate an unintended pregnancy. The main objective of the recent amendment to MTP is to reduce the rate of unsafe abortion by making legal abortions widely accessible. Lack of access to MTP services at the primary healthcare level has been cited as an important reason for the high rate of unsafe and illegal abortions. One of the main provisions of this amendment is therefore, to decentralise the authority for approval and registration of MTP centres from state to district level and to provide specific punishments for conducting illegal abortions. This is an important first step to reduce the toll of unsafe abortions.

Partnerships with NGOs

The Mother NGO (MNGO) programme of the Department of Family Welfare has been recognised by the Planning Commission as a model scheme for adoption by other Ministries/Departments of the Government of India for funding NGOs. Four Regional Resource Centres (RRC) for capacity building of NGOs have been set-up. It is proposed to increase the number of RRCs to 10.

To fill the gap in information available on public healthcare services, especially those provided by hospitals, Centre for Enquiry into Health and

Allied Themes (CEHAT) has brought out a directory of public health facilities that would provide comprehensive and portable information on public hospitals in Mumbai. This was done in active collaboration with the public health department of the Brihan-Mumbai Municipal Corporation and the Directorate of Medical Education. The directory contains both general and specific information, including information on various services provided by the hospitals and maternity homes.

The focus of work of the Support for Advocacy and Training to Health Initiatives (SATHI) cells in Mumbai is primary healthcare; supporting initiatives with a specific rights-based approach. SATHI cells aim at fostering a broad-based health movement by offering training and advocacy-related inputs to various organisations taking up health initiatives. Activities include continued collaboration with four people's organisations in Dahanu, Aajra, Badwani and Sendhwa for strengthening the ongoing Community Health Worker (Arogya Sathi) programmes and local advocacy on primary healthcare issues.

The Arogya Sathi Project (1998-2001) is an initiative in primary healthcare developing health programmes and health advocacy with people's organizations. The aim was to reduce medical deprivation and exploitation, support peoples' organization in their advocacy efforts to make public and private healthcare systems accountable.

Aarogyacho Margavar (Violence and Women's Health, 1998-2002) a women centred health project led to the establishment of community-based healthcare, through trained women community health workers. It included an outreach programme for preventive and promotive care, health education, a referral clinic in the community and networking with public health systems. The research component through qualitative group discussions and a household survey helped understand the extent and patterns of domestic violence, women's perceptions about its nature, causes, coping mechanism, help seeking behavour and community response to domestic violence.

Dilaasa, a crises for treatment and counselling of women victims of public hospitals has been set-up in collaboration with the Brihan-Mumbai Municipal Corporation (BMC). CEHAT provides the training inputs to BMC staff and presently runs the centre, which provides counselling and allied services to survivors of violence. CEHAT will run the centre for three years after which the BMC would take responsibility for it through the core team trained at the hospital. Through Dilaasa and CEHAT other public hospitals are also being exposed and oriented to incorporate this concern in their hospital.

The Ministry of Health and Family Welfare (MOHFW), initiated a project to train and disseminate health information among women's groups. This effort was initiated on a pilot basis in 15 states, aiming to address the information needs of 2500 women's groups covering 40000 rural women. The Centre For Health Education, Training and Nutrition (CHETNA) took a leadership role to collate and strengthen each topic by incorporating its two-decade long experience in the field of women's health. The manual was further critiqued by experts and field level NGOs. The state level manual became a rich reference material, based on which, CHETNA developed training modules to be used by the district and village level trainers. These modules cover 23 topics related to women's comprehensive health along with training design and description of the training methods.

Health Programmes

The Reproductive and Child Health (RCH) Programme (first phase 1997-2003, second phase starting 2003) has been designed to meet women's needs across their life span. The general objectives of the project include empowering women and children through providing high quality care to them, empowering the community as a whole to demand better health services, and improving substantially the performance of the healthcare delivery system. The RCH Project, Phase I, as built upon the success of the Universal Immunization Programme and Child Survival and Safe Motherhood Programme (CSSM). In addition, it covers all aspects of women's health across their reproductive cycle, from puberty to menopause. It gives due importance to male participation in the programme.

The Family Welfare Programme has adopted a Community Needs Assessment Approach since 1997, through a decentralized participatory planning strategy. The preparation of AAP at district and state levels based on the assessed needs of the people for family welfare services in one of the most vital activities under this approach.

The National Maternity Benefit Scheme (NMBS) provides for 100% central assistance to the States/UTs for extending financial benefit of Rs. 500 per pregnancy for first two live births to women who belong to households below poverty line and have attained nineteen years of age and above.

Health Infrastructure

An extensive healthcare delivery system has been created in the country by the government, voluntary and private sectors. However, paradoxically few hospitals are located in areas with high morbidity. The Tenth Five Year Plan (2002-07) proposes an appropriate reorganisation and restructuring of existing healthcare infrastructure at the primary, secondary and tertiary levels, to reduce such imbalances. Another initiative is the appropriate delegation of powers to Panchayati Raj Institutions (PRI) to ensure local accountability of public heath care providers. Through the National Disease (Control Programmes, an effort is made to provide additional support for essential primary healthcare and emergency life saving services.

Less than 20% of healthcare needs are currently met by the public sector. It has been recognised that there is a need to involve private sector providers in ensuring health services for all. However, forming such partnerships raises issues of accreditation, social franchising, quality control and improved regulation.

The Pradhan Mantry Swasthya Suraksha Yojana has been designed with the objective of reducing the gaps that remain in the availability of tertiary care hospitals/medical colleges by providing special/super specialty services across various states. Under the scheme, institutions on the model of AIIMS, are proposed to be set-up in the six backward states of Bihar, Chhattisgarh, Madhya Pradesh, Orissa, Rajasthan and Uttaranchal.

Health System Reforms

Health is a state subject. Faced with sub-optimal functioning and resource limitations, almost all state governments have introduced health system reforms. Several states have obtained external assistance to augment their own resources for initiation of health sector reforms. Almost all States have attempted introduction of user charges for diagnostics and therapeutic procedures from people above the poverty line. The funds, thus, generated could be used to improve the quality of care in the institution. Some ongoing health system reforms to improve healthcare services include:

- Strengthening/appropriately relocating sub-centres/PHCs e.g. Tamil Nadu, Gujarat.
- Merger, restructuring, relocating of hospitals/dispensaries in rural areas and integrating them with existing infrastructure—e.g. Himachal Pradesh.
- Restructuring existing block level PHC, Taluk, Sub-divisional hospitals, e.g. Himachal Pradesh.
- Utilising funds from BMS, ACA for PMGY and EAP to fill critical gaps in manpower and facilities—all States.
- District level walk-in-interviews for appointment of doctors of required qualifications for filling the manpower gaps in PHC, e.g. Madhya Pradesh and Gujarat with limited success.
- Use of mobile health clinics Orissa (for Tribal areas), Delhi (for urban slums).
- Handing over of PHCs to NGOs—Karnataka, Orissa, while Karnataka reported success.
- In Orissa as the NGOs did not have the resources and ability to run the institution, these were handed back to the Government after some time.
- Training MBBS doctors in specialization for 3-6 months (Obstetrics, Anaesthesia, Radiology) in a teaching institution and posting them to fill the gap in specialists in FRUs, e.g. Tamil Nadu and West Bengal.
- Improving logistics of supply of drugs and consumables.

One of the major initiatives of the Ninth Plan was the Secondary Health System Strengthening project funded by the World Bank in seven states (Andhra Pradesh, Karnataka, Punjab, West Bengal, Maharashtra, Orissa and Uttar Pradesh). The focus in this project is on strengthening

FRUs/CHCs and district hospitals to improve availability of emergency care services to patients near their residence and reduce overcrowding at district and tertiary care hospitals. The States have reported progress in construction works, procurement of equipment, increased availability of ambulances and drugs improvement in quality of services following skill upgradation training in clinical management, changes in attitudes and behaviour of healthcare providers; reduction in mismatches in health personnel/infrastructure; improvement in hospital waste management, and disease surveillance and response system.

Health Insurance

Public sector general insurance companies have been encouraged to design community based Universal Health Insurance Schemes. Upto March 2004, 417,000 families involving 1.16 million persons have been covered under the scheme. Some state governments have taken initiatives to formulate health insurance for families below the poverty line. Kerala has proposed a health insurance scheme administered through the Kudumbashree groups. Madhya Pradesh and Himachal Pradesh are in the process of launching community health insurance schemes.

Nutrition

Nutrition and health of women are a high priority. A number of policies, namely the National Nutrition Policy (GOI, 1993) under DWCD, the National Population Policy (2000), the National Health Policy (2001) and National Plan of Action of Nutrition (1995) gave higher priority to the nutrition and health of women.

Special emphasis was placed on the following:

- on nutrition and health education of women,
- improving nutritional status of adolescent girls,
- ensuring better coverage of expectant women in order to reduce the incidence of low birth weight in newborns,
- controlling micro-nutrient deficiencies related to vitamin A,
- iron and folic acid and iodine through intensified programmes, and
- implementing global strategy on infant and young child feeding giving due emphasis to women's health.

A multi-cultural strategy was advocated by the Nutrition Policy identifying a series of actions for various concerned sectors of the government. Direct nutrition interventions for vulnerable groups, as well as, indirect policy instruments for creating conditions for improved nutrition were recommended. To ensure policy outreach, all the district collectors in the country were addressed by the Secretary, DWCD on nutrition policy.

A pilot project was launched in 2002 in 51 backward districts in the country under which undernourished adolescent girls, pregnant and lactating women are provided 6 kg of wheat/rice per month per beneficiary free of cost.

The states have taken various initiatives for promoting nutrition of people. The Government of Megahalaya has taken an active interest in the implementation of nutrition policy instruments. The Government of Tamil Nadu launched a special drive in early 2002 to make Tamil Nadu malnutrition free.

The Government of Madhya Pradesh also undertook a malnutrition eradication drive, the special features of which were nutrition monitoring of pre-school children, Annaprashan Abhiyan through the Aanganwadis and the creation of nutritional awareness by intensifying the IEC activities. The Madhya Pradesh Government has also organised a state level consultation on infant and young child feeding to focus on eradication of child malnutrition. The Government of Haryana has utilised Mahila Mandals and Sanjeevanies in creating nutrition and health awareness amongst the people. The field units of Food and Nutrition Board (FNB) at Chandigarh and Delhi have provided training on nutrition to Sanjeevanies and Mahila Mandals on the request of the state government. The Government of Andhra Pradesh has adopted nutritious recipes provided by the field unit of FNB at Hyderabad in its Janmabhoomi Programme.

In order to address the widespread problem of malnutrition particularly among women and children, a National Nutrition Mission under the chairpersonship of the Prime Minister was set-up in July 2003 involving a two-tier supervisory structure. The basic objective of the mission is to address the problem of malnutrition in a holistic manner and accelerate reduction in various forms of malnutrition (including undernutrition anaemia, vitamin A deficiency, iodine deficiency disorders and chronic energy deficiency), especially among women and children. The mission is also responsible for policy direction and effective coordination of nutrition programmes being implemented by the Government. An Executive Committee has been set-up to aid and advise the ANM.

National Guidelines on Infant and Young Child Feeding were released during the World Breast Feeding Week in August 2004. This provides government and civil society with an opportunity as well as a practical instrument for protecting, promoting, and supporting safe and adequate feeding of infants and young children.

Immunisation

The Universal Immunisation Programme which was taken up in 1980 as a National Technology Mission, became a part of the SSM programme in 1992 and the RCH programme in 1997. Under the programme, infants are immunised against tuberculosis, diphtheria, pertussis poliomyelitis, measles and tetanus. As a result of the programme, the reported cases of vaccine preventable diseases declined post-independence but have remained largely stagnant in the 1990s.

Due to increased focus on campaign mode programmes in health family welfare, routine immunisation received a set back. States have been requested to formulate district specific strategies for improving routine immunisation. Under the Pulse Polio Programme, which was initiated in 1995-96, all children below five years are to be administered two doses of OPV in low transmission seasons every year until polio is eliminated. As a result, there was a substantial reduction in polio cases till 2001 but in 2002, there was a sudden increase in number of cases, seven times the previous years cases. To bring this down more rounds are being organised in high burden zones so that polio is eradicated by 2005.

Men's Participation in Planned Parenthood

Men play an important role in determining education and employment status, age at marriage, family formulation pattern, access to and utilisation of health and family welfare services for women and children. Their active cooperation is essential for the prevention and control of STI/RTI. Vasectomy was the most widely used terminal method of contraception in the 1960s and the 1970s but since then there has been a steep decline in its use. To promote their participation, No Scalpe Vasectomy (NSV) Project was launched in 1998 and as a result male sterilizations have increased from 1.8% in 1997 to 2.46% in 2002. Around 300 NSV training sessions have been held and 1156 doctors trained.

HIV/AIDS

HIV/AIDS has emerged as a formidable challenge to public health over the last decade. HIV prevalence in India among adults is estimated at 0.9% (or 4.58 million persons) in 2002; 25% of reported cases are women. The spread of HIV infection is not uniform across states. Six states have been categorised as high prevalence states. Key factors fuelling spread of HIV infection have been identified as labour migration from economically backward pockets to more developed regions, low literacy levels, particularly among marginalized and vulnerable sections of society, gender disparity, prevalence of reproductive tract infections and sexually transmitted diseases among both men and women. The following measures have been adopted to deal with HIV/AIDS:

- The National AIDS Control Organisation was set-up in 1992.
- Phase II of the National AIDS Control programme launched in 1999 has a specific focus on strengthening the capacity of the Central/State governments to respond to HIV/AIDS on a long term basis.
- The National AIDS Control and Prevention Policy, 2002 makes special mention about the protection of rights of HIV positive women in making decisions regarding pregnancy and childbirth.
- There has been a change in approach from seeing transmission mechanism as mother-to-child to seeing it as parent-to-child.

The Government commits itself to providing prophylaxis for prevention of parent to child transmission and the requisite counselling to all infected mothers. This facility will be voluntary, on the basis of informed consent.

- Safe blood transfusion is assured at district level.
- As per agreed guidelines of WHO and GOI, by 2005, 3 million persons with HIV will be covered by anti-retroviral (ARV) drugs. From April 1, 2004, free ARV drugs are being made available to mothers living with HIV.
- The Family Health Awareness Campaign is an effort to address the management of STIs and HIV/AIDS by generating awareness among the vulnerable groups, residents of rural and urban slums and vulnerable women.

The DWCD has been addressing the gender dimensions of HIV/AIDS. They have actively participated in high level round tables on Gender and HIV/AIDS organized by UNIFEM and NACO for the Ministry of Social Justice and Empowerment, Department of Elementary Education and Literacy and Ministry of Road Transport and Highways. The Department has been responsive to issues of positive women and their concerns.

In a unique partnership, Indian Railways, a large public sector undertaking, in collaboration with UNIFEM has initiated a pilot project in Vijayawada division in Andhra Pradesh to impart gender friendly HIV counselling and support services to railway employees and their families. Project interventions are through the railway schools, hospitals, training institutions, railway workers' unions and railway mahila samities. The project is working towards transforming gender relations and catalysing supportive roles of men within the family, community and work place.

Tuberculosis

Tuberculosis is a leading killer of women. It kills women more than all other causes of maternal mortality. In many parts of the country, women do not have adequate access to diagnosis and treatment of TB due to stigma and limitations on mobility. To increase access, under the Revised National TB Control Programme (RNTCP), microscopy centres for every 100,000 population in general areas and 50,000 in difficult tribal and hilly areas are being established. Treatment facilities have been decentralised by way of establishing Directly Observed Treatment Short Course (DOTS) centres nearest to the patients' residence and pro and anti-TB drugs are provided free of cost. Efforts are being made to involve more women SHGs in the programme. Emphasis is being given to IEC activities for removing stigma attached to TB patients.

Women and Disability

Roughly 2% of the country's population is disabled. According to the survey conducted by the National Survey Organisation in 58th round (July-

December 2002) there were 18.5 million disabled persons in the country. Of those 7.6 million were women in urban areas. Distribution of disabled women by type of disability indicates that 46% disabled women suffered from locomotor disability, 17% from hearing disability, 13% blindness, 10% with speech disability, 5% each with mental illness and low vision, and 4% with mental retardation. Policies of Government of India for welfare of disabled persons are gender sensitive. There has been recognition of the special difficulties faced by disabled women.

Resources

Public expenditure on health as a percentage of the GDP has declined from 5.3% in 1997 to 5.1% in 2001. The ratio of government to total expenditure on health has remained constant at around 18%. The increasing importance of private provision, skewed as it tends to be away from the health needs of the poor, poses important questions of regulation and direction.

Source: Deptt. of Women and Child, Ministry of Human Resource Development, GOI, New Delhi.

APPENDIX 9.2

Selected Gender Development Indicators

Sl. No.	Indicators	Female	Male	Total	Female	Male	Total
	Demography and Vital Statistics						
1.	Population (in million 1991 and 2001) (Census)	407.1	439.2	846.3	495.7	531.3	1027.0
2.	Decennial Growth (1981 and 2001) (Census)	24.93	24.41	24.58	21.79	23.93	21.34
3.	Sex Ratio (1991 and 2001) (Census)	927			933		
4.	Juvenile Sex ratio (1991 and 2001) (Census)	945			927		
5.	Life Expectancy at Birth (in years in 1991 and 2001) (Census)	58.1	57.1		65.3	62.3	
6.	Mean Age at Marriage 1981 and 1991 (Census)	17.9	23.3		19.3	24.0	
	Health and Family Welfare						
7.	Birth Rate (per 1000 in 1981 and 2002) (SRS)			35.6			25.0
8.	Death rate (per 1000 in 1981 and 2002) (SRS)	12.7	12.4	12.5	7.7	8.4	8.1
9.	Infant Mortality Rate (per 1000 lie bits in 1990 and 2002 (SRS)	81	78	80	65	62	64
10.	Child Mortality Rate (per 1000 live births under 5 yrs. of age in 1985 and 2001) (SRS)	40.5	36.6	38.4	71.6	70.5	71.1
11.	Maternal Mortality Rate per 100,000 live births in 1997 and 1998) (SRS)	408			407		
	Literacy and Education						
12.	Literacy Rate (1991 and 2001) in percentage (Census)	39.29	64.13	52.21	53.67	75.26	64.84
13.	Gross Enrolment Ratio (1990-91 and 2002-03)						
	Classes I-V (Ministry of HRD)	85.5	114.0	100.1	93.1	97.5	95.3
	Classes VI-VIII (Ministry of HRD)	47.0	76.6	62.1	56.2	65.3	61.0
14.	Dropout rate (1990-91 and 2002-03) in %						
	Classes I-V (Ministry of HRD)	46.0	40.1	42.6	33.7	35.8	34.9
	Classes I-VIII (Ministry of HRD)	65.1	59.1	60.9	52.3	53.4	52.8
	Work and Employment						
15.	Work Participation Rate (1991 and 2001) in percentage	22.3	51.6	37.4	25.6	57.9	39.2
16.	Organised Sector (number in millions in 1981 and 1999) (DGEandT)	2.80 (12.2%)	20.50	22.85 (17.2%)	4.83	23.20	28.11

17. Public Sector (number in millions in 1981 and 1999) (Employment review)	1.5 (8.7%)	14.0	15.5	2.8 (14.5%)	16.8	19.4
18. Government (number in millions in 1981 and 1997)	1.2 (11%)	9.7	10.9	1.6 (14.6%)	9.1	10.1
Women's Representation in Decision-making						
19. Administration (number in IAS and IPS in 1997 and 2000)	579 (7.6%)	7347	8036	645 (7.6%)	7860	846
20. PRIs (number in figures in 1985 and 2001)	318 (33.5)	630	948	725 (22.6%)	1997	2722
21. Parliament (no. in 1991 and 2004)	77 (9.7%)	712	789	72 (9.2%)	712	784
22. Central Council of Minister (number in 1985 and 2001)	4 (10%)	36	40	8 (10.8%)	66	74

Source: Office of the Registrar General of India.

APPENDIX 9.3

CHART 1

Projected Values of Expectation of Life at Birth 1980-2006

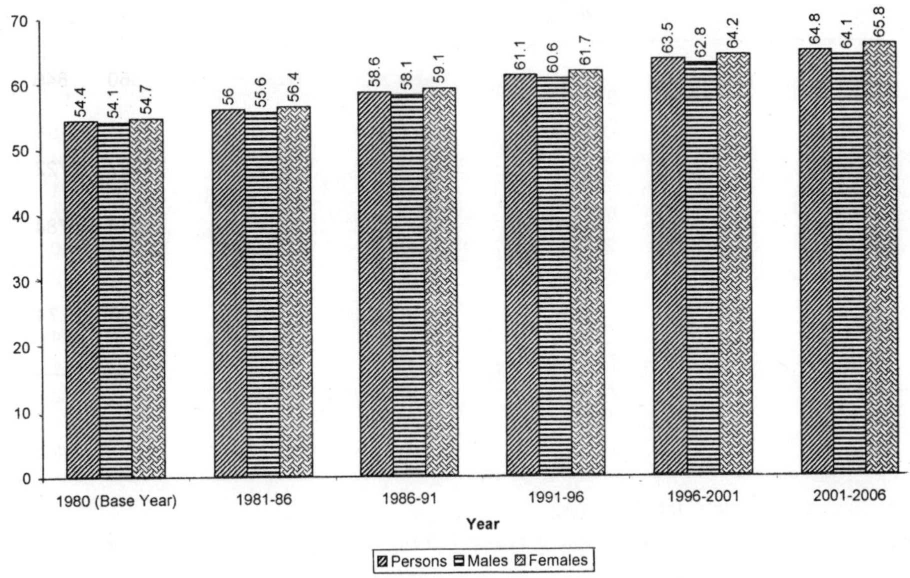

CHART 2

Birth Rate, Death Rate and Natural Growth Rate in India 1991-2002

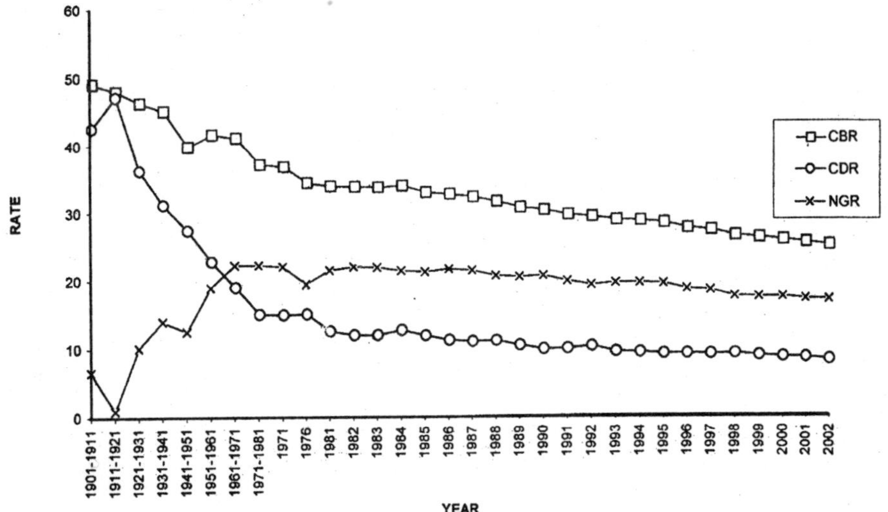

Appendix 9.4

Table I

Infant Mortality Rate by Sex for India

Year	*Female*	*Male*	*Total*
1985	98	96	97
1986	97	96	96
1987	96	95	95
1988	93	95	94
1989	90	92	91
1990	81	78	80
1991a	80	81	80
1992a	80	79	79
1993a	75	73	74
1994a	73	75	74
1995a	76	73	74
1996a	73	71	72
1997a	73	70	71
1998	73	70	72

(a) Excludes Jammu and Kashmir.

Source: Sample Registration System (Various Years), Office of Registrar General, India.

TABLE 2

Expectation of Life at Birth by Sex for India

Year	*Female*	*Male*	*Total*
1901-11	23.3	22.6	22.9
1911-21	20.9	19.4	20.1
1921-31	26.6	26.9	26.8
1931-41	31.4	32.1	31.8
1941-51	31.7	32.4	32.1
1951-61	40.6	41.9	41.3
1961-71	44.7	46.4	45.6
1970-75	49.0	50.5	49.7
1976-80	52.1	52.5	52.3
1981-85	55.7	55.4	55.4
1986-90	58.1	57.7	57.7
1987-91a	58.6	58.1	58.3
1988-92a	59.0	58.6	58.7
1989-93a	59.7	59.0	59.4
1990-94a	60.4	59.4	60.0
1991-95a	60.9	59.4	60.3
1991-96a	61.4	60.1	60.7
1993-97b	61.8	60.4	61.1

(a) Excludes Jammu and Kashmir.

(b) Unpublished (under printing).

Note: Figures for 1901-11 to 1961-71 are based on census Actuarial Reports and for 1970-75 onwards on the basis of estimates from Sample Registration System.

Source: Office of Registrar General, India, Census Actuarial Report and SRS based abridged Life Table 1986-90 (Occasional Paper No. 1 of 1994).

TABLE 3

Number and Percentage Distribution of Deaths of Expected Mothers due to Causes Related to Child-Birth and Pregnancy for India

Causes	*Number*					*Percentage*				
	1989	*1992*	*1993*	*1994*	*1995*	*1989*	*1992*	*1993*	*1994*	*1995*
Abortion	22	37	45	49	62	10.9	13.7	11.7	12.6	17.6
Toxaemia	16	34	49	51	35	7.9	12.6	12.8	13.1	7.9
Anaemia	41	53	78	75	60	20.3	19.6	20.3	19.3	17.0
Bleeding of Pregnancy and Puerperium	48	68	87	92	102	23.8	25.2	22.6	23.7	28.9
Malposition of child	22	23	21	25	14	10.9	8.5	5.5	6.4	4.0
Puerperial Sepsis	12	31	48	41	30	5.9	11.5	12.5	10.6	8.5
Not classifiable	41	24	56	55	50	20.3	8.9	14.6	14.2	14.1
Total	202	270	384	388	353	100.0	100.0	100.0	100.0	100.0

Source: Survey of Causes of Deaths, Office of Registrar General, India.

TABLE 4

Maternal Mortality Rate for States/Union Territories during 1998

State/Union Territory	*Maternal Mortality Rate*
Andhra Prudish	159
Arunachal Pradesh	NA
Assam	409
Bihar[1]	452
Goa	NA
Gujarat	28
Haryana	103
Himachal Pradesh	NA
Jammu and Kashmir	NA
Karnataka	195
Kerala	198
Madhya Pradesh[1]	498
Maharashtra	135.
Manipur	NA
Meghalaya	NA
Mizoram	NA
Nagaland	NA
Orissa	367
Punjab	199
Rajasthan	670
Sikkim	NA
Tamil Nadu	79
Tripura	NA
Uttar Pradesh[1]	707
West bengl	266
Andaman and Nicobar Islands	NA
Chandigarh	NA
Dadra and Nagar Haveli	NA
Daman and Diu	NA
Delhi	NA
Lakshadweep	NA
Pondicherry	NA
India	407

NA: Not available.

1. Figure is for undivided state. The states of Bihar, Madhya Pradesh and Uttar Pradesh here include the newly constituted states of Jharkhand, Chhatisgarh and Uttaranchal, respectives.

Note: Material mortality rate is the number of maternal deaths per 100,000 live births.

Source: Sample Registration System, Office of Registrar General, India.

TABLE 5

Prevalence of Anaemia among Women by Background Characteristics for India during 1998-99

Background Characteristic	*Percentage of women with anaemia*				
	Number of women	*Mild anaemia*	*Moderate anaemia*	*Severe anaemia*	*Total*
Age	7117	36.2	17.9	1.9	56.0
20-24	14560	34.8	17.0	2.0	53.8
25-29	15965	34.8	14.7	1.9	51.4
30-34	13595	34.8	13.7	1.9	50.5
35-49	28426	35.1	13.6	1.9	50.5
Marital Status					
Currently married	74830	34.9	14.8	1.8	51.5
Not currently married	4833	36.6	15.7	3.1	55.5
Residence					
Urban	20872	32.0	12.2	1.5	45.7
Rural	58791	36.1	15.8	2.0	53.9
Education					
Illiterate	45818	36.7	16.8	2.3	55.8
Literate < middle school complete	15735	34.4	13.8	1.9	50.1
Middle school complete	6718	34.0	12.6	1.3	48.0
High school complete and above	11381	29.7	9.7	0.9	40.3
Work status					
Working in family farm/business	11450	35.7	15.2	2.2	53.1
Employed by someone else	15671	35.8	16.2	3.0	54.9
Self-employed	3974	35.0	15.3	2.0	52.2
Not worked in past 12 months	48543	34.6	14.3	1.5	50.4
Total	79663	35.0	14.8	1.9	51.8

Note: The haemoglobin levels are adjusted for altitude of the enumeration area and for smoking when calculating the degree of anaemia. Total includes 10 and 26 women with missing information on education and work status respectively, who are not shown separately.

Source: National Family Health Survey-II, 1998-99.

TABLE 6

Prevalence of Anaemia among Women by States during 1998-99

State	*Percentage of women with*			
	Mild anaemia	*Moderate anaemia*	*Severe anaemia*	*Total*
Andhra Pradesh	32.5	14.9	2.4	49.8
Arunachal Pradesh	50.6	11.3	0.6	62.5
Assam	43.2	25.6	0.9	69.7
Bihar[1]	42.9	19.0	1.5	63.4
Delhi	29.6	9.6	1.3	40.5
Goa	27.3	8.1	1.0	36
Gujarat	29.5	14.4	2.5	46.3
Haryana	30.9	14.5	1.6	47.0
Himachal Pradesh	31.4	8.4	0.7	40.5
Jammu and Kashmir	39.3	17.6	1.9	58.7
Karnataka	26.7	13.4	2.3	42.4
Kerala	19.5	2.7	0.5	22.7
Madhya Pradesh[1]	37.6	15.6	1.0	54.3
Maharashtra	31.5	14.1	2.9	48.5
Manipur	21.7	6.3	0.8	28.9
Meghalaya	33.4	27.5	2.4	63.3
Mizoram	35.2	12.1	0.7	48.0
Nagaland	27.8	9.6	1.0	38.4
Orissa	45.1	16.4	1.6	63.0
Punjab	28.4	12.3	0.7	41.4
Rajasthan	32.3	14.1	2.1	48.5
Sikkim	37.3	21.4	2.4	61.1
Tamil Nadu	36.7	15.9	3.9	56.5
Uttar Pradesh[1]	33.5	13.7	1.5	48.7
West Bengal	45.3	15.9	1.5	62.7
India	35.0	14.8	1.9	51.8

1. Figure is for undivided states. The states of Bihar, Madhya Pradesh and Uttar Pradesh here include the newly constituted states of Jharkhand, Chhatisgarh and Uttaranchal, respectively.

Note: Figures give the percentage of ever-married women classified as having iron-deficiency anaemia by degree of anaemia. The haemoglobin levels are adjusted for attitude of the enumeration area and for smoking, when calculating the degree of anaemia.

Source: National Family Health Survey-II, 1998-99.

TABLE 7

Daily Average Intake of Energy and Proteins against Recommended Intake by Age/Sex/Physical Activity of Rural Population for India during 2001

Age (years)	*Sex*	*Activity*	*Energy (kcals/day)*		*Protein (g/day)*	
			Intake	*RDI*	*Intake*	*RDI*
1-3	Boys and Girls		729	1240	20	22
4-6	Boys and Girls		1066	1690	28	30
7-9	Boys and Girls		1294	1950	34	41
10-12	Boys		1524	2190	40	54
	Girls		1500	1970	39	57
13-15	Boys		1856	2450	49	70
	Girls		1689	2060	44	65
16-17	Boys		2114	2640	55	78
	Girls		1856	2060	49	63
>=18	Male	Sedentary	2225	2425	59	60
		Moderate	2371	2875	61	60
>=18	Females	Secondary	1878	1875	48	50
	(NPNL)	Moderate	2020	2225	52	50

RDI Recommended Dietary Intakes.

NPNL Non-Pregnant Non-Lactating.

Source: Based on National Nutrition Monitoring Bureau (NNMB) 'Diet and Nutritional Status of Rural Population', Technical Report No. 21 based on repeat surveys conducted during 2001 in rural areas of Kerala, Tamil Nadu, Karnataka, Andhra Pradesh, Maharashtra, Gujarat, Madhya Pradesh, Orissa and West Bengal.

TABLE 8

Percentage of Currently Married Women who know about any Contraceptive Method by Specific Method and Sector for India during 1998-99

Method	*Rural*	*Urban*	*Combined*
Any method	98.7	99.7	99.0
Any modern method	98.6	99.7	98.9
Pill	75.2	91.5	79.5
IUD	64.6	87.8	70.6
Condom	64.9	88.0	71.0
Female Sterilization	97.8	99.3	98.2
Male Sterilization	87.8	93.6	89.3
Any traditional method	44.9	60.3	48.9
Rhythm/safe period	41.0	56.7	45.1
Withdrawal	27.7	41.1	31.2
Other method	2.6	3.1	2.7
Number of Women	61761	21888	83649

A. Includes both modern and traditional methods that are not listed separately.

Source: National Family Health Survey-II, 1998-99.

TABLE 9

Family Planning Acceptors by Methods for India

(Figures in thousand)

Year	Sterilisation		I.U.D. Insertions	Equivalent C.C users	Equivalent oral pill users	Total acceptors
	Vasectomy	Tubectomy				
1990-91	2255	3871	5370	14735	3125	27356
1991-92	174	3916	4386	13875	3366	25717
1992-93	150	4136	4740	15004	3001	27031
1993-94	150	4347	6017	17283	4302	32099
1994-95	144	4436	6702	17707	4873	33862
1995-96	124	4298	6858	17297	5091	33668
1996-97	72	3798	5681	17214	5250	32015
1997-98	71	4167	6173	16796	6395	33603
1998-99	103	4104	6083	17448	6944	34682
1999-2000	87	4509	6200	18135	7748	36678
2000-01	109	4558	6027	18050	7556	36300

IUD : Intra-Uterine Device.
CC : Conventional Contraceptives.
P : Provisional.
Source: Department of Family Welfare, Ministry of Health and Family Welfare.

TABLE 10

Percentage of Couples Effectively Protected by Various Family Planning Methods for India

Year	Eligible couples (figures in thousand)	Percentage of couples protected by				
		Sterilisation	IUD	Oral Pill	CC	All methods
1990-91	145140	30.3	6.7	2.1	5.1	44.1
1991-92	148430	30.3	6.3	2.2	4.7	43.6
1992-93	151720	30.3	6.3	2.0	4.9	43.5
1993-94	155020	30.3	6.8	2.7	5.6	45.4
1994-95	158310	30.2	7.2	3.0	5.4	45.8
1995-96	161593	30.2	7.8	3.2	5.3	46.5
1996-97	164749	29.6	7.4	3.1	5.2	45.4
1997-98	165869	29.3	7.3	3.8	5.0	45.4
1998-99	168558	29.1	7.4	3.3	4.2	44.0
1999-2000	172298	29.0	7.3	4.6	5.3	46.2

IUD : Intra-Uterine Devices.
CC : Conventional Contraceptives.
Source: Department of Family Welfare, Ministry of Health and Family Welfare.

TABLE 11

Lifestyle Indicators of Addiction

Background characteristic	*Chew paan masala or tobacco*	*Drink alcohol*	*Currently smoke*	*Ever smoked*	*Number of household members*
			Female		
Age					
15-19	2.1	0.6	0.2	0.3	24602
20-24	4.3	1.1	0.6	0.6	22288
25-29	8.0	2.0	1.1	1.2	20761
30-39	12.3	2.5	2.2	2.4	32127
40-49	18.6	3.1	4.0	4.5	21253
50-59	22.8	3.8	5.7	6.4	15108
60+	25.0	3.1	5.3	6.0	18588
Residence					
Urban	8.8	0.5	0.9	1.0	43173
Rural	13.8	2.9	3.1	3.4	111554
Education					
Illiterate	17.4	3.5	4.0	4.5	83359
Literate < middle school complete	10.2	0.8	0.8	0.9	30563
Middle school complete	3.8	0.5	0.3	0.3	14217
High school complete and above	1.8	0.2	0.1	0.2	23529
Standard of living index					
Low	18.7	4.4	4.2	4.7	47225
Medium	11.7	1.7	2.2	2.4	71497
High	5.2	0.3	0.6	0.8	34144
Total	12.4	2.2	2.5	2.8	154726
			Male		
Age					
15-19	9.4	2.4	4.4	4.8	26297
20-24	20.3	7.7	13.7	14.6	21461
25-29	28.0	14.9	25.1	27.3	19641
30-39	34.1	23.6	37.6	41.2	33554
40-49	35.6	26.1	45.0	49.9	24151
50-59	35.4	23.9	45.3	52.3	15195
60+	37.6	18.6	38.2	46.6	20571
Residence					
Urban	20.8	12.4	21.4	24.5	46245
Rural	31.3	18.5	32.6	36.5	114626
Education					
Illiterate	38.0	26.7	44.8	49.6	44661
Literate < middle school complete	31.5	17.8	33.1	37.5	43328
Middle school complete	23.2	11.8	21.2	23.7	25376
High school complete and above	18.9	8.9	15.9	18.5	47485
Standard of living index					
Low	37.6	24.8	39.4	43.5	46887
Medium	27.7	15.0	29.1	32.7	76510
High	17.2	9.8	16.9	20.2	35463
Total	28.3	16.7	29.4	33.1	160871
Total (Male and Female)	20.5	9.6	16.2	18.2	315598

(a) Includes household members who currently smoke.

Note: The figures give the percentage of usual household members age 15 years and above who chew paan masala or tobacco, drink alcohol, currently smoke, or have ever smoked by selected background characteristics and Sex, India.
Total includes 23 males and 58 females with missing information on education and 2012 males and 1861 females with missing information on the standard of living index, who are not shown separately.

Source: National Family Health Survey-II, 1998-99.

Appendix 9.5

RECOMMENDATIONS

Tenth Plan (2002-07)
Working Group on Empowerment of Women
Report—Chapter XIV

Challenge in the New Millennium

The global setting of the Tenth Five Year Plan is completely different from the earlier Plans. It is characterized by new challenges of 'market driven forces' on the one side, and expectations of the people—women and men—fast getting sensitized to their rights and entitlements, on the other. This new scenario calls for an approach based on recognition of 'people's entitlements' and the responsibilities of the State to facilitate and provide the conditions for achieving these entitlements.

Approaches to Development

Limitations of earlier approaches to development that relied on 'trickle down effects' are well known. 'Access' to benefits of development was conditioned by the prevailing social environment of discrimination, which limited the outreach of the programmes. The ever-increasing population, the burden of 'diseases of poverty', limited supply of services, and even more pathetic absence of 'effective' demand, further smothered the advantages of relatively 'meagre' investments in the social sectors. The challenge, more than ever before, is to design strategic investments whose outcome will sustainably enhance social gains in terms of good health, education and capabilities and usher in social justice and equity in distribution, in effect holistically bringing about empowerment of women in the entirety of its connotation.

Social Development and Economic Progress

The inevitable link between social and economic development has emerged as an important factor to be reckoned. The Annual Economic Survey 2000-01 emphasizes the economic gains of investment on social sectors, particularly on women: "From the efficiency point of view, what is important is the social rate of return of investment in women, and in many cases, this can be greater than the corresponding rate for men."

Decline in Development Expenditure

The Economic Survey highlights that the total central plan outlay on social sector and rural development as percentage of total plan expenditure has declined from 29.27% in 1997-98 to 26.43% in 2000-01. Likewise, the percentage share of GDP on these sectors at current market prices has also

---

Department of Women and Child Development, Ministry of HRD, May 2001.

declined from 1.21% to 1.08% during the same period. Further, actual plan expenditure has shown a consistent downward trend as compared to the budget and revised estimates. This trend at a time when investment in development is very critical is a serious cause for worry. It is therefore urgent to sharpen the approach in the Tenth Plan to focus on strategies to optimize the very scarce public resources to increase gains for larger numbers of people and remove inequities. Government resources have to be supplemented from the corporate sectors as well as the community to reach the aspired goals of social development.

Correction of Regional Imbalances

Regional disparities continue to prevail in India, despite special efforts in the national process to bring up backward regions special economic incentives. The process of liberalization has exacerbated existing imbalances and deepened the schisms since investments under the liberalized regime tend to flow in the direction of regions and States, which have a head start in infrastructure development. The flagging economic situation of the less developed States has also slowed down the process of their social development further jeopardizing human resource development in those regions. Intra-state differences are equally marked creating pockets of prosperity amidst poverty and deprivation. It is urgent to evolve a new set of sustainable strategies to eliminate the regional imbalances in social and economic development.

Gender Equity

The planning process for the development of women has evolved through 'welfare' to 'development' to 'empowerment' to 'participation'. Despite the dynamism of the approach, the constitutional and legal provisions for affirmative action, the institutional build up and attendant step up in investments, gender discrimination continues to be a daunting challenge.

Significant gains have, however, been made in the life expectancy of women, literacy and representation in the local self-governing institutions. An active and grass-roots level leadership is emerging from among women. If properly harnessed this can be a very effective and catalytic agent for transforming the social conditions of women in the country.

The National Policy for Empowerment

National Policy on Empowerment of Women which was announced by the Government in April 2001 has outlined the approach to the whole gamut of issues for the empowerment of women and laid down a number of policy prescriptions for the national, state and local governments. The Nation has the mandate to implement this Policy and therefore nothing could be a better approach to the Tenth Plan than the National Policy itself. The Tenth Plan should essentially be in the nature of an Action Plan for the implementation of the National Policy.

Issues for Social Empowerment of Women: Declining Sex Ratio

Although the Census 2001 has registered a marginal improvement in the overall sex ratio in the country, the juvenile sex ratio (age group 0-6) has sharply declined from 945 per 1000 male in 1991 to 927 in 2001. It has declined in all the States and Union Territories except Kerala and Lakshadweep in the southeast, and Tripura, Mizoram and Sikkim in the northeast. The decline has been very sharp even in the prosperous States of Punjab, Haryana, Maharashtra and Gujarat. A massive awareness campaign involving the community, religious leaders and opinion makers at all levels is necessary to counter this trend.

Gender Asymmetry in Population

A strange gender asymmetry in population pyramid is taking place, with 'males outnumbering females' and 'females outnumbering males' at the lower and upper end of the pyramid respectively, while the middle is swelling, with numbers. This would create new demands for intervention at each level—protection and care of the girl child, social security for the aged, and training, capacity building and employment of more and more women in the working age group.

Rights of the Girl Child

Measures undertaken in the Ninth Plan do not seem to be having the desired impact on the condition of the girl child who is facing all round discrimination within the family and outside. The Pre-Natal Diagnostic (Regulation and Prevention of Misuse) Act, 1994 has completely failed to prevent the female foeticide. Balika Samridhi Yojana has also not much enhanced the value of girl child in society. The implementation of the scheme has been tardy as is reflected in huge unspent balances with the State Governments and a complete mismatch between the birth of girl child and disbursement of incentives under the scheme. A completely new strategy based on a holistic approach of awareness, incentives, education, nutrition and enforcement need to be worked out to protect the rights of the girl child.

Women's Health and Nutrition

The complex socio-cultural determinants of women's health have cumulative effects over a lifetime. Discriminatory childcare, under-nutrition and micronutrient deficiency in early adolescence is compounded by early child bearing and consequential serious pregnancy-related complexities. This is reflected in very high MMR (408 per 100,000 live births), IMR (72 per 1000 live births) and underweight babies (47%). Therefore, interventions for women's health and nutrition are extremely crucial not only for the health and the well-being of the women but of the nation as a whole. National Socio-Economic Goals of NPP 2000 aims, inter alia, to bring down MMR to 100 and IMR to 30 by 2010. These goals should be broken into certain achievable targets upto the year 2007 and measured by national level surveys.

Women should have access to comprehensive, affordable and quality 'health care' which should go beyond the 'reproductive health' to take into account their vulnerability to various endemic, infectious and communicable diseases. The social and health consequences of HIV/AIDS and sexually transmitted diseases also need to be tackled from a gender perspective.

Education and Training

Although the gender disparity in the level of literacy both in urban and rural areas continues, the urge for women's literacy has taken the shape of a movement throughout the length and breadth of the country. For the first time, the number of absolute female illiterates has come down, rate of growth of female literacy has out-paced that of male and the gap between female and male illiterates and dropouts is narrowing down.

The Sarva Siksha Abhiyan aims to provide useful and quality elementary education to all children in the age group of 6-10 and bridge the gender and social category gaps at primary level by 2010. This mission should also be broken into measurable goals to be achieved by the end of Tenth Plan in 2007. Tenth Plan should also further focus on reducing the gender gap in secondary and higher education and on the special category groups including SC/STs, OBCs and Minorities.

The vocationalisation of secondary education and vocational training for women is another priority area, which would require greater attention during the Tenth Plan. The existing network of regional vocational training centres should be extended to all the States and the women IITs with residential facilities be opened in all districts and sub-districts. More and more women should be trained on the emerging areas of technical education such as bio-technology, bio-engineering, food processing, electronics and computer systems and applications, fabric designing, communications, media, etc. which have high employment potential.

ECONOMIC EMPOWERMENT OF WOMEN

Employment and Work

Census 1991 had registered that only 22.3% of adult female population of India are workers, which may be a gross under statement since much of the work that women do, other than in the domestic and care sector, is not recorded in the work participation format of the Census. This format was revised for the Census 2001, which is expected to give a more realistic assessment of women's work. A pilot Time Use Survey conducted by the Central Statistical Organisation came out with the startling revelation that 51% of the work of women which qualify for inclusion in GDP are not recognized and remain unpaid.

Census 1991 further recorded that 95.8% of the women workers in India are employed in the unorganized sector where there are no legislative safeguards even to claim either minimum or equal wages, leave aside the other benefits that the women in the organised sector enjoy. The Report of the National Commission of Self Employed Women Workers (1988) gave a comprehensive account of the problem of women workers in the informal sector and recommended an intervention strategy which is largely valid even today.

Access to Resources

Traditionally women have been discriminated in her access to the productive resources. She has been denied coparcenary rights over the ancestral property. She has been denied ownership of land, cattle, trees, harvest and shelter. She has been discriminated in accessing credit and marketing facilities for her economic activities. Major interventions at the macro-economic and social policy levels are required to eliminate these age-old discriminations against women. While on the one hand there is the need to recognize women's economic activities in the domestic sector which largely go unpaid, on the other hand all the shackles should be removed for women's access to the productive resources so that she can be self-reliant and enjoy all the benefits of development. During the Tenth Plan various intervention strategy shall be required to improve the access of women to productive resources.

Women in Agriculture

The overwhelming majority of female workforce in the country are employed in the agricultural sector. Therefore, concerted efforts should be made to ensure that the benefits of training, extension and various programmes reach women in proportion to their numbers. Programmes for training women in soil conservation, social forestry, and other occupations allied to agriculture, horticulture, livestock including small husbandry, poultry, fishery, etc. should be expanded to benefit women workers in this sector.

Women in Industry

The important role played by women in electronics, technology, food processing, agro-industry and textiles has been crucial to the development of these sectors. They should be given comprehensive support in terms of labour legislation, social security and other support services to participate in various industrial sectors.

Women at present cannot work in night-shift factories even if they wish to. Suitable measures should be taken to enable women to work in night-shift in factories. This should be combined with support services for security, transportation, etc.

Equal Wages for Women

Although the twin legislations of the Minimum Wages Act and Equal Remuneration Act have granted equal means of livelihood and equal pay for equal work to the women, these rights are violated with impunity particularly in the informal sector. Administrative infrastructure of the Labour Department is not conducive to the enforcement of the provisions of the Act through the functionaries of the Department. Therefore, a new approach for involving women's groups and other civil society organizations for facilitating the enforcement of the laws is called for.

Women and Poverty

Women comprise nearly 70 per cent of the population below the Poverty Line. Many women like destitute, disabled and female-headed households face extreme situations of poverty. Although 40 per cent benefits of Swaran Jayanti Gramin Rozgar Yojana (SJGRY) and 30 per cent under Swaran Jayanti Shahari Rozgar Yojana (SJSRY) have been earmarked for women, various studies have shown that the actual benefits have not flown to them in the same proportion. It has been experienced that these programmes have a greater chance of success in a group approach rather than individual beneficiary approach and therefore the women's self-help groups should be fully mobilised at the block level and the programmes should be converged with the Block Level Action Plan of Integrated Women's Empowerment Programmes (IWEP).

Micro-Credit for Women

In order to enhance women's access to credit for consumption and production the micro-credit institutions in the country should be further strengthened and the actual flow of fund should be substantially enhanced so that self-employed groups of women have access to adequate credit for the income generating activities.

With the removal of all quantitative restrictions on import of various products the self-employed women's groups, mainly in the informal sector, have started facing competition of low price imported consumer goods which are invading the market. This has the imminent danger of throwing out a large number of women from their self-employment. At the same time the process of globalization has opened up opportunities for exporting the products to new markets all over the globe. Unfortunately the country has not fully geared itself to face the challenges of the globalization. It is necessary to identify the areas where skill and quality upgradation is required to make the informal women's groups more competitive. The training, infrastructure and credit requirement of all such activities should be fully arranged by the Government. The scope of the existing Women's Employment Programme (WEP) and Support for Training and Employment for Women (STEP) should be restructured and the allocation of resources under these two programmes substantially stepped up to meet the new requirement.

Women and Environment

Departmentalisation of forest management and commercialisation of forest extraction directly impinge on the interests of tribal and other women living in the vicinity of forest areas who depend on non-timber minor forest produce for their livelihood. The complementarities of relationship between the women and the forest can be strengthened and institutionalised through the proper implementation of the mechanism of Joint Forest Management. There are instructions that 50 per cent of the members of the JFM should be women and that the 50 per cent of women members should be present for holding the General Body meeting. There are reports that these instructions are not being followed in many States.

There is also a need for change in the silvi cultural practices in the forests so that trees and plants which generate a lot of fodder, fruits, nuts, twigs and branches are planted in place of timber and other conventional species. This will enable the local community driven by the women's groups to take greater role and interest in the management and conservation of the forests.

Women are the most interested group for consumption of domestic fuel and therefore their involvement for the spread of non-conventional energy sources like bio-gas, non-smoke chullahs, etc. are of critical importance for success of this programme. Air pollution arising out of conventional cooking system affects the health and the respiratory system of the women. The existing programme of smokeless chullahs and other non-conventional energy resources should be taken up on a massive scale for the benefit of women.

Drinking Water and Sanitation

This is an area of critical concern for the public health. Although 85 per cent of the villages have been covered under safe drinking water supply, the actual coverage of the hamlets and households have been much less particularly in the hilly, tribal, drought prone and desert areas where women have to travel a long distance for fetching the drinking water. The priority concern for the Tenth Plan should be to ensure that every woman could access safe drinking water in the neighbourhood.

More than 70 per cent of the population in India are not covered by toilet and sanitation facilities. The women, particularly living in the urban slums, are the worst sufferers since their privacy is disturbed severely. The low cost sanitation scheme for the liberation of the scavengers had unfortunately a very tardy performance. Even the meagre allocation of the Plan resources are not being fully utilised by the State Governments and the demeaning practice of manual scavenging of night soil by the female scavengers is still continuing in many urban areas. The Tenth Plan should have a fresh look into the entire issue of urban sanitation in the country which badly affects the interests of the women.

Housing and Shelter

Although the women are the house-keepers their perspectives are not generally considered in the planning of houses and housing colonies and provision of shelters in both urban and rural areas. The gender bias in planning of human settlements should be removed by necessary amendments in the building bye-laws and the rules and regulations of the town planning.

Special attention should be given for providing adequate and safe housing and accommodation for women including single women, heads of households, working women, students, apprentices and trainees.

Science and Technology

A number of women-specific technologies have been developed by the various research institutes to reduce the drudgery of women in their domestic and farm works. There is a need for dissemination of these technologies through the collaborative efforts of the research institutes, manufacturers and the women's groups. Research should be more focused for development of new technologies which would have greater chances of acceptability by the women.

Although more and more women students are taking up higher education in the fields of science and technology there is still a large gender gap in this area. Liberal scholarships and other incentives should be given to the girl students to pursue higher studies on scientific research and technology.

Women's Support Services

Department of Women and Child Development is implementing a number of schemes to provide social support services to the women. A number of State Governments have also initiated innovative schemes on support services which are duplicating the efforts of the Central Government. While on the one hand there is a need for merger and convergence of similar schemes and restructuring of many schemes according to the changing situations there is also pressing requirement of professionalisation of some of the services like Family Counselling Centres, Creches, and Short Stay Homes, etc.

Similarly, there are new areas of support services which require the attention of Government. The long awaited scheme on Women in Difficult Circumstances which is expected to be launched during 2001-02, should be expanded to cover various types of women in distress like widows in religious places, prostitutes, migrant women, women affected by natural calamities, disabled women, women ex-prisoners, mentally retarded and disordered women, women in conflict situations, etc.

Similarly, there is a dire need for introducing social security system for women in the unorganised sector which employ maximum number of women but do not provide them any protection or safety network.

The Personal Accident and Social Security Insurance Scheme of the LIC and GIC which provide compensation for disability and death should be extended to the women in the informal sector. The women in the BPL families should be covered by insurance benefit when the male earning members sustain disability or die and the families are pauperised further.

Women and Legislation

Although the Constitution of India has granted equality to women and further empowered the State to make positive discrimination in favour of women for neutralizing the cumulative socio-economic, educational and political disadvantages faced by them, there are still some areas where rights of women are not fully secured by laws and there are laws which are either discriminatory against women or provide a week enforcement and punishment mechanism which do not deter the recurrence of crimes of against women.

The entire gamut of laws on women or related to women need a comprehensive and thorough review. Some exercise has been done in the past by the National Commission on Women and some major legislative initiative has been taken in hand. This process should be continued and completed during the Tenth Plan

Media and Empowerment of Women

A carefully planned mass media strategy is of critical importance for women's empowerment. Men and women in decision-making position -in family, community, workplaces and society at large—can be gender sensitized through media intervention. The issues of women's rights, health and education, access to resources, sharing of domestic responsibility, girl child's right to be born, survive, develop and many other related issues can be packaged in interesting, viewer friendly programmes for assimilation and absorption in social psyche.

The Tenth Plan must consciously address to the need for a welt planned media strategy not only for bringing a massive awareness, and education on the gender issues but also preventing a derogatory and biased portrayal of women in the media. Such a Plan would not only cut across issues but also across agencies, Ministries and Departments. The Plan should also provide adequate resources for implementation of such a comprehensive and holistic media strategy for social change.

NATIONAL MACHINERY FOR WOMEN'S ADVANCEMENT

Considerable institutional development has already come about for facilitating women's advancement. Useful work has also been done by various institutions like the National Commission for Women, Central Social Welfare Board, NIPCCD, Rashtriya Mahila Kosh, Parliamentary Committee for Empowerment of Women, State Women Development Corporations, etc. While these institutions should be further strengthened and streamlined according to their felt needs, various grass-roots level institutions and initiatives should be involved with the process of empowerment of women.

Panchayats and Municipalities

Panchayati Raj institutions and the Municipalities, created under the

73rd and 74th Constitutional Amendments, have both the Constitutional mandate and potential as grassroots institutions to bring about a sea change of development in the social sector. They should be empowered with resource support for the purpose of enhancing the status of women in societal as well as developmental terms. A nation wide capacity building exercise should be taken up for all elected women members of PRI and Municipalities. They should be given responsibility of planning, implementation and monitoring, particularly in the areas of health services, primary education, child development programmes, drinking water, irrigation, management of all natural resources—land, forest and water, social security for women in BPL families, aged, disabled, deserted women de facto female headed households, etc.

Women's Self Help Groups

Self-help groups of women have been found to be very effective grassroots institutions in facilitating access for women to means of development, be it information, financial and material resources or services. The 'self-help group' mode should be encouraged, so that the groups become dynamic change agents in bringing about empowerment and socio-economic development of women.

Organizations of the Civil Society

Efforts of the governmental institutions have to be supplemented by the Organizations of the Civil Society (NGOs). Already a large number of such institutions have emerged in different parts of the country and they have to their credit significant contribution and experience at the grassroots level in projecting and addressing women's issues. The services of these institutions should be encouraged, supported and availed of, so that advancement of women becomes a truly national and people's movement.

Corporate World

The Corporate world, especially of late, has evinced significant interest in social development issues including women's development, transcending their limited business mandates. As employers, corporate bodies have strategic interface with the working people. Their services should be utilized for further gender sensitization of the corporate world as a whole as well as the working people. Their infrastructure and resources should also be drawn upon in implementation of women's development programmes.

UN and other Agencies

The United Nations and its various specialized agencies, as a matter of pro-active and coordinated in-house policies have taken very keen interest in women's development in their own respective areas of competence. They have been providing resource support for various gender-oriented programmes. More importantly, they have been facilitating sharing of international experience in addressing women's issues and catalyzing national action. Full support should be given to the efforts of these agencies at the national, regional and grassroots level. World Bank, Asian Development Bank and other multilateral as well as bilateral agencies are increasingly providing resource support for social development including gender development programmes. Their assistance should also be availed of to maximize investments in human resource development amongst women.

IMPLEMENTATION STRATEGY

Women's Component Plan

Ninth Five Year Plan adopted Women's Component Plan as one of its major strategies and directed both the Central and State Governments to ensure that "not less than 30 per cent of the funds/benefits are earmarked in all the women's related sectors." It also directed that a special vigil be kept on the flow of the earmarked funds/benefits through an effective mechanism to ensure that the proposed strategy brings forth a holistic approach towards empowering women.

Although 12 Ministries/Departments and 4 State Governments have confirmed their efforts to extend the benefits to Women's Component Plan, it has not been possible to exactly quantify the allocations, although substantial benefits from the core sectors of health and family welfare, education, labour and employment, rural development, urban development, agriculture, science and technology are stated to be flowing to the women.

The concept of the Women's Component Plan must not be abandoned or weakened merely because it was not operationalised effectively. Rather it should be further strengthened with comprehensive guidelines and instructions and an effective system for monitoring the progress should be developed both in the Planning Commission and in the Department of Women and Child Development.

Tenth Five Plan should also enlist the schemes and programmes of the various Ministries/Departments which will be covered under WCP. The estimates of allocation and expenditure of these schemes should be shown as a separate account head in the Demands for Grants on the pattern of Tribal sub-plan and Special Component Plan for Scheduled Castes. No reappropriation from WCP to the general schemes should be permitted without the prior approval of Women and Child Development Department. Various schedules and formats for reporting progress should also be devised to include separate columns on men and women so that the benefits flowing to women can be monitored more closely.

Gender Budgeting

Gender budgeting is not a separate budget for women; rather it isa dissection of the government budget to establish its gender-differential impacts and to translate gender commitments into budgetary commitments. The main objective of a gender-sensitive budget is to improve the analysis of incidence of budgets, attain more effective targeting of public expenditure and offset any undesirable gender-specific consequences of previous budgetary measures.

The Department of Women and Child Development has taken the initiative of starting a gender budgeting exercise from the current year. For the first time a separate section on Gender Inequality has been included in the chapter on Social Sector in the Annual Economic Survey of the Government. An analysis of the Budget 2001 from the gender perspective has been carried out and this should be continued as a regular feature every year.

Convergence of Services

Various Ministries/Departments and their agencies engaged in women's development have often tended to function in a compartmentalised manner, leading to duplication of services, escalation of costs and fragmentation of efforts at various levels. Strategies and mechanisms for bringing about coordination and convergence of services and sequencing multi-sectoral functions for social development have to be given priority in programme design and implementation.

Identification of best practices, critiques on failures and the analysis thereof of the causes leading to those failures and adoption of measures for mid-course corrections would need to be a continuous process. Various bottlenecks that have been exposed in the implementation of several well-intentioned projects and programmes have to be identified for specific scrutiny to strategize the elimination of those bottlenecks.

The Integrated Child Development Services (ICDS) is almost universalized. The units under this programme (Anganwadis) have become the ubiquitous grassroots level institutions. This infrastructure should be used for converged delivery of a variety of social services—immunization, health, nutrition, preschool education. life-long education of adolescent girls, adult literacy, population education, AIDS awareness, etc., apart from general Awareness Creation.

Resources and Priorities

The share of women specific programmes constitute a fraction of the total fund allotted to the DWCD. During the financial year 2000-01 out of the total expenditure of Rs. 1335.93 crores in the Department, expenditure on women specific programmes was only Rs. 115.71 crores. This constituted a meager 8.57%.

It is also a matter of concern that the central plan investment on women specific programmes has been shrinking over the years. The total outlay of Ninth Plan on women specific programmes of the DWCD was Rs. 1238.76 crores, but the actual budget allocation during these five years was only Rs. 851.49 crores (68.73%). The revised budget allocation for the first four years was Rs. 568.73 crores (45.91%), out of which only Rs. 472.35 crores (38.13%) could be actually spent. It is unfortunate that nearly one-fourth of the sanctioned budget allocation of the Department on women specific schemes could not be utilized during the Ninth Plan and had either to be surrendered or diverted to some other schemes due to limited capacity of absorption of funds under existing strategy.

Both these trends must be reversed during the Tenth Plan.

Delivery Mechanism

The existing mechanism of implementation of most of the schemes of the Department of Women and Child Development, either directly by the Department or through the Central Social Welfare Advisory Board, severely constraints the capacity of the system to reach the target women. This model had its relevance when no institutional machinery existed at the State level for the delivery of services to the women. Today every State Government has its Department of Social Welfare, besides Women and Child Welfare Department and Women Development Corporation. Panchayat Raj institutions with one-third women members and a large number of women self-help groups have come up at the grassroots all over the country. These new institutions can take up the responsibility of the implementation of most of the schemes on women. The Tenth Plan must recognise this changed scenario and accordingly restructure the entire institutional mechanism for the delivery of the programmes of women.

Integrated Women's Empowerment Programme

This programme has been designed to create a synergy of women's self-help groups, panchayati raj institutions, NGOs and the State administration at the block level for preparation of block level action plan for the development of women. This action plan shall essentially be in the nature of convergence of schemes of the State Government, DWCD and other Ministries/Departments of Government of India. This programme should be universalized in all the 5025 plus blocks of the country. This would require an investment of Rs. 1043.80 crores during the Tenth Plan.

Universalisation of IWEP will significantly augment the outreach of the women's programmes. This will also generate substantially additional demands for women's training and skill upgradation, which should be fully met in the Tenth Plan.

Restructuring of the Programmes

With the introduction of Swaran Jayanti Gramodaya Yojana, Sarva Siksha Abhiyan, and success of National Literacy Mission and National Open School, etc. some of the existing schemes like Socio-Economic Programme, Condensed Courses for Women's Education and Vocational Training, etc. have completely lost their relevance and should be converged with the new institutions and programmes. The women specific programmes of the Department should be completely restructured. There should be two main programmes, (a) Women's Support Services Programmes, and (b) Women's Economic Programmes, which should offer a wide range of choices according to the specific situations in particular States, regions and sub-regions.

Role of CSWB and State Boards

CSWB should specialize on the schemes on women's support services such as Awareness Generation Programme, Short Stay Homes, Family Counselling Centres, Women in Difficult Circumstances, etc. The State Social Welfare Advisory Boards are often duplicating the efforts of the State Government and its agencies without any coordination with them. Therefore, there is a need to redefine the role of the State Boards. The DWCD has constituted a Committee under the Chairmanship of Shri T.N. Chaturvedi to look into the whole gamut of issues regarding the future role of CSWB and the State Boards. The recommendations of the Committee should be taken into account while taking any decision in this regard.

Gender Development Index

Gender segregated data on the various indices of human development at the State, district and sub-district level are not available for preparation of region specific projects for empowerment of women. DWCD had taken an initiative for preparation of 18 minimum indicators on gender development at the district level throughout the country. There should be further discussions on these Indices for establishing certain uniform and comparable indicators at the national and international levels. The statistical system of the country should be strengthened for generating such data at district and sub-district levels at a regular intervals.

Monitoring and Evaluation

Monitoring systems and mechanisms need to be developed both at the community and Panchayat level at one end and State and National levels at the other end to ensure allocations, expenditure and implementation of programmes and projects as per the Component Plans. Evaluation and midcourse correction of the gender-budgeting and monitoring system should be done systematically and the experience gained there from should be applied to evolve and establish fine-tuned institutionalized procedures. The critical mass of technically qualified persons should be positioned in the Planning Commission, Ministries/ Departments and States to undertake this task on a half-yearly basis.

The system of concurrent evaluation of the major schemes through independent organisations should be built into the programme itself. Important State and national level research organisations and other academic institutions and societies should be involved for the regular evaluation of the major programmes of the Department.

Research

Any developmental plan to be realistic is to be based on information on ground truths in terms of cultural traditions, practices, problems and their magnitude as well as developmental experience itself. Reports and feedbacks on all these factors have to be obtained through field level research conducted on credible and scientific basis. For the purpose, scientific researches would be undertaken on women's issues and concerns through various governmental and non-governmental institutions having competence and credibility.

APPENDIX 9.6

CHALLENGES IN WOMEN'S HEALTH IN THE 21ST CENTURY AND WHO STRATEGY

Review of Progress

Considerable progréss in improving the status of women's health has been made over the last two decades. Politics and programmes based on gender considerations have been developed in several countries. Gender action plans to promote and protect the health of women as fundamental human rights have been drawn up. Initiatives have been taken to promote the participation of women at policy and decision-making levels. Public awareness of women's health issues has also increased considerably, along with pressure to convert policy statements and legislation into effective action. There is increased awareness in countries in relation to gender-based violence, including harmful traditional practices such as female genital mutilation. More programmes are looking into ways of encouraging men to take responsibility for their own and their partners' sexual and reproductive health. And, most importantly, all these activities have advanced the prospects of establishing a participatory process and approach, which is at the heart of the women's health agenda.

Despite these remarkable advances, overall progress on women's health has been altogether unsatisfactory. Globalization and the current economic crises in some regions have had adverse effects on national health systems which in turn, have affected health services for women. Furthermore, in some countries, recently made gains in improving infant, child and maternal survival have been lost and even reversed as a result of social unrest, war, and the epidemic of HIV/AIDS. Globally, we are also witnessing a feminization of poverty in which most of the one billion people who live in extreme poverty are women. The consequences of poverty are serious at the level of the individual and the family. The health consequences are disastrous to women because poverty restricts women's choices in so many ways that are basic to good health. It is widely acknowledged that poverty remains a root cause of women's ill-health. Regardless of this fact, the shrinking public resources for healthcare are cushioned by the voluntary contributions of women, for whom the care for ailing family members is an additional burden.

There is a growing demand for reproductive health services and for access to a wide range of contraceptive methods, including the need for informed choice. Adolescent's health and, in particular, teenage pregnancy, remain a serious concern. With regard to male fertility regulation, attitudes are changing, and younger men and couples are now volunteering for clinical trials. The pharmaceutical industry, which had not shown interest in research in the 1980s, has recently become involved in studies on male contraception. The burden of infertility on couples, in particular on women, is of concern to some countries. The lack of information on the causes of infertility and the effects of biomedical research, including cloning, have been expressed as areas of concern in women's health. The physical, psychological and social effects of medically assisted reproduction technology on the health of women, and the risks involved, must not be underestimated.

The dramatic increase in HIV/AIDS infection among women, in particular, the high risks for adolescents aged 15 to 25 years, now representing half of recent HIV victims, is alarming. Infection in young girls is often related to forced sex and rape. Migration, trafficking and sexual exploitation contribute to the spread of the disease among young women. The taboos surrounding the disease and the stigmatization of the victims cause further violence and isolation. Of particular concern are the mother-to-child infection and the dilemma surrounding breast-feeding for HIV positive mothers. Countries are calling for greater protection of women from infection, including access to the female condom and improved treatment of HIV/AIDS patients through affordable access to anti-retroviral therapy and drugs. Several countries have reported campaigns and legal action taken to accelerate the elimination of harmful practices such as female genital mutilation.

The negative impact of violence on women's mental health, one of the major reasons for psychiatric disorders, anxiety and depression among women, is well recognized. Mental disorders in women seem to be caused more by social problems than by hereditary and hormonal processes. Mental healthcare for women needs to be integrated into primary healthcare services to make it more easily accessible. With regard to substance abuse, women face discrimination in treatment and rehabilitation that are not gender-sensitive. Women are increasingly being singled out in the marketing of products associated with certain lifestyle patterns. The increasing number of women smoking, and their difficulties in abandoning the tobacco habit, as shown by research, is also of concern. The rising rate of lung cancer among women is one of the consequences of changes in lifestyles. Another is the association of alcohol abuse and unemployment with increases in domestic violence against women and children. In relation to the environment, occupational and environmental health suffers from lack of attention to pollution and to the risk factors of certain lifestyles. Women react to certain hazards at work which include stress, trauma and physical reactions. Occupational health regulations need to address women's health issues. Steps must be taken to safeguard the health of pregnant and breast-feeding working women in particular.

Bridging the gap between policy and implementation on one hand, and between awareness and attitudinal changes on the other hand, is the challenge at this stage. The creation of an enabling environment that includes a supportive legislative framework and political commitment at the highest level is a prerequisite for effective social change and improvement in women's health. In connection with this, several countries have made modifications to the legal framework that are beneficial to women's health.

These modifications relate to health insurance, patients' rights, and healthcare and social security systems. Some progress has also been noted in the collection of health statistics disaggregated by sex and age and the awareness of the need for the development of gender-specific indicators on health. Special emphasis needs to be placed on the importance of mainstreaming the gender perspective into all fields of health. This should include a focus on the role of men and the importance of partnership, specifically in reproductive health. A gender perspective is also needed for integration in medical education and research. This would lead to changes in the health sector at the decision-making level, where women still do not have a decisive presence. There is a need for more gender-sensitive training, but the unavailability of training materials, trainers and training opportunities represents a serious obstacle to creating greater gender sensitivity among health professionals and policy-makers in particular.

Wellness and Women's Health

Women's health is an expression of relationships. The term "social-developmental model of women's health" implies three elements: the biological determinants, the process of human development and the social and cultural context in which health and disease are expressed. The central theme of these three dimensions of health are the ever changing, hopefully maturing relationship of the woman to her physical, ecological, personal, social and cultural environment.

These changes involve the relationship of a woman to her own body and physiology, and her relationships to parents, family, intimate partner, peers, community and the broader society.

The Life Span Approach

Reducing women's health to women's reproductive health has had numerous negative consequences for the state of scientific knowledge which include:

- An inadequate understanding of gender differences in health.
- A paucity of information pertaining to basic physiology and pharmacokinetics in women.
- Pervasive gender bias in research such as less attention being paid to conditions to which women are more vulnerable and the assumption that health through the lifespan follows the same course for women as it does for men.
- The neglect of social factors, discrimination and gender specific negative life events and stress in favour of reproductive and endocrinological explanations of women's higher rates of depressive and other psychological disorders.
- An emphasis on the health, including the mental health of women as mothers and a relative neglect of other aspects of women's health and other periods of the lifecycle.

The life span approach to human health and development brings one important conceptual ingredient to our understanding of health. Health is the sum total of our successful attainment of a state of wellness at earlier stages, our acquired capacity to resist disease, and our success in achieving the series of developmental tasks in the sequence of mental and social development at each stage of the life span. Because biological and social aspects affect women's health throughout their lives and have cumulative effects, it is important to look at the entire life span in examining the causes and consequences of women's health. The grouping of these stages varies with the focus and purpose. For purposes of an analysis of women's health, the following groupings are proposed: childhood (with sub-groupings of under-five years of age and up to adolescence, sometimes referred to as early and middle childhood), adolescence, reproductive years, post-reproductive years and the elder years (including, for those in the work force, the period of retirement, as well as that of death and bereavement, i.e., widowhood).

Infancy and Childhood

Scientific advances in reproductive technologies have allowed couples to have the number of children they want, when they want them. While these technologies are also appropriate in ensuring that carriers of serious genetic disorders are able to improve their chances of bearing a healthy infant, there is also evidence that they are being abused through sex selection of conceptions and sex selective abortions. Historically, cultures with a strong bias against girl births have resorted to infanticide or neglect as a means of limiting the number of girls in a family. More recently, sex-selective abortion is believed to be the cause of the "missing females in several countries."

Sex ratios of births serve as the first measure of gender discrimination. In developed countries with reliable and complete birth registration, the male-female birth ratio (M:F-BR) normally falls between 1.03 and 1.08. The M:F-BR is less reliable as a "true" measure in the developing world, where a large proportion of births occur outside institutional settings and the registration of births may not occur for months or years, if they are registered at all. Deaths that occur in the interim would not be registered. If gender discrimination is sufficient to increase the mortality among girl children, the M:F-BR would be abnormally high, as is apparently the case in rural China, the Republic of Korea, Azerbaijan and probably other countries with strong son preference, but which lack reliable M:F-BR data.

Comparison of the female:male ratios (F:M-MR ratio) of neonatal, infant and under-five child mortality is even more sensitive as a measure of sex and gender differences. The F:M-MR ratio serves to measure differential care received by girls which negates their innate biological advantage relative to boys. This ratio of rates is consistently 20 to 25% lower among girls in developed countries in which there is no identifiable preference for boys or girls. Several factors contribute to better survival of female newborns. Because the fetal lungs of girls mature earlier, male newborns are at a greater risk of developing and dying from respiratory distress. And because the latter have higher levels of serum ferritin, a lower incidence of neuro-developmental morbidity and very low birth weight, girls have much higher rates of survival.'

Evidence of a mortality disadvantage for the girl infant and child attributable to gender discrimination was found in the analysis of the infant and under-five child F:M-MR ratios in 35 countries. On the average, 5% of the infant mortality of girls was attributable to gender discrimination. The figures for the countries of the Middle East Crescent were 17%, three times greater than the differences in Latin America and Africa. The figures for the under-five F:M-MR ratios were 15% in sub-Sahara Africa and Latin America. Based on the mortality data reported to WHO, the mortality disadvantage of the girl child in rural China was similar to that in the Middle East Crescent. Limited data on long-term trends over time have shown a decrease in the mortality disadvantage of the girl child in Bulgaria, Ireland and Sri Lanka. However, in India, in over a 20-year period until the 1970s, there was an increase in the mortality disadvantage for the girl child.

More than one-third of the world's children suffer from stunting or wasting. In Asia, where 70% of the affected children live, most countries have high or very high prevalence. But only in Africa, where 25% of the affected children are, does one find an increase in stunting both in the absolute number and percentage of children affected. However, in an analysis on sex differences in stunting in 81 countries, in only ten, including Nepal, Bangladesh and Sri Lanka, was the frequency of stunting in girls more than 7% higher than in boys. Despite the anthropological reports of discriminatory feeding patterns to the disadvantage of the girl, the aggregated national data from 61 countries in other regions either showed no difference or higher stunting prevalence in boys. Despite the strong son preference, and a markedly higher mortality disadvantage of the girl child in China, over the last few decades of national and provincial nutrition surveys, none show a significant difference in stunting by sex. Furthermore, in the WHO databases on breast-feeding, there is no consistent evidence of a sex advantage for boys during breast-feeding even in countries with a strong son preference.

It was generally assumed that the response of girls to infectious diseases did not differ from that of boys until recent observations in several countries following vaccination of children using high-titre live measles vaccine. The observation showed an excess of non-specific mortality, particularly among females and those receiving the highest titre vaccine." Since vaccination with live measles virus results in a temporary depression of the immune response to other antigens, the female predominance in subsequent non-measles mortality may be due to sex differences in response to live measles vaccines, and may possibly be indicative of other immunological differences between girls and boys. With normal doses of vaccine, measles immunization appears to accelerate and increase the advantage of the girl child.

In many countries, parents with limited resources may be less willing to pay the school uniform or other fees for a girl's education. Yet, in the 35-country analysis of the DHS data, the factor most strongly correlated with female mortality disadvantage was the male:female differences in primary school enrolment. Fortunately, primary school attendance rates for girls are increasing, but completion and secondary school attendance lags far behind that of boys.

Poverty again becomes a major actor in creating disproportionate obstacles and even greater harm to girls as they become women, and as they bear and care for the next generation of children, both boys and girls. Girls are removed from school to assist in household chores and to care for younger siblings. Rural poverty, limited education, lack of work and a pattern of bonded labour draw children into the labour market. In India and Nepal, girls in rural areas from the age of six through fourteen, spend less time than boys in leisure, in study and reading, and more time in work. Girls 6 to 9 years of age spend three or more hours per day working, while boys of the same age spend less than two hours. By the time they are 10 to 14, Nepali girls are working nearly 8 hours per day, while boys work half that time.

One is left with the hypothesis that gender specific healthcare seeking behaviours have a major impact on the mortality disadvantage of the girl child, particularly when compounded by poverty and its consequences. Health behaviours may change in negative, positive or paradoxical ways under the pressures of economic change or other crises. For example, several years ago, wasting and stunting among girls increased far more than in boys during times of famine and among the poorest population. Families were probably more likely to delay seeking medical care and limited their expenditures for the care when a girl became ill in comparison to when a boy became ill. Given the enormous mortality disadvantage of girls in the regions of the world with the largest population, it would seem that testing of this hypothesis should be of high priority on the international research agenda. If this hypothesis proves to be correct, addressing it would add another challenge and priority for targeted strategies in health education. It also would be important to determine whether the cultural presence of sons is also influencing the treatment decisions of health workers, possibly under parental pressure.

Adolescence

Adolescence is the period of transition from childhood to adulthood, and is characterized: (a) biological development from the onset of puberty to full secular and reproductive maturity, (b) psychological development from the cognitive and emotional patterns of childhood to those of adulthood, and (c) emergence from the childhood state of total socio-economic dependence to one of relative independence. WHO considers 10-

19 years as the period of adolescence, noting that it generally encompasses the time of onset of puberty to the legal age of majority. However, it also acknowledges that there are wide discrepancies between chronological age and biological and psychosocial stages of development, as well as wide variations due to personal and environmental factors. These discrepancies are particularly noteworthy among adolescent girls/women.

The dynamics of social change present adolescents with major challenges. In traditional societies, young people can be fairly sure that their lives will be substantially similar to their parents. In modern societies, they can be confident that they will be substantially different. In transitional societies, young people find themselves in two cultures: the traditional one in which their parents grew up and which they may still value, and the modern one which they learn in school and is portrayed in an increasingly globalized media. A similar clash of cultures may be found among young people whose families have migrated either from another country or from rural to an urban area.

The biological changes of adolescence are somatic and hormonal, with marked individual variation in the timing and tempo of changes. The growth spirit in height and weight is closely linked to sexual maturation. As the nutritional status of girls improves, the onset of menses occurs at an earlier age. From 1860 to 1960, the age of menarche declined from 16.5 years to 12.2 in industrialized countries. Virtually all developing countries have been going through similar changes in a shorter period of time. Completion of bone growth in both height and pelvic size and shape does not approximate adult status until two years after the onset of menses. Thus, the adolescent girl is capable of conception, but unlikely to delivery safely. Furthermore, the competing demands of her own growth and that of the fetus will result in a slowing or cessation of her growth, thus compromising the woman's health and that of future conceptions, unless appropriately, and nutritionally treated, therapeutically and prophylactically.

The long-term health of women is also influenced by the changes in the patterns of menarche and nutrition. The typical high fat, low fiber diet of the industrialized West, particularly when associated with inadequate exercise, is likely to advance the onset of puberty. This will manifest in girls as an earlier menarche, earlier onset of breast development, and an earlier growth spurt. Both early menarche and adult tallness are markers of increased risk to breast cancer. Earlier menarche in the West is usually associated with earlier onset of hyperinsulinaemia, which is also thought to be a marker of increased breast cancer risk. The time from puberty to the first pregnancy is particularly important for breast cancer risk. Girls who had menarche before they became 12 years old, have a more rapid onset of ovulatory menstrual cycles, than girls who have a later menarche. Significantly higher serum oestradiol and lower sex hormone binding globulin concentrations are seen in women who had an early menarche, and the differences still remain at 20-30 years of age. Thus, increased oestrogen and progesterone secretion might induce higher degree of breast epithelial proliferation. Further research is required concerning the possible role of physical exercise and nutrition in modifying breast cancer risk.

There are additional physical and mental health consequences that are associated with the rapid physiologic changes of reproductive maturation and appearance of secondary sexual characteristics. Despite the decline in the age of menarche, there is little evidence that this has been accompanied by a comparable shift in the cognitive, psychological and emotional capacity. The lack of synchronization in physical and emotional maturity will often put increased pressures on the adolescent who physically matures at a relatively younger age. Later maturation is generally associated with better affective adjustment.

During childhood and the transition to adulthood, the reproductive tract of girls is particularly vulnerable to infection. The cells and secretions of the immature reproductive tract are much less able to resist invasion and damage by sexually transmitted micro-organisms than in adults, including those associated with pelvic inflammatory disease and its consequences of infertility and ectopic pregnancy and those associated with cervical cancer. A later age of onset of menarche, but an earlier onset of sexual activity, greatly increases the immediate and long-term consequences of STDs in the young women. Because the presence of other STDs will also increase the likelihood of HIV infecting an individual, adolescent girls who have a later onset of menarche, but early onset of sexual activity will be at even greater increased risk of AIDS as well. Repeated C. Trachomatis which causes erosion of the normal cervical barriers, further increases the hazards of human papilloma virus infection and its subsequent risks of cervical carcinoma. Malnutrition greatly increases these risks.

Although women aged 10-19 are generally healthy, specific behaviours and cultural practices can jeopardize their well-being. In most traditional societies, sexual activity of girls is normally initiated within marriage, albeit in many, before or soon after the onset of menses—at times as young as 10 or 11 years of age. In an adolescent clinic population in Ethiopia, premenarche sexual initiation was noted to occur in 40% of the girls. The hazards of sexual activity and child-bearing before biological and social maturation have been well documented. In some settings, particularly when outside of marriage, the man engages in sexual activity with other women, including prostitutes, the child-wife in such marriages has an increased risk of acquiring sexually transmitted diseases on two counts: the increased likelihood of acquiring such infections from the husband and the increased vulnerability of the immature reproductive tract. Data from several countries in Africa, for example, have shown that the earlier the age of the onset of sexual activity, the higher the level of infertility becomes.

In cultures that practice child marriage, girls are catapulted to adulthood, by passing the period of biological and social maturation of adolescence as they are married off before or just after menarche. Although many countries have raised the legal age for marriage, it is rarely enforced, and generally shows little correlation with the actual age of marriage.

Marital discord is also more common with a younger age of marriage, and both circumstances are in some settings associated with child prostitution, often as consequence of the child-wife running away and having no other means than prostitution for supporting herself. For example, in one study, nearly 70% of the women engaged in prostitution were sexually active before menarche compared to half that number among a control group. Noting that half of all prostitutes were married for less than 5 years, a large number began prostitution as children. In some countries child prostitution has its roots in historical, social and religious traditions. Poorer families would dedicate their daughters to be wedded to a temple goddess, or would send them to be prostitutes for the ruling elite. Traffickers have found it easy to lure large number of girls to brothels, even with the collusion of their parents.

For many girls, adolescence is a period of sexual debut, leading to the health risks associated with early pregnancy, unsafe abortion, and STDs, including AIDS. Nutritional requirements increase during adolescence. Adolescents also adopt behaviours that affect their health, such as smoking and substance abuse. There also is an exacerbation of young women's susceptibility to STDs through the social acceptance of male promiscuity, social expectation of young women's passivity, and social assignment of greater value to what is masculine. Those who start having children early generally have more children than those who embark on parenthood later. Early marriage, pregnancy and child bearing are likely to limit the education and immediate and long-term employment prospects of an adolescent girl.

In the absence of adequate maternity care, maternal mortality among young adolescents is several times higher than those who are a few years older. In a large part of the world, the highest incidence of pelvic inflammatory disease is among women of 15 to 24 years of age, and the consequences of STDs are measured in rising rates of ectopic pregnancy and tubal infertility. There are also the silently suffering young women who have survived a traumatic delivery but are left with livelong morbidity of vesiculovaginal fistula. In addition to their physical injuries, women who have experienced prolonged obstructed labour often develop serious social problems, including divorce, exclusion from religious activities, separation from their families, worsening poverty, malnutrition, and almost unendurable suffering.

Women are much more likely than men to develop eating disorders. Regardless of the type, all eating disorders are rooted in emotions, often traced to problems during adolescence. Dieting is the most important predictor of new eating disorders. Differences in the incidence of eating disorders between sexes were largely accounted for by the high rates of earlier dieting and psychiatric morbidity in the female subjects. In adolescents, controlling weight by exercise rather than diet restriction seems to carry less risk of development of eating disorders. While the problem is widely found in North and South America, and Europe, it is also described in Asia as well. It is associated with a significant excess mortality in some groups.

There is limited evidence that some of the possible differences in immunological function of childhood may also be manifested during adolescence. Response to immunization booster doses may be lower in adolescent and adult women, and, when the incidence of tuberculosis is high, the incidence rate in adolescent women is much higher than would be expected. In industrialized countries in the middle of this century (1930s to 1950s), females aged 15 to 34 years had higher tuberculosis notification rates than males of the same age. However, as notification rates in these countries decreased in time, rates in males became higher than those of females for all ages over 15. The absence of comparable patterns now in the developing world among young women raises questions as to possible gender influences on reporting of such cases.

Throughout adolescence, self-esteem appears to be affected by the competence in certain valued domains—physical attractiveness, peer acceptance, and perceived support from peers, family or others. Identity is critical during adolescence. It reflects the formation of a stable, coherent picture of oneself that includes an integration of one's past and present experiences and a sense of where one is headed in the future. The process according to Erikson involves a series of selective narrowing of choices in the realms of sexual, occupational and social roles and a progressive commitment to the choices one makes. It remains to be seen as to the extent to which this model is applicable in other cultures, particularly those with a strong interdependent communal orientation.

For the adolescent, these developmental phases can be spoken of in terms of the need to attain or resolve a number of developmental tasks, *inter-alia*:

- adaptation to the physiological and anatomical changes associated with puberty and the integration of a mature sexuality into a personal mode of behaviour,
- the progressive resolution of earlier forms of attachment to parents and family, and the development through peer relationships of an enhanced capacity for interpersonal intimacy, and
- the establishment of an individual identity, incorporating a sexual identity and adaptive social roles.

In achieving these developmental tasks, the adolescent needs to make choices, and making choices involves having information, support and area, with a life services adapted to their needs and perceptions, expectancy of and recognizing their evolving capacities.

To entirely reduce women's health during this period to reproductive health does a disservice to women's needs that are not reproductively based. Where fertility rates are low and life expectancy is around 80 years, a woman will spend around 2% of her lifetime in childbearing. In contrast, in a high fertility area, with a life expectancy of around 52, a woman will spend over 11% of her lifetime in childbearing. Even in the absence of the "big killing and disabling" diseases, women suffer from a large number of conditions and sets of symptoms that are so common that they are not considered as complaints, but instead are perceived as part of the "burden of being a woman." A study from two rural communities in India 10 years ago, demonstrated that over half the women studied had gynaecologic complaints, but only 8% had sought care and were examined in the past. Multiple conditions were present and 40% of those with diagnosed diseases did not complain of any symptoms.

It is at this time in life that women frequently take the triple roles of reproduction, productive work, and begin to take important roles in the life of their community. Formal work can be hazardous to health via certain occupational and environmental hazards including pesticides, toxic chemicals, radiation, extreme temperatures, excessive noise and violence, women are more likely to work in agriculture, industries and small enterprises that are poorly regulated with exposure to unsafe working conditions. These hazards may affect unborn children and the level of health in later years of life.

The role of work in women's health is grossly neglected—often because it is largely invisible, or because attention is limited to legislative action to protect the woman in her reproductive role. As noted in women and Occupational Health—

> "Much of women's work remains unrecognized, uncounted and unpaid: work in the home, in agriculture, food production and the marketing of homemade products. . . . Within the paid labour force, women are disproportionately concentrated in the informal sector, beyond the scope of industrial regulations, trade unions, insurance. . . [they) may . . . combine . . . paid work with household work and the care of children, the sick and the elderly. . . "

Domestic work can also be hazardous for women. For example, a large proportion of the world population, especially women in developing countries, are exposed to indoor pollutants produced by inefficient biomass stoves. The levels of pollutants, including toxins and carcinogens in the kitchen are usually very high. An increase has been noted in the entire spectrum of diseases associated with tobacco in people who never smoked but who were exposed to wood smoke. Women exposed to wood smoke had a five-fold risk of chronic bronchitis and chronic airflow obstruction.

Smoking as a health problem is increasing in women in some countries. In developed countries, the highest rates of smoking occur among women with the most socio-economic disadvantage, such as single mothers. Smoking; in turn, is significantly more common among women who are depressed and have a history of violent victimization and smoking typically coexists with a number of other high risk health behaviours such as drug and alcohol use and poor PAP smear attendance. In addition to the risk of cancer, cardiovascular disease and chronic obstructive pulmonary disease, smoking has other health risks for women, including, reduced fertility, ovulatory dysfunction, ectopic pregnancy, spontaneous abortion, and earlier menopause. Tobacco smoking may also be associated with an increased incidence rate of adult-onset asthma, especially among women, in whom the prognosis is generally poorer.

For the most part of this century, scientific interest in the problem of violence against women and its links to poor mental health, has been negligible. However, the rise of second wave feminism and activism around women's rights engendered an upsurge of interest in the widespread social problem of violence against women. Women who have experienced violence, whether in childhood or adult life, have increased rates of depression and anxiety, stress-related syndromes, pain syndromes, phobias, chemical dependency, substance use, suicidal tendencies, somatic and medical symptoms, negative health behaviours, poor subjective health and changes to health service utilization. Accumulating evidence suggests that the relationship among violence and depression and anxiety is causal. Controlled studies from a variety of settings have consistently found increased rates of depression and anxiety in women who have experienced childhood sexual abuse, childhood psychological abuse and/or physical and sexual violence in adult life.

Depression has a significant impact on women's well-being and productivity (Paltiel, 1993b). Depression, aside from being the most prevalent psychiatric condition, is making an increasingly heavy contribution to the global disease burden. Depression is not only the most frequently encountered women's mental health problem, but it also ranks as the most serious women's health problem overall. There is approximately a 2:1 ratio of depression in women as compared with men, while early research sought a biological basis for this difference, current research suggests that environmental stress such as life events and chronic difficulties contribute to this condition. Factors that put women at risk of depression include their inferior status, physical or sexual abuse, infertility, and conflicting demands of their domestic and income producing roles. Depressive symptoms are a significant risk factor for cardiovascular and non-cancer, non-cardiovascular mortality in older women, whether depressive symptoms are a marker for, or a cause of life threatening conditions remains to be determined.

To focus entirely on DALYs, a measure of disease, as an indicator of women's health—both in its biologic and gender dimensions—is to loose sight of the definition of health including well-being as a quality of health. Increasingly, as one examines the gender aspects of how health and disease are perceived by women, and how the healthcare system and professionals perceive the health needs of women, one sees the discordance of the medical and the social model of health.

Too often it is the negative dimensions of a phenomenon that draw the most attention, almost to the complete neglect of the positive. For example, the issue of women and work needs further study, better insight as to how work and income can be advantageous and when work becomes a health disadvantage. There are no measures of the satisfaction for successfully assuming an adult role, earning a decent living, contributing to the well-being of one's family, and the satisfaction of sharing the responsibilities and pleasures of parenthood, a close intimate relationship with one's partner and the companionship of friends.

The inter-relationship of work and breast-feeding and the economic advantage to the family of continuing breast-feeding also need further analysis. The role of occupational health services, trade unions and other formal workplace arrangements can all contribute to the health of women of this age, such as the concentration on the principles of a "woman friendly environment" that may mean the reducing of respiratory problems through an improved stove design, or enhancing women's use of health services by increasing the number and status of women healthcare providers at all levels of care. The important socializing role of the older women on younger women who are entering the childbearing stage and their role as mother substitutes need to be recognized and supported as key factors in the development of the next generation.

Finally, the accumulated ill-health and inadequate care of women up to and during their reproductive years take its toll not only on the continued health of the women, but also on the next generation, not only during childhood, but through the adult life. In protecting her own health and nutrition, a woman is also protecting the health of an unborn or yet to be conceived child. There is increasing evidence that suggests that pen-conceptual and intrauterine malnutrition, known to increase the risk of low birth weight, is also associated with an increased risk of coronary heart disease, hypertension and non-insulin dependent diabetes. In addition, aside from the effects on her own health, exposure to toxic elements before conception, during pregnancy or while breast-feeding, may affect the health, survival or future development of her offspring. Even if the woman's health is not directly affected, disability or impaired function in her child is bound to affect the woman's mental health. Most industrialized countries have occupational health standards which limit a pregnant woman's exposure to known teratogenic agents. But some toxic substances, such as dioxins may build up in her body fat over a lifetime, and then be excreted largely from the body in breast-milk.

Post-reproductive Years

The context of women's health in the post-reproductive years still carries the residue of the burdens of earlier reproductive ill-health to which is added the physiologic changes associated with menopause, which lead to skeletal, cardiovascular and other problems. The expectations of youth are worn down by the fatigue of chronic illness, anemia and other deficiencies.

The energy spent in the multiple roles of production, reproduction and care, not to speak of low self-esteem, leaves the woman physically and mentally frail. Widowhood and abandonment often leave them destitute, isolated and with increased risk of mental health problems. Not infrequently, the perceptions of healthcare providers to the problems of men and women at this and the older age differ. The number of women who presented themselves into an emergency department because of acute asthma, was almost twice the number of men. Although men received less outpatient care and had worse pulmonary function, women were more likely to be admitted to the hospital and to report an ongoing exacerbation at follow-up. Further studies are needed to better understand the complex relationship between sex and acute asthma.

There is very limited information available on the health problems and priority needs in the developing world of women who have entered their post-reproductive years. For women aged 45 and above, the majority of problems are chronic: cancer (especially of the cervix), cardiovascular and cerebro vascular diseases, osteoarthritis, and diabetes particularly in people in the Indian sub-continent. Diabetes mellitus, is a major cause of morbidity and can lead to blindness, kidney damage, and damage of lower-limbs. Injuries and infections (particularly tuberculosis) also contribute to women's disability in later years. Loss of visual acuity, malnutrition, and anemia contribute to morbidity. Yet, the health problems of post-menopausal women have been largely ignored. Menopause -the cessation of menses -leads to alterations in the skeletal, cardiovascular, nervous, skin, genitourinary, and gastrointestinal systems and can affect women's capacity to perform everyday activities. There are gynecological sequelae to damages occurring in childbirth in earlier years. In this age group, women continue to fare badly with post-traumatic stress disorder, endocrine disorders, and rheumatic heart disease. There is growing awareness that women are less likely to have adequate health insurance in their older age.

Osteoporosis, for example, varies widely in incidence in different countries. Hip fractures, an indicator of osteoporosis among the elderly, is 10 to 20% higher in incidence in the United States as compared with Singapore or the non-white South Africa. In general, the higher the overall rate, the higher the proportion of women affected. In the US, it is estimated that one in three women over the age of 50 will sustain a fracture due to osteoporosis, and in at least 10% of the cases, the fracture or its complications will be fatal, and half of those who survive will need long-term nursing care.

The Old-elderly

It is estimated that the number of women over the age of 65 will increase from 330 million in 1990 to 600 million in 2015 (WHO, 1996) and that an aging society is evolving, which for the most part is female. As a result of urbanization, migration and changing family structures, women are increasingly neglected in their older years. Because women marry men older than they are, and since they live longer, women are more likely to be widowed than men. with the shift of support away from extended families, elderly women are increasingly being left on their own. Loss of a partner and living alone have important consequences on health.

Feminization of old-age is advancing rapidly. Current demographic data give a clear "statistical snapshot" of the aging population. By the year 2020, the number of people over 65 is projected to increase globally by 82%, or to more than 690 million. In 1995, UN estimates for the population aged 60 and over (almost one-tenth of the world's population) showed 302 million women and 247 million men. In the developed countries, women aged 60 and above, represented 20% of the total female population while the figure for men was only 16%. Projections suggest this divergence is accelerating at the global level but it is even more rapid in the developing world. This is largely explained by the fact that among people aged 80 years and over, the proportion of women is increasing faster than at the lower ages. Today, 61% of the world's women aged 80 live in developing countries, where most of them will be staying by the year 2025.

The greater longevity of women is offset by a higher sickness rate than that of men. Women need care for both physical and psychological infirmity and for social conditions such as widowhood, poverty and isolation. There is evidence that disability in old-age is related to the burdens of overwork and to under-nutrition that continues to occur as a result of poverty. But sadness must be distinguished from depression although both are possibly associated with the accumulation of losses—personal loss of autonomy, mobility, vision and hearing, and of losses of family members and companionship. Treating depression at this stage of life can have a profound effect on the quality of life and encourage the elderly to live in dignity until the end.

It is very clear that women's lives, especially in old-age, become quite different from those of men. Two principal trends can be seen: In the developed countries, women who have greatly improved their social standing and have moved towards more equality with men (for instance, in literacy, healthcare, social security and wages in old-age), are living longer than men and the longevity gap is widening as their social status becomes more equal with men. In the developing countries, women who remain deeply disadvantaged in relation to men, due to reasons of high illiteracy rates, poor earning levels, high fertility rates and high rates of early marriage (between 15 and 19 years of age), become highly dependent on their children and grandchildren as they grow older.

Disability and the increasing number of mental disorders in the old-elderly, which originate in the earlier stages of life and are often avoidable, will become more common. Dementia causes more disability (DALYS) in women over sixty than in men of the same age group. Depression is the single most serious mental problem for women in every age group (Paltiel, 1993b). And one of the factors that puts women at risk of depression includes isolation in elderly women. Women are disproportionately represented among the oldest-old, not just as those in need of care but also in the unpaid caregiver roles, caring for the oldest-old and the most socially and economically disadvantaged. Social support systems are needed, as those who provide care are often young elderly women. The intervention needed is not just medical but social, economic, and environmental. They must all be applied if we are to improve the health of the current and future generations.

The health of women is hidden behind many masks—social, economic, cultural and religious, and political. Gender so complicates and increases the diversity of settings in which women find themselves as to blunt the efforts to address women's health needs. The social dimension of the women's health model includes both men and women. It also includes the economic and environmental circumstances of women. Although the latter may be independent of gender in terms of underlying causality, gender often accentuates the disease burden of the economic and environmental impact on women's health. The constraints of customary and statutory law on women are also linked to gender, while the impact of poverty—while not attributable to gender—is nonetheless often disproportionately borne by women and increases their burden of disease.

The impact of poverty in an urban environment is increasing as factors affecting women's health. Three groups of health hazards are generally recognized as simultaneously operating on the urban poor, particularly women. The first includes low income and education, overcrowding, lack of personal security and insufficient diet. The second includes man-made conditions such as pollution, traffic, noise, stress, alienation and unhealthy behaviours which may lead to cardiovascular and mental diseases and to accidents in the home, at work and on the roads. The third is related to social instability, promiscuity and prostitution which, in a context of poverty and low education, can lead to alcohol and drug abuse and sexually transmitted diseases especially HIV and AIDS. In addition, particularly for poor women, anxiety, depression, and violence are common features of the urban environment.

A significant proportion of urban households are headed by women who have to work to support their family. These women often have limited education and job skills; which limit them to low-income occupations or to the service sector with long working hours. They are often malnourished and exposed to mental stress, sexual harassment and abuse in searching and maintaining a job.

Lack of social status of women is expressed in several forms, including limitations on their legal status (particularly in relation to land ownership, inheritance, divorce) or failure to enforce laws that do exist. In addition, lack of decision-making, and poor and lack of participation in the household are other factors particularly affecting younger women. However, as women go through the different stages of adult life, the decision-making power may change dramatically. In many societies, older women can be very influential in household decision-making so it is important that they understand the health and development needs of family members. However, even if young mothers have such decision-making privileges, when complications occur in the course of an illness, decision-making may shift away from the mother. Also undermining women's status is the fact that women's work is often "invisible." "Work" defined as paid labour in the private sector, seldom acknowledges the unpaid family worker—women, children, and the aged. Women are not valued for their work as managers of natural resources, food growers or wage earners. In truth, working women take responsibility for a multitude of health-related activities, all of which affect the quality of life for the family and community. In developing countries, rural women grow and process food, raise small animals, and provide the main labour for transporting water and fuel.

Violence against women, in its many forms, is a cross cutting determinant of ill-health in women. Violence is often chronic and prolonged rather than acute. It usually occurs in the family, and in severe cases, it is likely to be reported to health or judicial authorities; it is often associated with sexual abuse and has long-term as well as immediate physical and psychological consequences. Domestic violence, rape, and sexual abuse are widespread in all regions, classes and cultures. Violence takes a heavy toll on women, causing death, broken bones, internal injuries, miscarriage, and cuts and bruises. Psychological after-effects include depression, fear, anxiety, fatigue, sleeping and eating disorders, and past traumatic stress disorder. Many battered wives and rape victims attempt suicide. Homicide and suicide motivated by the stigma of rape, pregnancy outside of marriage, or beatings or dowry problems have been noted to make a significant contribution to maternal mortality.

Prostitution is another form of woman-oriented violence which perpetuates the low status of women and may result in unwanted pregnancy and STDs, as well as physical assault and low self-esteem. Preventing violence against women would raise the quality of life of women, help to reduce healthcare expenditures for both short and long-term consequences as well as address this violation of basic human rights. Domestic violence and sexual abuse are among the factors contributing to child prostitution and the commercial sexual exploitation of children.

Civil conflicts and war exacerbate women's health problems. Most refugees are women and children. They may suffer isolation, abuse, severe stress and poor access to healthcare. The consequences of civil unrest, ethical, religious and national conflicts have taken a disproportionate toll on the health and development of women and children, as increasingly, the majority of those killed and disabled are non-combatants. Such conflicts undermine nutrition by disrupting and destroying food production and distribution. They destroy the infrastructure of schools and health services, forcing large populations to move as refugees or as internally displaced persons in communities already strained to meet the needs of their own population. Refugee women have particular needs, such as protection against sexual and physical abuse and exploitation, and against discrimination and violence to women and girls have become weapons of war, considered now as a war crime.

Economic migration, while potentially opening new economic opportunities to women and families, may pose serious risks of exploitation and ill-health. Migration takes many forms. In one scenario, it is the woman left behind in a rural setting, coping with the care of children and the elderly and in ensuring adequate and nutritious food production. The woman faces a number of potential health problems as a result of the change of family structure and social support systems. Increasingly, in these and other settings, monogamous women bear the consequences of acquiring sexually transmitted diseases from the migrant male who returns to the family periodically.

In other settings, it may be the single or married woman who migrates, either to an urban industrial setting such as trade zones or into the domestic labour market or the informal economy. An increased participation of women in the paid labour force has accompanied economic growth and globalizations, thus putting increased disposable income in the hands of women which increases their self-esteem. Yet, the effects may not necessarily be positive. Special trade and economic zones which rely heavily on a female work force, have been created as part of the globalization trends. Such zones which are often exempted from following the national labour, health and social welfare standards and legislation, subject the women potentially to exploitation and denial of certain rights such as healthcare and protection from hazardous substances. Similarly, women in the domestic service and the informal economy are not given the protection and benefits that are given to those in the formal labour market.

It is estimated that 10 to 15% of the rural population of developing countries live in environmentally degraded or ecologically vulnerable areas. Both women and men are involved in environmental degradation, but women—particularly poor women—are the first to suffer due to their closeness and dependency on the environment and work burden and the time entailed in the collection of water and fuel gathering. Women more than men will be burdened by fuel scarcity. Women in some developing countries spend much of their time cooking with biomass—wood, straw and dung—in poorly ventilated areas, thus making them likely to suffer the consequences of indoor pollution.

Lack of access to health services ranks among the more important factors influencing women's health. Several factors combine to produce inequities in the access that directly undermine the ability of women to maintain good health. These include the time involved in obtaining care, deficiencies in the health system, health service fees and cultural factors. The family is one of the most important social contexts within which illness occurs and is resolved and should serve as a primary unit in health and medical care.

Cultural and social factors often interfere with the indigenous and other minority groups accessing to health services. Too often the perception of the indigenous people and minority groups do not correspond with the understanding of their specific health needs from the health agencies and professionals. There is no doubt that cultural and social concerns have made these groups of people less willing to improve their health status and seek access to mainstream services. As a consequence, they generally have very poor health status in comparison with the general population.

Educational attainment of women is one of the most important predictors of the health and well-being of women and children. Female school enrolment and completion and/or adult women's literacy programmes have consistently shown an impact on child and women's health. In every economic setting, the children of literate women have a better chance of survival than those of illiterate women. Educated women tend to marry later, delay the onset of child-bearing and are more likely to practice family planning. They generally have fewer children with a wider spacing between births. They have better nutrition, manage household resources better for the benefit of all members of the family and make better use of health services for themselves and for their children.

The interactions of women, gender and family have important implications for women's health. Gender roles are initiated within the family but are derived and are parallel to those within the society. These include the distribution of power and influences within the two entities. Both within and outside the household, the system of gender relationships includes sexual relations between adults, division of labour and gender socialization. These relationships not only affect such health issues as sexually transmitted diseases, including HIV/AIDS, and violence against women and children, but also the division of health decision-making. Many societies, both "modern" and "traditional" are now paying the price of inequality in negotiating sexual relationship between male and female partners in a family, and the double standard applied to the expression of male sexuality within and outside the family. One expression of this inequity is the burden and blame for infertility which is placed on women even though up to 40% of infertility may be attributed to a male factor. The term "barrenness" is applied to women, not men, and it has strong negative connotations and is the basis of divorce in many traditional societies and religions. Another consequence of the inequality in negotiating sexual relationship in a family is the increasing burden that AIDS is placing on women and children. The vast majority of women with new HIV infections are monogamous and acquire the infection from their partners. The inequity must also be measured in terms of the greater risk of HIV transmission from a man to a woman than from a woman to a man.

Cultural and religious values and traditions are often considered as the anchors that provide stability and continuity for a community and society. Women play a critical role in the day-to-day maintenance of these values and practices in the family and the community. At the same time, these values and institutions that sustain them provide moral and spiritual sustenance. The largest group of attendance of religious services is elderly women. Well-being is improved in the elderly women who have religious links. At the same time, there are a number of traditional practices to which women are subjected, which are decidedly harmful. These include such practices as child marriage before the biological and social maturity of the girl (and less often, the boy), and female genital mutilation.

It is very clear that women's Health is "everybody's business" but initiatives lack coherence and a framework to show how they can link together. There are many approaches that will bring improvement to Women's Health. In fact, seven spheres of influence on women's health can be identified, WHO and the Women's Health Department will take a leadership role in demonstrating how Women's Health can be improved through partnerships with governments, other UN agencies, the health and social sciences research community, and non-governmental organizations, particularly those working at the community level.

Seven Spheres of Action

- **Sphere 1** is action on the environment (e.g. distance to water, access to firewood and other biomass fuels, fuel saving stoves and energy for cooking).
- **Sphere 2** is legislation, advocacy and the political environment.
- **Sphere 3** covers the economic influences on Women's Health both macro-economic such as the impact of the implementation of structural adjustment policies and micro-economic in the sense of access to resources both formal and informal. This includes work influences on Women's Health (formal work, informal work including caring, and also household work).
- **Sphere 4** covers Healthcare.
- **Sphere 5** identifies the influence of education (schooling) and lifelong learning on Women's Health.
- **Sphere 6** focuses on the socio-cultural factors influencing women's Health.
- **Sphere 7** is the biological influence on Women's Health.

Singly, none of the above approaches is sufficient to lead to the improvement of women's health. But they can be combined. The new approach needs to build partnership in each sphere with all the organizations contributing to improve

Women's Health and the determinants in each sphere. In addition, each of these seven spheres can influence Women's Health through its own action in each decade of the life span.

Overall Goal of WHO in Improving Women's Health

WHO's goal is to improve the quality of women's lives and decrease their burden of disease by addressing the aspects in women's health that arise as a consequence of gender inequalities at the social, economic and cultural levels, in health and nutrition services, and in the setting of national and international priorities for research. A focus on human relationships at each stage of development and women's situation within the social-developmental model of health will be critical in addressing the gender inequities in health. Improvements in women's health are imperative if women are to achieve an acceptable quality of life at each stage in their life, if they are to achieve their economic, social and cultural goals, and, if with their partner, they are to rear and care for the next generation. The development of a policy and strategy by the Department of Women's Health is in the consultative stage.

The immediate goal within the new framework is to identify evidence and opportunities for action to improve women's health by promoting and supporting wellness and action on determinants of illness at each stage of the life span. Working on the seven spheres of determinants of women's health, WHO will take a leadership role in demonstrating how women's health can be improved through forging partnerships with governments, other UN agencies, the health and social sciences research community, and non-governmental organizations, particularly those working at the community level.

Twelve conceptual, programmatic and operational principles can be used in the development of the strategies for achieving women's health and development:

Principles to Improve Women's Health

- Taking a life-course approach to women's health by recognizing inter-related stages across the life span.
- Recognizing biological, social, cultural, economic, educational, healthcare, political and legislative, and environmental determinants of Women's Health.
- Forging Partnerships to tackle the seven spheres of influence on Women's Health.
- Seeking partnerships in developing the evidence base and in service provision, e.g. joint Initiatives for Women's Health as part of Health For All and Agenda 21 action on the environment.
- Collation of data and developing the Evidence Base particularly for the effect of earlier health on later women's health, and the effectiveness of interventions in each of the 7 spheres.
- Ongoing debate on policy development with communities, districts, national and regional bodies.
- Networking and support for Women's Organizations.
- Exploring and "unpacking" cross-cutting key determinants of Women's Health, particularly poverty, ethnicity or social exclusion, age, and the exacerbation of problems by conflict and migration.

Bibliography

Anita, N.B. and Bhatia, Kavita, Peoples Health in People's Hand-A model for Panchayati Raj, FRCH, Mumbai. 1993.

Basch, P.E., Vaccines and World Health, New York, Oxford University Press, 1994.

Bhatnagar, S. and Goel, S.L., Development Planning and Administration. New Delhi. Deep & Deep Publications (P) Ltd., 1992.

Bhattacharjee P.J. and G.N. Shashtri, Population in India, A Study of Interstate Variation, New Delhi, Vikas, 1976.

Bosh, Ashish, From Population to People, Delhi, B.R. Publication, 1988.

Brown, Esther, Newer Dimensions of Patient Care, Russell Sage Foundation, New York, 1961.

Cartwright, A., Patients and their Doctors, A Study of General Practice, Routledge Kegan Paul, London, 1961.

Chanawongse Krasal, Rural Development Management, Research and Development Institute, Khon Kaen University, Thailand.

Chandra, R.C., A Geography of Population, Concepts, Determinants and Patterns, New Delhi, Kalyani, 1987.

Chauhan, Devraj, Anaita, N.H. and Ramdan, Sangita, Healthcare in India: A Profile, FRCH, Mumhai, 1996.

Das, K., Civil Service Reforms and Structural Adjustment, Oxford, Delhi 1998.

Duggal, R., Nandaraj, S. and Shetty, Sahana, State Sector Health Expenditure-A Database All India, FRCH, Mumbai, 1992.

P. Jurfelds, G. and Lindbergs, Pills against Poverty—A Study of Introduction of Western Medicine in a Tamil Village, Curzon Press, London, 1975.

FRCH, Panchayati Raj Information Resource Book, Mumbai, 1996.

Ghai, Sandhaya, Bursing Services Administration: A Case Study of Nehru Hospital, PGI, Chandigarh (Doctoral Thesis, Panjab University, 1998).

Ghosh, Brindra Nath, A Treatise on Hygiene and Public Health, Scientific Publishing Company, 1970, Calcutta.

Gill, Sonya, Health Status of the Indian People, FRCH, Mumbai, 1987.

Goel, S.L., Healthcare Administration Policy-making and Planning, Sterling, Delhi, 1981.

———, Healthcare Administration Levels and Aspects, Sterling, Delhi, 1981.

Goel, S.L., Healthcare Administration Ecology, Principles and Modern Trends, Sterling, Delhi, 1981.

———, Family Planning Programme and Beyond, New Delhi, Deep & Deep Publications Pvt. Ltd., New Delhi, 1990.

———, International Administration: WHO, South-East Asia Regional Office, Sterling, New Delhi, 1977.

———, Modern Management Techniques, Deep & Deep Publications Pvt. Ltd., New Delhi, 1987.

———, Public Health Administration, Sterline, New Delhi, 1984.

———, Public Personnel Administration, Sterling, New Delhi, 1984.

———, Hospital Administration and Management, Deep & Deep Publications Pvt. Ltd., New Delhi, 1903.

———, Distance Education in 21st Century, Deep & Deep Publications Pvt. Ltd., New Delhi, 2000.

Hanlon, John, Principles of Public Health Administration, C.V. Mobsy, Sthouis, 1969.

ICSSR & ICMR, Health for All-an Alternative Strategy—Report of a Study Group set-up Jointly by ICSSR & ICMR, Pune, Indian Institute of Education, 1981.

Govt. of India, Annual Reports of the Ministry of Health and Family Welfare, Delhi.

———, Committee on Multi-purpose Workers under Health and Family Welfare Programme (Kartar Singh Report), Delhi, Ministry of Health and Family Welfare, Delhi, 1973.

———, Govt. of India, Health in Independent India (G. Borkar Report), Delhi, 1961.

———, Health Survey and Development Committee (Bhore Committee), Delhi, 1946.

———, Lok Sabha Secretariat, Estimates Committees and Public Accounts Committees Reports.

———, Planning Commission, Five Year Plans, New Delhi.

———, Report of Health Survey and Planning Committee, (Mudaliar Committee) Ministry of Health, August-October, 1961.

———, Ministry of Information and Broadcasting, India, 1999, A Refresher Manual, New Delhi, 1999.

———, Initiatives and Best Practices of Government of India for Effective and Responsive Administration, New Delhi, Ministry of Personnel, Public Grievances, and Pensions, 1997.

———, Deptt. of Family Welfare, Reproductive and Child Health (World Bank Component), Vols. I and II, New Delhi, 1997.

———, Report of the Working Group on Health for All by 2000 A.D., New Delhi Ministry of Health and Welfare, 1981.

Gunaratne Herat, V.T., Challenges and Response Health in South-East Asia Region, New Delhi, McGraw Hill, 1977.

Hardon, A., et. al., Monitoring Family Planning and Reproductive Rights, A Manual for Empowerment, London, Zed Books, 1997.
Indian Society of Health Administrators, Bangalore.

Annual Conference Reports

Health for all by 2000 (AD 1980).
The Role of Hospitals in Healthcare (1981).
Health Manpower Requirements for 2000 (1982).
Role of the Health Administrator in India (1983).
On Growing Needs of Urban Health Management (1985).
Cost Reduction in Hospitals and Healthcare (1986).
Health of the High Risk Groups Mothers, Children and Elderly (1985).
Health of Women and Children for Development (1988).
Healthcare for the Villages and Urban Slums (1989-90).
Health of the Youth and the Female Child.
Role of Voluntary Organizations in Healthcare in India (1992).

Books

Stress and Health of Executives and Professionals.
Hospital and Health Administration.
Modern Technology for Hospitals and Healthcare.
Management for Nursing Administrators.
Community Participation in Health and Family Welfare-Indian Experiences.
Health of the Metropolis-Bangalore-A Guide to Health Planning and Development of Urban Cities in India.
Leadership and Human Resources Development for Healthcare.
Managerial Effectiveness for Organizational Excellence.
Computer Applications to Hospitals, Healthcare and Medical Education.
Health and Development of the Tribal People in India-A Guide for Professionals and Administrators.
Retirement Planning, Adjustment and Health.
Janovsky, K., Health Policy and Systems Development on Agenda for Research, WHO/SHS/NHP/96.1, Geneva, 1996.
Jesani, Amar & Ganguly, Shilpi, Some Issues in Community Participation in Health Services, FRCH, Mumbai, 1993.
Khandewale, Shreekant V., Health Administration and the Weaker Sections in an Indian Metropolis, Devika Publications, Delhi, 1996.
Klinoboul Krienkrai, Health and Family Welfare Administration in Thailand—A Case Study of Lampang Province (Doctoral Thesis).
Kumar, R., Child Development in India, Ashish, New Delhi, 1988.
———, Environment Pollution and Health Hazards in India, Ashish, New Delhi (Year not mentioned).
———, Youth Health, Problem, Planning and Development, Deep and Deep Publications Pvt. Ltd., New Delhi, 1986.
Lane, S.D., From Population Control to Reproductive Health: An Emerging Policy Agenda, Social Science and Medicine, 1994.

Lush, L., Integrating Services, from Rhetroic to Action, Development Research Insights, 1997.

Mattoo, P.K., Project Formulation in Developing Countries, Macmillan, Delhi, 1978.

Meher, C. Nanavaty and P.D. Kulkarni, NGO's in the Changing Scenario, New Delhi, Uppal, 1998.

Miller, George E. and Tamas Fulop, Educational Strategies for the Health Professionals, Geneva, WHO, 1974.

Mishra, R.P., Medical Geography of India, NBT, Delhi, 1970.

Murray, C.J.L., Lopez, A.D., The Global Burden of Diseases, WHO, Geneva, Switzerland, 1996.

Myrdal Gunnar, Asian Drama, An Enquiry into the Poverty of Nations, Vol. III, Penguis, London, 1968.

Naik, J.P., An Alternative System of Healthcare Service in India Some Proposals, Allied, Bombay, 1988.

National Institute of Health and Family Welfare, New Delhi

Management Training Modules for District Health Offices.

Management Training Modules for Health Offices.

Management Training Modules for Health Assistants (Male and Female).

Management Training Modules for Health Workers (Male and Female).

Management Training Modules for TBA.

Management Training Modules for Health Guide.

Park, J.E. and K. Park (1990), Textbook on Preventive and Social Medicine, Banarasidas Bhanot Publishers, Jabalpur.

Pai Panadiker, V.A., et. al., Organizational Policy for Family Planning, New Delhi, Uppal, 1983.

Pathak, Shankar, Social Welfare, Health and Family Planning in India, Marwah Publications, Delhi, 1979.

Rao, C. Hayavandana, Mysore Gazetteer, Vol. IV, B.R. Publishing Corporation, Delhi, 1984.

Ramanathan, S. (ed.), Landmarks in Karnataka Administration, New Delhi, Uppal, 1998 (Published for Indian Institute of Public Administration, Karnataka, Regional Branch, Bangalore).

Rafei, Dr. Uton M., Primary Healthcare in Changing World South-East Asia Regional Perspectives, WHO Regional Office for South-East Asia, Delhi, India, 1993.

Ranga, R.K., Admn. of Family Planning Programmes in India—A Case Study of Haryana (Doctoral Thesis, Panjab University, 1998).

Rao, V.K.R.V., Food, Nutrition and Poverty in India, Vikas, New Delhi, 1982.

Rifikin, S.B., Health Planning and Community Participation, Crown Helm, London, 1985.

Sahni, Ashok, The Third Force in Healthcare—Voluntary Sector, Bangalore Indian Society of Health Administrators (1992).

Scott-Samuel A., Total Participation, Total Health, Scottish Academic Press, 1990.

Sarjivi, K.S., Planning India's Health, Orient Longman, Delhi, 1971. Shenoi, P.V. (ed.), Contours of Social and Economic Development Political Issues, Concept, New Delhi, 1997.

Sharma, R.D., Advanced Public Administration, New Delhi, H.K. Publishers, 1994.

Singh, Sarabjit, Management Information System in a Hospital—A Case Study of General Hospital, Chandigarh (Doctoral Thesis, Panjab University, 1991).

Taori, Kamal, People's Participation in Sustainable Human Development (A Unified Approach), New Delhi, Concept, 1998.

Vaeth, R.M., A Theory of Medical Ethics, New York, Basic Books, 1981.

Vettivel, S.K., People's Participation in Social Development, Role of NGO, New Delhi, Vetri Publishers, 1992.

World, Health Organisation Alma Ata Revisited, WHO/SHS/CC/ 94.2, WHO, Geneva, 1994.

Werner, D., Where there is no Doctor?, The Voluntary Health Association of India, Delhi, 1984.

World Bank Financing of Health Services in Developing Countries, Washington, 1987.

World Bank, Development Report, 1993, New York, Oxford University Press.

World Bank, World Development Report, 1997, New York, Oxford University Press, 1997.

World Health Organisation, Annual Report of South-East Asia Regional Office, Delhi, 1997.

———, Bulletin of Regional Health Information, Regional Office for South-East Asia, Delhi, 1980, 1981, 1982, 1983, 1984-85, 1986-87, 1988-90, and 1991-93.

World Health Organization, Collaboration in Health Development in South-East Asia, 1948-88, Fortieth Anniversary Volume (Revised), Delhi, 1992.

———, Community Action for Health, SEA/HSD/185, Regional Office for South-East Asia, Delhi, 1993.

———, Development of Indicator for Monitoring Progress Towards Health for all by the Year 2000, Geneva, 1981.

———, Eighth General Programme of Work—Covering the Period 1990-95, Geneva, 1987.

———, Evaluation of the Strategy for Health for All by the year 2000, Regional Office for South-East Asia, Delhi, 1986.

———, Formulating Strategies for Health for all by the year 2000, Geneva, 1979.

———, Global Strategy for Health for all by the year 2000, Geneva, 1981.

———, Health in Development—Prospects for 21st Century, WHO! DGH/ 94.5, Geneva, 1994.

World Health Organization, Health Situation in the South-East Asia Region, 1991-93, Regional Office for South-East Asia, Delhi, 1995.

Index